Psychological Problems in General Practice

Oxford General Practice Series 15

A. C. MARKUS
General Practitioner
Clinical Tutor in General Practice
Oxford

C. MURRAY PARKES
Senior Lecturer
Department of Psychiatry
London Hospital Medical College

P. TOMSON
General Practitioner
Hon. Senior Lecturer
The Medical Colleges of St Bartholomew's and
The London Hospitals

M. JOHNSTON
Senior Lecturer in Clinical Psychology
Royal Free Hospital
London

OXFORD   NEW YORK   TOKYO   MELBOURNE
OXFORD UNIVERSITY PRESS
1989

Oxford University Press, Walton Street, Oxford OX2 6DP
Oxford   New York   Toronto
Delhi   Bombay   Calcutta   Madras   Karachi
Petaling Jaya   Singapore   Hong Kong   Tokyo
Nairobi   Dar es Salaam   Cape Town
Melbourne   Auckland
and associated companies in
Berlin   Ibadan

Oxford is a trade mark of Oxford University Press

Published in the United States
by Oxford University Press, New York

British Library Cataloguing in Publication Data
Markus, A.
Psychological problems in general practice.
1. Medicine. Psychiatry — For general
practice
I. Title
616.89
ISBN 0-19-261529-7

Library of Congress Cataloging in Publication Data
Psychological problems in general practice/A. Markus . . . [et al.]
p. cm. — (Oxford general practice series; 15)
(Oxford medical publications)
Includes index.
1. Family medicine.   2. Psychiatry.   I. Markus, A. (Andrew)
II. Series   III. Series: Oxford general practice series; no. 15.
R729.5.G4P89   1989   616.89'156 — dc19   88-8650
ISBN 0-19-261529-7 (pbk.)

Phototypeset by Dobbie Typesetting Limited, Plymouth
Printed in Great Britain
at the University Printing House, Oxford
by David Stanford
Printer to the University

OXFORD MEDICAL PUBLICATIONS

Psychological Problems in General Practice

OXFORD GENERAL PRACTICE SERIES

Foreword

DR JOHN HORDER

This book can help in that part of clinical practice which most GPs find the most challenging. In it are discussed the range of psychological problems which they meet — from severe and obvious illness of mind to mental aspects of physical illness and to those difficulties in daily living which commonly bring people to the consulting room. The authors set out to show that these problems, though complex, are sufficiently understandable that exploration of them together can be therapeutic for the patient and fascinating for the doctor.

The book particularly helps understanding of those forms of response, inevitably used by GPs and others working in primary care, but needing skill — call them counselling, psychotherapy, behavioural therapy, or just the use of the doctor-patient relationship in the consultation. Precise techniques are discussed, as for the treatment of phobias, and also 'attitudes' — habitual ways of regarding people — thus bringing insights which can contribute to the care of people with any disorder, even the most seemingly mechanical.

Other forms of response are not neglected — psychotropic prescribing, influencing the environment of family, work, or school, mobilizing other services for a variety of purposes. But pride of place in this book is given to listening, observing, understanding how patients see their own situation, helping them to see it differently and to solve their own problem whenever possible.

Why then start with animal behaviour? Like the chapters on psychology and social influences, this can help us to recognize some of the roots of human behaviour. Together these chapters put forward a range of models — based as far as possible on the evidence of observation or experiment — which illuminate the disorders and personal difficulties about which GPs are consulted. But equally they throw light on the influences which foster mental health. The book is concerned throughout with the aim of preventing disorders and helping people to live healthily, within the limits of our understanding.

Authorship shared between two general practitioners, a psychologist, and a psychiatrist brings together experience of common problems with special knowledge and skills in a mixture which makes it difficult to attribute any particular section of the book to a particular writer or background. They all share a concern for prevention and for the psychological approaches to treatment. They have written a very interesting and useful book.

Preface

The authors believe that general practice psychiatry is a different specialty from hospital psychiatry. Textbooks of psychiatry derived from hospital practice rightly lay emphasis on the diagnosis and treatment of the major psychoses, and relatively little emphasis is given to the less bizarre but equally complex psychological problems which loom so large in general practice. More important, the hospital-based psychiatrists find it easier to maintain an 'illness model' of psychiatry simply because many of the people whom they see are unequivocally sick. By contrast the GP is more often faced with people who have 'problems in living' and for whom the reassurance that they are not mentally ill may be more important than the making of a psychiatric diagnosis.

The boundary between mental health and mental illness will never be clear, and it is often inappropriate and misleading for us to label people who come to us for help in this way. This does not mean that theories and practices derived from an illness model are of little use; they may well be useful. But an approach to psychological medicine confined to the diagnosis and treatment of mental illness will be of limited use to the GP.

What other models are available to us? GPs frequently have to devise management plans in response to problems presented to them, without going through the intermediate stage of attaching a diagnostic label to the patient, and this problem-oriented model is, in our opinion, the model which is most appropriate here. It is not simpler or less sophisticated than the more traditional approach, nor is it less scientific or less well supported by good theory. In fact we hope to show that there is a great deal known about the kinds of problem which are met with in general practice and that a proper understanding of these problems can sometimes enable the primary care team to prevent psychological and psychosomatic disorders as well as treat those that occur.

To prevent psychological disorder it is necessary to understand the circumstances that foster mental health as well as the circumstances that bring about mental illness. These include the factors which foster the development of basic trust (appropriate trust of others as well as self-trust), the factors that bring about an accurate view of the world and which enable that view to be changed in the face of changing circumstances, and the factors which enable a person to develop and maintain a personal network of human relationships. They are considered in Chapter 1 of the book. The authors believe that these factors are often more important in preserving mental health than the biochemical and endocrine factors which receive such prominence in the literature provided by drug companies. Not that biochemistry and endocrinology can be ignored, for, quite apart from anything else, it is particularly important for us to know what we are about when we set out to modify their effects by means of drugs. However, drugs are too often the easy option. Depressed — prescribe an antidepressant, anxious — an anxiolytic, sleepless — a sedative; it cannot be as easy as that, and it is not. General practitioners, more than other doctors, have to cope with the consequences of the misuse of psychotropic drugs and their lay brother, alcohol. It is in their interest to prescribe these drugs with caution and respect.

Psychological problems play a very large part in general practice; how large is considered in Chapter 2. They are very common, very varied, and at times very complex. They are also very fascinating, but their fascination can itself be a problem if it causes GPs to take on more than they should. The handling of psychological problems can be very stressful to the doctor, and take a lot of time, a commodity that is in short supply. It follows that the management of psychological problems in general practice must involve taking a hard look at the logistics of the practice team. At one extreme is the single-handed practitioner whose large list and lack of support make it impossible to tackle more than a fraction of the psychological problems met with; at the other extreme is the larger group practice whose sheer efficiency of organization may create an impersonal conveyor belt which matches the anonymity of a modern hospital and militates against the personal relationships that are the touchstone of successful psychological care.

We believe that there are other alternatives. It is perfectly possible for a GP to remain fascinated by psychological medicine without being overwhelmed by all the sorrows and stresses of the world. A general practice can be organized in such a way that personal medicine as well as significant preventiv : work is possible. The results of treating most mental illness in general practice are likely to be better and more humane than the results of referring the majority of such patients to hospital.

The contents of the book are divided in such a way that theory and practice are linked. We hope that the index will make it easy for the busy reader who wants help with a particular problem to find the relevant section quickly.

In Chapter 3 we describe a number of theoretical models which represent different ways of viewing prevention and therapy, and in Part II the practical implications of these models for the primary care team are considered, and illustrated by means of examples taken from clinical practice.

Models should not be confused with the reality itself. A map is not the landscape that it represents even though some maps are better models of reality than others. Nor should we be surprised if the models appear to simplify the complexities of human psychology — it is the function of models to simplify the objects that they represent. The test of a good model is its utility, and it is this criterion that we have adopted in deciding what to include in this book.

Wherever possible we have relied on models whose implications are consistent with the findings of well-conducted research, but there are many areas of human behaviour and thought which cannot yet be tested in that way. Nevertheless the GP, faced with a person who is, say, suffering the hopelessness of depression, must make use of the best conceptual tools that can be mustered, and these will often turn out to be derived from clinical practice rather than research. In place of the precision and clarity of most other areas of scientific medicine, the GP has to 'guess and test'.

We have tried to avoid discussing the points of difference between the various schools of dynamic psychology and psychoanalysis. Many of the apparent conflicts between these various models boil down to differences in the way words are used, or differences between points of view. In the end the 'right' convention to use is the one which proves most useful in practice.

Psychoanalysis provided a generation of psychiatrists with a frame of reference which we believe has now outlived its usefulness, but which, however controversial its detail, did focus attention on a range of problems which had previously been ignored and enabled us to begin to think constructively about them. The technique to which Freud's theoretical models gave rise is of little use in general practice and a more useful and consistent paradigm will be developed in this book.

This model is based on the assumption that human beings are themselves model-builders. We are born with a propensity to perceive and to learn certain things which enable us to reach out to our environment and to build, within our minds, complex models of the world which soon become our most important mental equipment. It is by using these internal models that we recognize the world that we meet, solve problems, and, with luck, achieve our aims — aims that are not, in essence, different from those of other animal species. But, unlike other species, we have developed methods of communication which enable us to share our models with each other and, by so doing, vastly increase the size and complexity of these models. Also, we use our model-building capacity to plan and construct a man-made environment.

With this degree of complexity it is no surprise that things can go wrong. A model which fits one situation may not fit another, changes in the world and in ourselves may render our internal models obsolete, the models employed by one person may conflict with those of another, and the environments which were created to solve one set of problems may themselves give rise to a new set of problems.

Medicine has traditionally been concerned with problems arising out of malfunctions of the body and the mind, but these malfunctions, as we shall see, are often themselves reflections of another set of problems whose origins lie at the interface between internal and external worlds, and at the interface between one person's internal world and that of another. It is these areas that constitute our frame of reference.

ew frame of reference is only now beginning to become established
a figure-head of Freud's stature to hold it together. One reason
be the enormous increase in published research in this field which
d in the past half-century. Another is the diversity of related
siology, ethology, anthropology, cybernetics, sociology, etc. —
w.... ....ributions need to be included in the paradigm. No one person
can be expected to provide an authoritative perspective on all of these topics.
We have involved four people, two are general practitioners and the other
two, a psychiatrist and a psychologist, work closely with primary care teams.
We have met together often to agree on the basic philosophy of the book
and, although the chapters are written by individual authors, we have each
commented on each other's contributions, and we accept collective
responsibility for them. The editor has tried to harmonize styles, without
altering the substance, in such a way that the original authors can 'own' their
chapters. We have tried to avoid jargon or, if that is unavoidable, to define
what we mean.

Our choice of models is obviously a personal one. No doubt other models
will one day replace the viewpoints put forward here, but the knowledge
of that fact should not deter us from making the best of what we have.
Physicians who make use of no theory, for fear of being wrong, should not
be surprised if their patients stop making use of their help. Agnostics make
poor pastors.

In accepting a pastoral role for general practitioners we are not claiming
something that they do not already have. General practitioners today find
themselves faced with people whose problems require the exercise of skills
which range from that of father confessor to moral tutor. It is no use our
refusing to accept these roles. The dividing lines between curing and caring,
between medical problems and social problems, and between problems of
health and problems of living are never clear. More than any other doctors,
we must work at the fuzzy interface. It is often important not to back away
from those who have 'nothing wrong' in the conventional medical sense.
Conversely, problems must not be medicalized and labelled in order to justify
the decision to offer help.

This leaves the general practitioner in a difficult position, one in which
the hard-earned skills which were acquired in medical school often prove to
be of limited value. We have set out to give something rather different which
will, we hope, be more helpful in everyday practice.

Oxford
1988

A. C. M
C. M. P
P. T.
M. J.

Acknowledgements

The authors would like to express their thanks to Dr John Horder for his valuable comments while we were grappling with the final drafts of this book, and also for agreeing to write the Foreword. We are also very grateful to Jane Morbey and Ann Tyrrel for their cheerful help and patience while typing and re-typing the various stages of the manuscript.

Acknowledgements

Contents

Part I Background

1 Sciences basic to psychological problems in general practice

1.1 ETHOLOGY: THE STUDY OF ANIMAL BEHAVIOUR

It may seem strange to start a practical book on psychological problems in general practice with a chapter on animal behaviour. Yet human beings are animals and much human behaviour becomes easier to understand if we view it from an ethological perspective. The behaviour of psychiatric patients is often deemed 'unnatural' but we believe that knowledge of the 'natural' roots from which our behaviour evolves explains a great deal. Problematic behaviour may turn out to be a 'natural' reaction to an 'unnatural' situation.

The world in which most people now live is very different from the world in which we evolved. To some extent the greater degree of control which we can now exert over our environment makes it easier for us to satisfy our basic needs, but it also increases the risk that, in solving one set of problems we may create others.

Observation of the similarities between the behaviour of different species helps us to identify the fundamental laws which govern the complex patterning of human behaviour and to sketch in the inborn tendencies which underlie it. Observation of the differences between species warns us of the dangers of over-generalizing, for there are many distinctive patterns of human behaviour which have few, if any, similarities to the behaviour of other species.

In other words, comparative behaviour is like comparative anatomy; behavioural tendencies are just as distinctive as physical structure. Similarities in behaviour between species point to fundamental mechanisms which have evolved because they ensure the survival of genes.

Instinct and learning

Innate instinctive behaviours are modified by learning from the moment of their inception. Once learned they soon become patterned and habitual. These behaviour patterns can then be repeated without the need for much thought. Many behaviour patterns (e.g. the complex co-ordination of muscle groups used in walking) can be carried on outside conscious attention, leaving the higher realms of cerebral activity available for less routine matters.

The concept of instinct as a predisposition to pay attention to, and to learn, particular things, has now replaced the earlier view which emphasized the rigid fixity of certain patterns of animal behaviour. Almost all behaviour is modified by experience.[1]

The hierarchical organization of behaviour and the problem of mental energy

Innate instinctive tendencies may determine the ultimate goals but learning soon modifies the routes by which these are attained. Since some goals are more important to survival than others, the behaviour patterns which lead to them have priority. Thus, animals engaged in exploration or play (both activities having low priority) can easily be switched to food-seeking or sexual pursuit if appropriate stimuli are perceived. These have moderate priority but can themselves be superseded by alarm (high priority) when triggered by the perception of threat.

Human goals—ranged in likely order of priority

(The hierarchy is not fixed and will change with maturation and experience.)

- perception and removal of threats to young;
- perception and removal of threats to self;
- perception and removal of threats to other dependants;
- obtain water and food;
- maintain proximity to and contact with parent (in childhood);
- obtain sexual partner and maintain proximity with him/her (in adult life);
- attain sexual orgasm;
- obtain and maintain proximity to children (particularly one's own);
- obtain and maintain proximity to home and possessions;
- obtain and maintain proximity to allies;
- attain the highest possible status in the dominance hierarchy;
- explore and learn to control or adjust to unfamiliar aspects of the environment;
- maintain optimal temperature;
- empty bladder and bowels;
- maintain body surface;
- obtain rest, sleep, and shelter.

These represent ultimate goals. In order to achieve them people set-up and move towards a wide range of intermediate goals, they make plans, rehearse behaviour, and play at solving problems of varying degrees of complexity.

Goal-directed behaviour is, of course, switched off by the attainment of a goal and the individual then normally turns to behaviour of a lower hierarchy.

Stimuli from within and from outside the body form the switches which release and terminate behaviour patterns, but these include the stimuli arising out of mental activities such as anticipation and planning which, in human beings, can be very complex and time-consuming.

The existence of memory banks of the cerebral cortex enables human beings to learn a great deal about the world in which they live. In fact it is not going too far to suggest that each of us, in the course of childhood, will build up an internal model of the world of such complexity that it can act as both a template by which we recognize the world we meet and a rehearsal ground in which we plan our own future. The internal model contains everything which we assume to be true on the basis of our previous experience. For this reason it is sometimes termed the Assumptive World. It is probably the most important mental equipment which we possess. Without it we become as helpless a new-born babes, but with it we can anticipate events, plan our responses and prepare for most eventualities. Hence human behaviour is less obviously determined by minute-to-minute changes in the environment than is that of other species. But, even if it is possible in this way for humans to have a measure of free will, they are nevertheless not immune from the vagaries of survival needs.

Goals, and the behaviours by which they are attained, change in the course of maturation, and young animals pass through a series of critical learning periods in the course of which they show an instinctive predisposition to add certain specific skills to their stock of behaviour patterns. Thus, learning to feed usually comes before learning to run, and finding a mate comes relatively late in the sequence.

This model of a hierarchy of behaviour patterns, which can be switched on by one set of circumstances and switched off by another, differs from the traditional model of drives which were assumed to release 'mental energy' (libido) which would persist until the energy was used up. In fact, only very small amounts of physical energy are needed to perform mental functions, and mental fatigue (which is usually taken to reflect exhaustion of reserves of such energy) can more easily be abolished by the perception of novel or threatening stimuli than by resting: the vigour with which mental activities are pursued is governed by the hierarchical level of the behaviour and the proximity of a goal rather than by the strength of 'libido'. Hence it is not always appropriate to treat complaints of mental (as opposed to physical) tiredness by advising a person to rest.

Attachment behaviour

Once learned, a behaviour pattern usually remains open to modification, but there are some behaviours which become relatively fixed. Thus, in many species there is a critical period during which the image of the principal caregiver (usually the mother) is learned. This image thereafter has the capacity to provoke highly specific 'attachment' behaviour which has the function of reinforcing the caregiver's tie to the infant and the infant's tie to the caregiver.

In human babies this behaviour soon comes to include smiling, cooing, babbling, and all the other charming tricks by which small babies captivate their mothers. It also includes the cries and yells by which they attract her attention when she goes too far away and, in time, the following and clinging which enable them to stay close to her.

The caregiver, in turn, finds that the perception and behaviour of an infant switches on an urge to cuddle and care which soon comes to occupy a high priority over most other behaviour. The baby's babbles produce reciprocal crooning and 'baby talk' in the caregiver, to the mutual delight and advantage of both.

Once an attachment has been made it is not easily reversed. In geese the critical period for learning attachment occurs soon after the chick has hatched from its egg. It will then become attached to any large moving object in its vicinity. In nature this is normally the mother, but in the laboratory an entire brood of goslings can be induced to become attached to a man wearing a white coat. Heinroth, who termed this 'imprinting', would walk into his lecture theatre followed by a line of goslings; he would then switch coats with his assistant who would lead the goslings out again.[2]

Originally it was thought that imprinting was irreversible. More recent research indicates that, even in goslings, imprinting can be modified by experience. The concept of imprinting has been used to explain the equally bizarre attachments that sometimes take place in human beings (e.g. in those who are abnormally attracted by leather, hair, or other fetishes).

Although some psychoanalysts have suggested that the child's first attachment is to its mother's breast, feeding and attachment are two different classes of behaviour. The new-born babe will suck with enthusiasm from any suitable object but attachment behaviour is to the whole mother and takes several months to mature. At five weeks most babies will smile at a balloon with two 'eyes' painted on it, but by five months they will only smile if it also has a 'mouth' whose corners go up. By nine months nothing short of a human face will evoke a smile. Even so, most babies are able to distinguish familiar from unfamiliar faces by the age of four months and they show a distinct preference for one person (usually their mother).[3]

It does seem that the first year of life is a critical period for the learning of human parent–child attachments and that, once learned, these ties are difficult to sever. Human beings are less inflexible than geese (who will surely perish if they don't stay close to Mum) but their survival also depends upon a firm bond which will persist throughout the long period of childhood dependency which is characteristic of our species. Recent research even suggests that physical contact with her child during the period immediately after its birth evokes stronger nurturant behaviour in the mother than will occur if contact is delayed.

The effects of learning on the attachment bond

How this bond develops depends on both partners. Thus Ainsworth's important research into the behaviour of young children in a standard 'Strange Situation' shows how patterns of insecure attachment can develop early in life.[4] Factors in the mother (e.g. unresponsive or punitive reactions to the child's cries or clinging) or factors in the baby (e.g. sluggish or hyperactive behaviour) can undermine the confidence which each feels in the other, and may result in excessively anxious clinging or in avoidance and rejection. Once established, such attitudes tend to persist, and there is reason to regard them as one of the major causes of lack of 'basic trust' throughout life. Erickson's term, 'basic trust', can be taken to include both trust in oneself ('self-trust'), and trust in others ('other-trust').[5] A reasonable degree of basic trust is essential to the development of autonomy and the capacity for making and maintaining satisfactory relationships with other people.

Not that the aim of parenting is to produce complete independence. Nobody is so strong or so clever that they need never rely on others. It is part of the function of parents to teach their offspring what to fear. The survival value of anxiety (a general reaction of alertness to danger) and fear (a specific reaction to particular danger) is self-evident. A child that is not taught that roads, open windows, and electric fires are dangerous will be less likely to survive than one who is apprehensive of these things. And because signals of danger are a matter of life and death, they tend to be learned very strongly.

It follows that the view which a child gets of the world, as a safe or a dangerous place, will be determined largely by the views of its parents and that abnormal fears, both general and specific, are easily passed on from parent to child. This enables us to add a third component to 'basic trust' — 'world-trust'. Upon the triad self-trust, other-trust, and world-trust, the developing child will build a set of attitudes and expectations which will tend to persist and to colour their whole personality.

Effects of separation and loss of parents

In the light of these considerations it is no surprise to find that children vary widely in their reaction to separation from their parents. If the separation is acute, they will probably cry, search restlessly, and lose interest in other pursuits, but their age and basic trust will decide how intense these behaviour patterns are. In most instances, the effects of short separations are not harmful, in fact they teach the child that when people go away they *do* come back and this enables them to tolerate increasing periods of time alone. More lasting separations, however, can give rise to lasting problems. They do this partly because of their effects on the child and partly through secondary effects on the caregivers.

Bowlby's work, by emphasizing the importance of mothering, sparked off considerable controversy at a time when women were asserting their rights to autonomy.[6] It also triggered a great deal of research in this area, so that it is now possible to be reasonably confident in our conclusions. Few people now regard even lasting separations from mother as always and necessarily harmful. But a great deal depends upon the circumstances.

Factors which make separation less harmful are:

(1)   the acquisition by the child of secure attachments and basic trust;

(2)   the provision of a consistent, caring person who is capable of acting as a substitute for the person lost;

(3)   a safe familiar home which does not present too many new challenges to an anxious child.

Conversely, the absence of any or all of these factors will militate against satisfactory adjustment. For instance, a young child who becomes sick and is admitted to hospital may suffer from the combined effects of physical discomfort (which evokes intense attachment behaviour), separation from parents, and removal from home. Robertson's film *A two-year-old goes to hospital* illustrates the consequences. Not only do such children suffer from severe grief, but their subsequent capacity for attachment may be impaired, and they may become either excessively clinging or compulsively self-reliant. This, in turn, may create further difficulties for the caregivers, who may react in such a way as to perpetuate the problem (e.g. by punishing a child for clinging).

Other behaviour patterns

Other behaviour patterns which are learned early in life and for which an instinctual basis can be assumed in most social animals are feeding, seeking warmth or shade, and grooming. Only the first of these is a major behavioural issue in human beings whose lack of hair makes grooming less important than in other species and who remain dependent on society to provide a man-made environment and clothing within appropriate limits of climate. Feeding, on the other hand, becomes a crucial activity involving parent–child interaction and one in which problems can easily arise.

In most instances the infant's need to suck is matched by the mother's need to suckle until such time as the child is mature enough to share the parent's food. Thereafter it needs to be protected from poisons and contaminants until it has learned what is safe to eat. But even these simple needs can create great problems in the minds of reluctant or over-anxious mothers and meal times easily become a battleground in which conflicting needs are repeatedly acted out. Small wonder that the roots of later eating disorders can often be traced to early childhood.

Contaminants are a particular source of danger to nest-building and home-making animals. For them, disposal of excreta outside the home is essential, and it is important for the infant to learn to control the timing and disposal of its own excretions as soon as it is physiologically able to do so. Freud's dictum that faeces are a child's first gift to its mother should, perhaps, be rephrased to acknowledge that control of its faeces is a major developmental step which is much appreciated ('There's a good boy!'). Conversely, the conflicts and anxieties which easily complicate parent–child interactions can give rise to special problems in the area of bowel and bladder control.

Autonomy

As time passes individuals must become increasingly autonomous if they are to survive without the continuing support of their parents. Competition for limited environmental supplies lends survival value to strength, assertiveness, and the ability to achieve high status in the dominance hierarchy. But it also gives survival value to the ability to make alliances and to switch appropriately from threat to retreat; 'He who fights, then runs away / Lives to fight another day'. Ethologists and sociobiologists delight in studying the complex laws which govern such issues as the distances which are maintained between individuals and the circumstances which determine whether an approach leads to greeting, threat, or retreat. These laws must be learned by the young animal and much childhood play is devoted to testing out the consequences of an increasing repertoire of aggressive and other behaviours. One consequence of this is the establishment of status hierarchies which reduce the need to spill blood every time a conflict of interests arises. In a remarkably short period of time every child in a pre-school playgroup knows who can be safely challenged and who should be submitted to. The same applies to a group of free-living chimpanzees or a flock of geese. Such hierarchies are not completely fixed, and from time to time a young adult who is gaining in strength and courage will successfully challenge and supplant one of higher status. Similarly, allies may act together to increase their joint standing by mobbing or jointly threatening one or more of the others. This is most likely to occur when strangers approach an established group, but it can also occur within groups.

Conversely, accident, illness, or the loss of allies may cause an individual to decline rapidly in status, and it has been suggested that the passivity and 'depression' which so often accompanies losses of these kinds may serve as a signal system to others to inhibit their aggression, while a new status hierarchy is established without sick individuals being attacked by everyone who is to overtake them. A new status, similar to that of a child, is accorded the sick or bereaved during the period of sickness or mourning, but will soon be lost once they recover their strength and are again seen as potential allies or potential threats.

Sexuality and bonding in adult life

The formation of bonds between adults is, of course, important to the protection of their young, and it takes different patterns in different species. Pair bonding, in which a mother and father mate for life, and rear their young together, is common in birds, but uncommon in other genera. More often, dominant males father children by several females, forming a living group which they then protect while the females rear and protect their own children. In many species the females in oestrus are impregnated by several sexually active males who jointly protect the living group, and do not form exclusive bonds with their own children.

These differences between species make it dangerous to assume that, in human beings, the bonds of matrimony are ordained by instinct rather than by society. Even so it would be surprising if sexual behaviour, which is found in all vertebrates, did not have a strong instinctive basis.

But sexuality and bonding are two different things. It is quite possible, and indeed common, for humans to be sexually satisfied by people to whom they are not attached, and attached to individuals to whom they are not sexually attracted. Sexual behaviour plays a part in bonding by creating the conditions in which attachments between adults can arise (proximity is perhaps the most important of them), but it is not the sole determinant of attachment.

Sexual behaviour has no biological value prior to the onset of puberty and normally becomes apparent at this time. However, like other behaviours which develop after birth, aspects of it may appear before the pattern is fully developed, either by imitation of adults or as a reflection of the incipient onset of the full pattern (few biological changes take place suddenly). Freud observed that many of the patients who sought his help for the treatment of neurotic problems in adult life had had intense feelings of ambivalence towards their parents throughout their childhood. When directed against the parent of the same sex, this was seen as evidence of sexual rivalry, with all the guilt which incestuous urges can be expected to evoke. He termed this 'The Oedipus Complex'. We share the view that mixed feelings of anger and guilt towards one or both parents are often associated with vulnerability to neurosis later in life, but we believe that these findings are a reflection of the insecure attachments which can easily develop early in life and which, for the reasons given above, often persist. Freud's concept of 'infantile sexuality' remains an unproven and unlikely theory.

Homes and territories

The safety of the young depends not only on their attachment to particular safe adults, but also on their tendency to stay close to one particular safe place, home. Most non-nomadic species locate their nurseries in the safest part of their territory, and even nomadic species commonly settle in a particular safe place during periods of child-rearing. Human territories are centred on the home, which remains the place in which people usually feel most secure, even in adult life.

Attachment to home is most obvious in small children for whom going to nursery school may be a terrifying experience. To some extent mother and home are interchangeable and a child who can not have one may be content with the other. At times of sickness, threat, or loss, people of all ages usually prefer to stay home.

Exploratory behaviour

Although home, parents, and other familiar places and persons are a source of security, it is also necessary for the young to learn to cope with unfamiliar and novel individuals and places as they grow up and become more autonomous. Exploratory behaviours occur in all species and curiosity would not have persisted if it did not have survival value (even in cats). By exploring the unfamiliar world we make it familiar, and add it to our internal model of the world. This model can then be used as a means of rehearsing possible events and planning responses—an activity which the human brain is particularly well able to perform.

Exploration of the outside world provides material to improve our internal model of the world, which is then used in another type of exploration, play. In play, young animals try out and develop the skills that will eventually ensure autonomous survival. Fighting, running, hunting, nurturing, robbing (with and without violence), and mollifying are just a few of the skills which can be observed in many social animals at play.

How a young animal responds to a novel situation depends upon the extent to which it perceives the situation as dangerous. Taking its cues from the adults to whom it is attached, the youngster may approach or avoid the stimulus. Insecure youngsters explore and play much less than those who feel safe. This can seriously impair learning, and the competence which would enable them to become more autonomous and secure. An animal which does not learn about the world and practise how to cope with it is at a strong disadvantage. Seligman[7] sees this as the root of feelings of helplessness which in humans, and possibly other species, predate depressions later in life.

Aggression

Aggression has been the topic of much study in animal societies because of its assumed danger to the human race. In animal societies even the noisiest territorial battle seldom leads to anything more serious than a scratch on the nose.[8] Courage is inversely proportional to distance from home, and a nice set of laws can be drawn up to predict which combatant will eventually give way in any given conflict. Only in very special circumstances, as when an individual or its young are trapped and under attack by a supposed predator or mortal enemy, will an animal fight to the death.

Human beings show similar discretion, and it is rare for a battle for promotion to leave the boss dead on the carpet. However, our ability to train people to kill at a distance without witnessing the consequences of their actions introduces a new element into the situation, and the ability to project images of death and destruction into the living room of every home may contribute to feelings of loss of control over one's own safety and that of one's children. This may itself raise the overall threshold of anxiety and increase vulnerability to stress.

The knowledge that normal tigers don't eat people is of limited value if we have no means of knowing if a given tiger is normal. Likewise, it is safer to treat strange people as a threat until they have proved themselves worthy of trust. The more unfamiliar they are, and the more they deviate from our social norms, the more difficult they will find it to become accepted. Sadly, this often leads to rejection or alienation of many of those who are most vulnerable, notably those who are deformed, mentally disordered, or disabled.

Sex roles

It would be surprising if the large anatomical differences between men and women were not reflected in equally large psychological differences. A controversial issue at the present time is the extent to which sexual roles are genetically determined. Assuming that human beings are likely to feel most fulfilled when they have learned how to satisfy in-built behaviour tendencies, it is arguable which tendencies are carried by the X and Y chromosomes.

Most of the psychological differences between the sexes do not become apparent until puberty, by which time a long period of schooling has inculcated a set of goals and behaviour patterns which often seem to conflict with the emerging priorities of mate-selection, home-making, and child-rearing. Women bear the brunt of this conflict and commonly find themselves in a no-win situation in which one set of goals, those concerned with achievement of an acceptable place in the dominance hierarchy, can only be achieved by giving up another set of goals connected with child-rearing. Continued attempts to achieve both goals produce dissatisfaction and can be disastrous to the entire family. It seems very likely that problems of this kind explain the greater vulnerability of women to depressive illness by comparison with men.

Conclusions

The behaviour of human beings may be more flexible than that of other animals but it is not always as flexible as we would like it to be. Patterns of behaviour which proved effective during the critical period of life in which they were first learned, may be quite inappropriate at a later stage, yet these patterns of behaviour are so important to survival that we do not readily relinquish them. This explains why so many of the ways of thinking and behaving which, in later life, are termed 'irrational' or 'neurotic' only become comprehensible when we explore the circumstances in which they first arose. It also explains the peculiar intensity of the feelings which accompany these patterns of behaivour. Patients who cling to counsellors as if their lives depended on them are expressing feelings which arose in a situation in which this might literally have been true.

It follows that any attempt to modify such behaviour, together with the attitudes and feelings that accompany it, will require patience and understanding, Blaming people for these character traits is only likely to increase their insecurity. We need to concentrate on their strengths, and build on these. In this way we can demonstrate our commitment to helping them.

References

1. Thorpe, W. H. (1956). *Learning and instinct in animals*. Methuen, London.
2. Heinroth, O. (1910). *Beitrage zur Biologie, nomentlich Ethologie und Physiologie der Anatinden*. Verkl. 5 Int. Orn. Kongr. 589–702.
3. Ahrens, R. (1954). Beitrage zur Entwicklung des Physignomie und Mimikerkennens. *Z. exp. Angew. Psychol.* **2**, 412–54.
4. Ainsworth, M. S. (1982). Attachment: retrospect and prospect. In *The place of attachment in human behaviour* (ed. C. M. Parkes and J. Stevenson-Hinde), Chapter 1. Basic Books, New York.
5. Erikson, E. H. (1950). *Childhood and society*. Imago, London.
6. Bowlby, J. (1982). *Attachment and loss*, Vol. 1, *Attachment*. Hogarth, London.

7. Seligman, M. E. P. (1975). *Helplessness: on depression, development and death*. University of Pennsylvania.
8. Lorenz, K. (1963). *On aggression*. Methuen, London.

1.2 PSYCHOLOGY

Ethology helps us to understand inborn goals and the roots of human behaviour. Psychology is more concerned with thoughts and feelings which relate to current behaviour. Our thoughts, feelings, and behaviours are influenced by both external and internal factors. External factors include the behaviour of others (the advice they give and what we observe them doing), as well as physical stimuli such as noise and warmth. The internal factors can be psychological, for instance our memories, or physical, such as the activation of different nerve fibres from pain receptors. Given this mass of stimuli, we select and interpret before responding.

Thinking

Perception and attention

Even the simplest external stimuli are processed before being interpreted. This is well documented by the Müller–Lyer illusion (Fig. 1.1) where the line appears longer with outward than with inward facing arrows. Ambiguous figures which can be perceived in two different ways, as the goblet and faces (Fig. 1.2), demonstrate that the same sensory input can lead to two different perceptions, and to two different sets of information entering the thought processes. More complex stimuli, or stimuli with social or emotional significance, are subject to even more elaborate interpretation. This makes it difficult to guess what information the individual has received from the

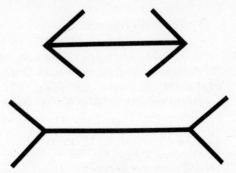

Fig. 1.1.   The Müller–Lyer illusion.

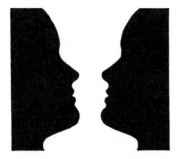

Fig. 1.2.   The goblet and faces illusion.

external environment to lead to a particular interpretation, and may need sorting out during a consultation.

The uptake of information is limited by the capacity of our sensory system. In addition, we selectively ignore or attend to some parts. Otherwise we could not cope with the amount of information presented at any one time. This is obvious in a crowded room where we can usually attend to one conversation while ignoring many others—the 'cocktail party phenomenon'. Experimental psychologists have studied selective attention by presenting two competing messages—for example, one in each ear, or one visual and one auditory—to identify factors which influence selection. It is not simply a passive process, but one that is determined by other information available which helps us to assign priority amongst our hierarchy of goals; for example, while attending to one conversation, one might hear one's own name in another conversation which one had previously ignored. Similar selective processes apply to our perception of pain, and, indeed, to doctors' selection of material which patients offer them.

The organization of thought

Previous learning and experience are obviously important in determining how new information is interpreted. Various researchers have used different terms to indicate how our thoughts are organized. Some talk of 'schemata' as the tools of structured thinking, and others use the term 'personal constructs'.

We each have our own model of the world which enables us to incorporate and interpret new information. At the same time, these models may be modified by new information which does not quite fit our previously held ones. If people are asked to remember information which does not fit an existing assumption, then they are likely to forget parts which do not fit— they may even fabricate new parts to the message to make it compatible with the existing assumptions. For example, an Englishman in France was given suppositories for the treatment of his sore throat. His assumptions about medical treatment only allowed for medication by suppository for constipation or piles. On returning to England he told his GP that his sore throat was the result of being constipated as a result of eating French food. The GP then had a splendid opportunity to expand the medical models available to this patient.

Each of us construes the world in a different way. Subjects might be asked to look at pictures of three famous people, and then to identify in what way two are alike, and different from the third. One subject might say 'two are kind but the other is cruel', whereas another might state 'two are weak but the other is strong'. These answers give a clue to the different constructs used, and to the different ways in which the two people attempt to analyse and interpret situations. Even where people use the same word it may imply different assumptions. When asked to say why he had ranked lung cancer as less serious than heart disease, a patient with lung cancer replied 'Because you do not die immediately'. Another patient might use different criteria for seriousness, such as the amount of pain, the degree of disability, the likelihood of death, whether the disease is treatable, or whether it affects young people.

Boyle[1] found in a multiple-choice test that when doctors and patients had to choose one of four pictures best depicting an anatomical structure, doctors agreed that the stomach was situated where the anatomy texts suggest. On the other hand, patients also showed considerable agreement but they agreed that the stomach was the whole of the lower abdomen. It is easy to conclude that others are using the same assumptions as we are, but clearly a GP and patient who do not share the same construct of 'seriousness' or 'stomach' could have a very muddled consultation. Such possibilities are elaborated in Section 4.2.

These models function as methods of exploring the world, allowing each of us to develop our own unique ideas about the world, based on experience. We use the assumptive world to make predictions in new situations. If our predictions are confirmed, then our model of the world is confirmed; if not, our model is challenged and may result in modification of the model or resistance to the new data. Those assumptions which are learned early in life, which are concerned with high priority goals, and/or which affect a large number of other assumptions can be termed 'basic assumptions'. In a familiar world, our basic assumptions are unlikely to be challenged, but at times we may be faced with important changes which necessitate a radical revision of our internal model of the world. Going blind, developing a terminal illness, losing a spouse, or even being promoted above our level of competence can all face us with the need to reorganize basic assumptions. What then happens is one of the major themes of this book and will be developed in several sections, but especially in Chapter 5 when we look at the changes which occur in the course of the life cycle.

Memory

Memory is not random and one can predict that certain items will be emembered and recalled better than others. If someone is given a list of words to memorize and recall, the words at the beginning of the list will be est recalled. If recall occurs immediately after hearing the list, then the final ew items will also be well recalled, but this does not happen if there is a elay, even of a few minutes, before attempted recall. Ley[2] has shown imilar effects in recall of information in medical consultations. He ecommends that doctors should introduce important items early in the onsultation and be careful not to overload the patient with too many things o remember. He has also shown that patients recall what they consider to e important; typically patients recall the diagnosis better than the advice iven. This may be because the diagnosis is seen as more important than the dvice, or because the diagnosis is usually mentioned earlier in the onsultation.

Two main models of memory have been described, one dealing with stages f processing and the other with levels. The *three-stage model* suggests that ll information is initially stored in a 'sensory store' where it is retained very riefly in a simple form. Sperling[3] demonstrated this type of memory by resenting a 3×3 matrix of letters very briefly and asking subjects to recall s many as possible. On average they recalled four or five. However, if mmediately after presenting the matrix he indicated which row or column vas to be recalled, subjects could report all three required letters, indicating hat all letters were available at least for a brief period. Items from the 'sensory tore' can be selected for processing at the next stage, labelled 'short-term nemory'. This is limited to about six items which are usually remembered or 15–20 seconds, or for longer if the material is rehearsed. For example, telephone number can be retained in the memory store and dialled mmediately after reading it in the directory. It can also be retained in short-erm memory for a couple of minutes by frequent repetition of the number. Anything which interferes with rehearsal, such as the arrival of new data, nterferes with recall. From this stage, information can be selected for more ermanent storage in 'long-term memory', which has a larger, though limited, apacity. Information in 'long-term memory' is organized according to its neaning for the individual, with the result that it can only be retrieved by ppropriate cues. The Englishman referred to previously might retain the vord 'suppository' in his long-term memory, but might not be able to retrieve if given the clue 'a cure for sore throats'.

The *level of processing model* suggests that we recall material better if we ave processed it more deeply. Obviously, if we do not attend, we will be nable to recall. If we attend to the meaning, we are more likely to recall nformation than if we only attend to physical characteristics, such as typeface n words or loudness of sounds. Better recall will be achieved if the material s actively processed, and associated with other material already present. Hence, individuals will tend to recall information which has more meaning or *them*. This explains some of the biases of memory.

The recognition that there are memories and assumptions which are not readily available to introspection is part of the concept of the unconscious mind, an idea fundamental to some schools of psychotherapy. While this is a reasonable enough hypothesis it is difficult to study 'the unconscious' simply because it is not open to introspection. This has not prevented psychoanalysts from building a complex theory which is largely based on the assumption that repressed or unconscious ideas and memories are responsible for many of the symptoms and behaviours which we term neurosis. By making the unconscious conscious, the therapist hopes to uncover the roots of neurosis and to cure it.

The problem with this therapy is that it is untestable. A psychoanalyst can attribute any symptom to unconscious forces without any chance of being proved wrong (or right). If patients accept the attribution, they are thought to be achieving 'insight'; if they do not, they are showing 'denial'. Either way, the analyst can retain his or her belief-system unaltered. While it would be going too far to dismiss the entire psychodynamic theory, we have attempted in this book to avoid attribution of symptoms or behaviours to unconscious forces unless we can indicate the evidence for such attributions.

Memory performs the important function of bringing previous experiences, information, and opinions back into the flow of consciousness and is thus an important internal stimulus. What is retrieved from memory in conjunction with other current stimuli from the internal and external environment will be subject to further processing as we form opinions, explain events, make decisions, and solve problems. It should be clear by now that the information we have available is limited, having been selected at many levels, and having been subject to bias and distortion at each stage.

Problem-solving and judgements

A thinking person can usually form a hypothesis based on the information already available, and collect further information to confirm or disprove this hypothesis. Studies of human problem-solving show that the first hypothesis considered is likely to be very influential, as the average person only seeks evidence to confirm that solution, rather than to test alternatives. Similar results are found in clinical problem-solving, with doctors seeking confirmation for early diagnostic hypotheses and a tendency to overlook conflicting evidence which might support alternatives. Experienced clinicians may be more efficient at using alternative hypotheses than newly qualified doctors, as has been shown in a study of interviews with patients complaining of abdominal pain.[4] Where the patient's problem is partly or wholly psychological, the potential for seeking confirmation is inevitably more difficult, making it even more important that the doctor should not focus on any one hypothesis too early in the consultation.

Other factors lead to distortion in the decision-making process. When faced with the need to make judgements on the basis of incomplete information we use 'rules of thumb', methods which help us to reach the right solution on most occasions, but which can lead to serious distortions. For instance, we might estimate the likelihood of an event by the number of examples that we can bring to mind. On the whole this helps us to reach good decisions based on probability, for instance that a patient's cough is more likely to be due to a common cold than to lung cancer. However, this approach could lead one to miss lung cancer. Again, there are some situations in which the instances that can be brought to mind are an unreliable index. For example, when lay people are asked to estimate the death rate from various diseases they over-estimate the number of deaths from murder, car accidents, and house fires, and underestimate the number due to asthma and diabetes. This can be explained by the tendency of the media to report newsworthy but infrequent events. Similar effects have been shown in American doctors who were more likely to over-estimate the frequency of diseases which had recently been given greater coverage in prestigious medical journals.[5] Thus both doctors and patients may be unduly influenced by their own experiences and by media-reporting in estimating the likelihood of disease. This may play a major part in leading patients to suspect serious illness when they experience minor bodily changes which have no agreed name, and which cannot therefore be grouped and recalled as instances of some common disease. Alternatively, it may lead them to underestimate the seriousness of conditions such as diabetes or asthma.

While such biases can influence all our judgements, there are additional systematic biases which influence our judgements about people. Work in the field of *attribution theory* shows that we give different kinds of explanation for other people's behaviour than we do for our own. We are much more likely to attribute the behaviour of others to an enduring trait or disposition, and to attribute our own behaviour to some feature of the situation. For example, if patients complain about treatment or fail to comply with medical advice, we as doctors are likely to explain this as due to them being difficult, inadequate, aggressive, or ignorant. However, the patients might think of this as due to the doctor's failure to give proper treatment, to fully comprehend the nature of the symptoms, or to the side-effects of the treatment. This type of bias is common in doctors' thinking about patients, and in patients' thinking about others in their environment. For example, a patient may be depressed at other people's success, attributing this to their being clever, rich, strong, attractive, or possessing some other unattainable, unchangeable feature. If the success were attributed to hard work, being two years older, or having completed a course, it would become attainable for the patient. If the behaviour of others is due to personality attributes, then little can be done to change it; if the explanation lies in situational factors, then change is possible. Attributional errors can be explained by noting the

different information we have about our own behaviour and about others —
there is a general actor–observer bias. A further aspect of this bias
is seen in our attributions for success and failure. We are much more
likely to attribute success to our own efforts and failure to external factors
or to chance.[6] Thus we tend to think that patients get better because
of the treatment we prescribed rather than to spontaneous remission;
or that they failed to improve because they took the drug incorrectly or
the drug was ineffective, not because we made the wrong diagnosis. To
correct for this bias we would need to allow failure to be due to ourselves
and success to chance, or to others, but such a correction might be
dispiriting. This bias in thinking may serve an emotional function by
protecting our own self-esteem. Again, this shows how important it is for
us as doctors to be aware of our limitations and not to think of ourselves
as omnipotent.

In addition to these cognitive sources of distortion, information selection
and decision-making may be influenced by the individual's emotions and
attitudes.

Feelings

Emotions

Emotions are described as having four components: the subjective feelings,
the cognitions, the physiological changes, and the behavioural aspects. When
we feel anxious we may be aware of the threat of the impending examination,
and of the heart beating faster, as well as being able to read more rapidly.
These changes do not necessarily occur together.[7] Some individuals may
experience little fear, and behave in a fearless manner, but display major
physiological changes, whereas others may show subjective and behavioural
evidence of fear, but little physiological response.

Many different emotions are experienced and they can broadly be divided
into positive emotions, such as happiness, joy, love, and excitement, and
negative emotions, such as sadness, rage, fear, and disgust. Emotion is usually
accompanied by increases in autonomic nervous system activity — producing
increases in heart rate, blood pressure, pupilary dilatation, and palmar
sweating — and the release of endocrine hormones — such as adrenalin,
noradrenalin, and cortisol. Psychophysiologists measure changes in
laboratory subjects by noting changes in electrical conductance of the skin,
and by measuring muscle tension and respiratory change. Ambulatory
monitoring devices allow the response to emotional stimuli in everyday life
to be measured. For more enduring emotional states, such as those resulting
from chronic stress in real life, endocrine changes or evidence of disease can
be monitored.

Several observable behaviours commonly accompany emotion, including
facial expressions such as scowls or smiles, trembling, fidgeting, postures

such as sitting upright or bowed, stammering, voice quivering, and tremor of the lips. These can serve as cues to other people that one is emotionally aroused, and in non-human animals they may be quite reliable indicators. Human beings, however, are masters at the art of simulation and we tend to attempt to control emotional expression to show only what is socially acceptable. Even so, during a consultation, a patient who professes no problem may have, for instance, moist eyes. This discordance may be used by the doctor to help the patient talk. 'You say one thing but your eyes tell me another.'

Emotional arousal may alter the efficiency of performance — it is a familiar experience that anxiety can ruin success in an exam. The Yerkes–Dodson law proposes that there is an inverted U-shaped relationship between arousal and efficiency so that maximum efficiency is achieved at moderate levels of arousal but that further increases in arousal may lead to a drastic fall in efficiency. This fits the common experience that some degree of anxiety helps us to function well, but that severe anxiety can be disabling. The optimal level of anxiety varies with the task. The more complex the task the less arousal is required.

Stress causes two main physiological response patterns: that due to activation of the sympathetic–adrenal medullary axis and that due to the hypothalamus-pituitary–adrenal cortex axis. These two patterns may be associated with different types of environmental stressor and with different types of subjective experience (see Fig. 1.3), and so, perhaps, with the development of different types of disease (see Chapter 6).

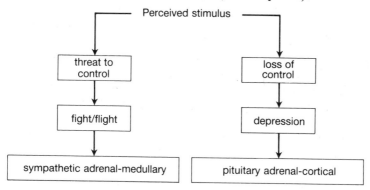

Fig. 1.3. The physiological response patterns to stress.

Schachter[8] has emphasized the role of thought in emotion. Physiological arousal alone does not produce emotion. In order to experience an emotion, an individual must not only experience physiological arousal but must also perceive or imagine a situation which justifies the emotion. In some well-known studies, Schachter and colleagues gave subjects injections of adrenaline or of placebo and gave varying information about the effects of the injection.

Both the adrenaline and the interpretation were found necessary for emotional arousal. While there have been problems in fully replicating Schachter's studies, there is enough evidence to point to the importance of the individual's interpretation of both events and bodily processes in forming an emotional response. A phobic person who experiences an unexplained increase in heart rate is likely to interpret it as a sign of fear and to look around for the likely cause of that fear. When we cannot sleep, we may think that worry kept us awake even though the more correct explanation may be the strong coffee we drank late in the evening, which caused a response to caffeine similar to that which we normally get with adrenaline.

It is a familiar experience that the thoughts that give rise to emotions also influence our perception of events. In one experiment, subjects were hypnotized to produce a post-hypnotic state of happiness or sadness. Both groups of subjects were then told a story about two characters, one happy and one sad. On being asked to recall as much of the story as possible, those with the happy post-hypnotic mood recalled more about the happy character whereas those in the sad mood recalled more about the sad one. This occurred even though the original story had the same amount of information about each.[9] This experiment, and many others by Bower and by other investigators, show that our mood alters our selective attention, our processing, and our recall of information. It may offer an explanation of the tendency for depressed patients only to have gloomy thoughts and only to recall the unfortunate aspects of their lives. Their reports may convince us that we, too, would feel depressed if we had had to contend with such difficult circumstances, but when such a patient's mood lifts, the same life may be described in a much more positive light. The effect of mood in the interpretation of events may also explain why those who are depressed may perceive ordinary bodily changes as 'symptoms'. Cognitive therapy for depression is based on the assumption that the depressed individual's thinking distorts the interpretation of events; therapy challenges some of these interpretations and guides the individual to more effective thinking.

Attitudes

The influence of what we think or how we feel is also apparent in the development of attitudes. Attitudes are the tendencies to respond less or more favourably towards people, objects or events. We are more likely to develop a favourable attitude towards someone whom we believe to be helpful, to work hard, to sing beautifully, or to cook well, than if we believe the person to be a nuisance, to be idle, to spoil the choir, or to give hopeless dinner parties. Similarly, our attitude toward alcohol consumption will be different if we think that alcohol makes us cheerful, gets parties going well, and facilitates good conversation, rather than if we think it causes brain damage, destroys family life, and can lead to cirrhosis of the liver or death.

Since we can hold a large number of beliefs about a topic such as alcohol, the cognitive and emotional factors which lead us to think selectively and distortedly can influence the attitudes we develop.

A number of theories, the best known being that of *cognitive dissonance*, deal with the organization of our beliefs and attitudes — how we deal with facts that conflict with our beliefs, and how we reconcile conflicting opinions. It would appear that we modify or distort information that does not fit our pre-existing beliefs and attitudes, or our knowledge of our own behaviour. If, for example, a class of teenagers is given information on smoking and told that the estimated number of deaths due to smoking in the UK is 100 000 per year, then the smokers are more likely than the non-smokers to distrust the source of the information and the validity of the estimates and also to recall a lower death rate. In this way they can maintain a consistent set of beliefs and attitudes — their existing model of the world can be maintained. Sometimes we pursue consistency unnecessarily and create a 'halo' effect. If we have a positive attitude towards someone, we may attribute many positive characteristics that are not related. For example, we may expect someone who is clever to be a good cook, or vice versa; or we may expect someone who is deaf to be stupid.

It has been shown that altering one word in the description of someone can alter opinions. Two groups of students were given a description of a new teacher and embedded in many other identical descriptive features were the adjectives 'warm' or 'cold'. Even after meeting the teacher, students showed quite different attitudes towards him, depending on whether the description they heard contained 'warm' or 'cold'. Such adjectives often feature in patients' descriptions of their relatives or in doctors' letters about patients, and may exert significant influences on the attitudes engendered.

Attitudes may predict behaviour, but not in the simple one-to-one manner that is often assumed. A patient with a positive attitude to the treatment prescribed will not necessarily comply with the doctor's prescription; the advice may be forgotten, the patient may not know how to comply, the prescription may be too expensive, the timing may be incompatible with hours of work, or family members may disapprove of the medication. Some attitudes may predict two incompatible behaviours. A patient with an unfavourable attitude towards doctors may avoid them as useless or attend regularly to prove that they are useless. Fishbein[10] has rejected the simple model that predicts an attitude from a belief and behaviour from an attitude. He has proposed that multiple beliefs determine one's attitude toward an object or person and that attitudes, in turn, lead to multiple behavioural intentions. These intentions are the best predictor of whether the behaviour will occur. Thus, if we wish to know if an obese patient will diet, it is the overall intention to eat less that is critical, not the attitude toward fatness or the single belief that being overweight may carry a health risk. Even so, other factors may intervene to determine actual behaviour.

Behaviour

While we can know about our own thoughts and feelings by introspection, we can only know about the subjective experience of others by what they say, or by their observable behaviour. This has led some psychologists, most notably B. F. Skinner, to assert that observable behaviour is the only thing that can be studied scientifically by psychologists. Others believe that it is possible to deduce thought processes by observing behaviour; for example, if we are slower in producing a happy association to a given word than a sad association, then we deduce that more unhappy than happy thoughts are available.

Thoughts and feelings can be used to predict and explain behaviour. Ley[2] has shown that patients frequently do not comply with medical advice because they do not understand it or cannot recall it. The Health Belief Model[11] explains failure to comply in terms of the patients' beliefs about the seriousness of the condition, personal vulnerability, the likely success of the recommended advice, and the barriers to, and benefits of, compliance (see also p. 92). Thinking processes in comprehension, recall, and interpretation of information can offer useful explanations of behaviour.

Similarly, emotional and attitudinal processes may explain approach or avoidance behaviour; one approaches what one has a favourable attitude towards or what elicits a pleasant emotional state, and one avoids the unpleasant. Emotions such as fear may have a disruptive effect on behaviour either by a simple reduction in efficiency or by directing behaviour towards fear reduction or avoidance. Leventhal[12] postulated that in a threatening situation one engages in fear control and/or danger control. For example, when faced with major surgery, one might engage in fear control by seeking reassurance that the risks are small, or one might engage in danger control by learning about post-operative procedures to control pain. Sometimes fear control may be incompatible with danger control, as when a woman ignores a breast lump rather than seek medical attention.

Our behaviour is also modified as a result of experience. Three well-known approaches to learning associated with Pavlov, Skinner, and Bandura deal directly with changes in behaviour. Pavlov showed that if one stimulus reliably precedes a second, the first stimulus gradually comes to elicit the behaviour normally elicited only by the second. This procedure is called *classical conditioning*. In his experiments, dogs were 'conditioned' to salivate in response to a bell or light which reliably preceded food. In a more complex experiment, a dog learned that a shock to one paw preceded food. After repeated trials the normal pain response, including withdrawing the paw, was gradually replaced by the responses related to anticipating food. When shock was administered to the trained paw salivation and tail-wagging resulted, but a similar shock to another paw resulted in paw withdrawal. This experiment indicated that the stimulus had to be localized and interpreted before the response occurred.

Medical treatments may produce unfortunate conditioning effects, and it has been noted that out-patients coming to hospital for chemotherapy may experience nausea or vomiting on the journey—a response which would normally be elicited by the treatment.

Skinner described and demonstrated *operant conditioning*, showing that behaviour which is followed by reward, i.e. is 'reinforced', increases in frequency, while punished behaviour becomes less frequent. Behaviour which terminates an unpleasant stimulus also increases in frequency, the opposite being true for behaviour that reduces a pleasant stimulus. It has been shown that doctors can influence what patients tell them by selectively reinforcing what they say. In one study, patients who were reinforced by agreement, head nods, etc. when they said they had symptoms, were then more likely to describe having symptoms 'often' than patients who were reinforced when they said they had symptoms 'rarely'. Thus the doctors' behaviour led to one group of patients complaining of more symptoms than the other. Some behaviour is carried out in order to avoid an unpleasant stimulus which has been anticipated. The 'reward' here is a non-event. Thus, a patient may be able to avoid back pain by walking in a particular way. The problem with avoidant behaviour arises from the fact that the only way people can discover that it is no longer needed is by deliberately doing the thing that they have learned not to do. Hence, the patient's peculiar walk may persist long after the injury which caused it has healed.

For both classical and operant conditioning, repetition increases the strength of the learned response. In each case the learned response is reduced in strength by extinction, i.e. presenting the first stimulus without the second or eliciting the response without giving the reward. The predictable relationships between the two stimuli and between the stimulus and the resulting response appear to be the necessary features of classical and operant conditioning respectively.

Learning can occur when predictability is not necessarily 100 per cent, if, for example, the critical response is only rewarded half the time. Responses which are learned by such *partial reinforcement* are particularly resistant to extinction. If a mother occasionally gives in to a tantrum by giving the toddler the requested sweet, it will take longer to break the tantrum habit by ignoring it than if she had always given a sweet. This kind of inconsistency is a common cause of behaviour problems in childhood.

It seems unlikely that these theories explain all of our learning, as the process would take too long. Bandura has proposed that much of our behaviour is learned by observing others. In an elegant series of experiments he showed that without further prompting we imitate the behaviour of others and that we may suppress or release behaviours if we see others punished or rewarded for similar actions. This work is the basis of *social learning theory*.

While cognitive and emotional factors may explain how experience influences behaviour, these three theories offer explanations without recourse to unobservable processes and postulate instead that we learn by association, by the consequences of our actions and by the observation of others. Some of our more undesirable habits may arise in these ways and it may be difficult to stop them simply by explaining them. It is generally agreed that the best predictor of behaviour in a given situation is previous behaviour in the same situation.

Individual differences

Differences in how people behave may also be attributed to differences in personality. People may be described as having certain traits such as sensitivity, hostility, anxiety, warmth, reliability, or introversion. They may also be described as high or low on any given dimension such as extraversion or hostility, and tests have been developed to measure these traits.

One approach to individual differences which has proved useful in the health field has been the study of 'locus of control'. Individuals displaying an 'internal locus of control' tend to believe that what happens is the result of their own efforts. Those with an 'external locus of control', believe that other people with power, or the forces of fate or chance, are responsible for what happens to them. It is reasonable to expect that patients with external loci of control will be content to receive very controlling medical care which involves authoritarian advice but might not fully participate in methods of care which depend on their own efforts.

The results of studies using personality tests as predictors of behaviour have been disappointing, because of people's inconsistency. Hostile individuals in one situation have not necessarily proved hostile in another. It seems important to keep a balance between personality and situational explanations, and psychologists have moved from an overuse of personality explanations to a greater recognition of situations as the determinants of behaviour. If we want to predict what X will do in situation A, it is not enough to know what kind of person X is—it may be more important to know what other people do in situation A. Thus, knowing that a patient is about to have complex diagnostic tests allows us to predict that they will experience anxiety regardless of who they are, but knowing whether the person is of anxious or calm disposition helps us anticipate whether their anxiety level will go up a lot or a little.

Differences over time

Behaviour changes over time, not simply because the situation changes, but because of changes in the maturation level of individuals, in their diurnal rhythms and brain functioning, and in their health in the broadest sense.

Changes with age are considered in more detail in Chapter 5, but it is important to note here the changes in perception, thinking, emotion, and social behaviour which are part of normal development during childhood. Children are not simply adults without the accumulated information and experience; they have different ways of processing information gained from their environment. Equally, it is inappropriate to see ageing as just a gradual erosion of thinking skills.

Changes in psychological functioning occur with the physical state of the individual. Our state of health, the time of day, and our wakefulness are all important. Many aspects of human performance follow a 24-hour cycle — a circadian rhythm — reaching their peak at the same time every day. Body temperature peaks in the late afternoon or early evening, and psychological efficiency tends to reach a peak about the same time. Laboratory studies in which subjects perform tasks of attention, memory, and reasoning, at varying times of the day, all show best performance at that time, assuming that we control for tiredness by only asking them to do the task once each day. Obviously, there is some variation between individuals, and personality and environmental factors may alter the typical circadian pattern. Each individual is likely to have an optimal time of day and, as stated above, most people find this to be late afternoon. We should not be too surprised if we perform poorly outside this 'peak' time, e.g. on night shift, or 'on call', or after a change of time zone.

Sleep and wakefulness are regulated by the reticular formation in the brainstem, which operates in conjunction with the hypothalamus, thalamus, and higher cortical regions. Changes in the functioning of these parts of the brain due to brain tumours, CVAs, metabolic disorders, or other causes can influence sleep, just as changes in other areas can affect, for example, attention, thinking, or emotion. Experimentally induced lesions in monkeys have shown the role of the limbic system in emotional reactions. In a stable colony of monkeys with an established dominance hierarchy, the amygdala in the top monkey were damaged surgically, with the result that he became less aggressive and dropped to the bottom of the hierarchy, being attacked and beaten by all the others. The same trauma to the other animals had various effects but always influenced aggression, either increasing or decreasing it. Thus, changes in behaviour can give a clue to the site of brain pathology. Finally, other forms of disease, not primarily caused by brain pathology, can lead to temporary changes in thoughts, feelings, and behaviours and these changes may well be relevant in diagnosing some conditions.

References

1. Boyle, C. M. (1970). Differences between patients' and doctors' understanding of some common medical terms. *B. Med J.* **2**, 286–9.

28   *Sciences basic to psychological problems*

2. Ley, P. (1982). Satisfaction, compliance and communication. *Br. J. Clin. Psychol.* **21**, 241–54.
3. Sperling, G. (1960). The information availability in brief visual presentations. *Psychol. Monogr.* **74**, (11).
4. Leaper, D. J. *et al.* (1973). Clinical diagnostic process: an analysis. *Br. Med. J.* **3**, 569–74.
5. Christensen-Szalanski, J. J., Beck, D. E., Christensen-Szalanski, C. M., and Koepsell, T. D. (1983). Effects of expertise and experience on risk judgements. *J. Appl. Psychol.* **63**, 278–84.
6. Antaki, C. and Brewin, C. R. (1982). Attributions and psychological change: applications of attributional theories to clinical and educational practice. Academic Press, London.
7. Rachman, S. and Hodgson, R. (1974). Synchrony and desynchrony in fear and avoidance. *Behav. Res. Therapy* **12**, 311–18.
8. Schachter, S. and Singer, J. E. (1962). Cognitive, social and psychological determinants of emotional states. *Psychol. Rev.* **69**, 379–99.
9. Bower, G. H. (1981). Mood and memory. *Am. Psychol.* **36**, 129–48.
10. Fishbein, M. and Ajzen, I. (1975). *Beliefs, attitudes, intentions and behaviour: an introduction to theory and research*. Addison-Wesley, Reading, Mass.
11. Becker, M. H. and Maiman, L. A. (1975). Sociobehavioural determinants of compliance with health and medical care recommendations. *Medical Care* **13**, 10–24.
12. Leventhal, H., Nerenz, D. R., and Steele, D. J. (1984). Illness representations and coping with health threats. In *Handbook of psychology and health* Vol. IV (ed. A. Baum, S. E. Taylor, and J. E. Singer). Lawrence Erlbaum, Hillsdale, N. J.

Further reading

Atkinson, R. L., Smith, E. E., and Hilgard, E. R. (1987). *Introduction to psychology* (9th edn). Harcourt–Brace–Jovanovich, Orlando, Florida.
Weinman, J. (1987). *An outline of psychology as applied to medicine* (2nd edn). Wright, London.

1.3 SOCIAL SCIENCE

If ethology focuses on the roots of animal behaviour, and psychology on the nature of the thoughts, feelings, and behaviour of the human individual social science views that individual in relation to the society of which we are all a part.

Every person is a member of several social groups, and that membership determines much of an individual's behaviour, the possible social relationships, the controls exercised by society, the events that occur in his or her environment, the circumstances in which he or she lives, and even the health risks incurred.

In this chapter we examine first how social relationships develop in the growing child. We then consider ways in which individuals and groups protect themselves by establishing boundaries and by sharing assumptions about the world which ensure a reasonable stability of social organization.

We move on to look at how the homeostasis of such groups can be disrupted by change, and by threats from within or outwith the group. Health professionals are seen as agents of change and specialists at helping people with the rites of passage which facilitate change.

Finally, we consider the social influence which can undermine or bolster mental health and the support systems which exist in every community.

Social development

'There is no such thing as a baby' wrote Winnicott in one of the most seminal of nonsense statements. What he meant, of course, was that the baby can only be understood in terms of the mother–child unit of which it is a part. Humans are social animals. Their survival depends upon their propensity to associate with others of the species for their joint benefit. Like the pterodactyl, the ant, and other social creatures, we are equipped with a set of inborn tendencies which enable us to interact in order to survive.

As the child develops, its view of the world extends progressively. At first it may be aware of little save the presence or absence of its mother. Soon other family members become familiar, and before long it begins to distinguish between peers and adults, friends and foes.

By the second year of life a baby is already fearful of strangers. Attempts to distinguish between potential allies and potential enemies, and to win friends and avoid or defeat foes, will remain a preoccupation throughout life.

The attachment behaviour by which we make alliances with others was described in Section 1.1. Although these attachments are essential for mutual defence and offence, they serve many more complex functions. Co-operation in a wide variety of activities is essential and, in most species, some forms of communication makes this possible. Among human beings communication becomes an important way of extending our view of the world, and the complex system of assumptions which makes up our internal model of the world is mostly acquired second-hand.

This makes it possible for us to speak of the shared assumptions of a group as if the group had one mind. Jung's theory of 'archetypes' rests upon the idea that there are certain basic assumptions which are shared by all human beings and that these are communicated by means of symbols which have universal significance. For example, since all children have experienced their mother in both angry, rejecting moods, and in loving, nurturant moods, they share highly charged memories about her which easily become linked to group myths about witches and princesses, female devils and goddesses.

Boundaries

Boundaries around the self are necessary for survival. These are numerous and of varying strength, like the skins of an onion. Most obvious are the coverings of our bodies and the walls and fences with which we secure our homes, but many more subtle barriers exist. Just as a home can include and defend more than one person, so the barriers are often shared barriers.

The comfortable dichotomy between friends and foes soon dissolves when we acknowledge that there are degrees of trust. Some individuals are permitted access to our most intimate places; others are not allowed to enter our country.

The safety regulations which are developed to govern the crossing points are finely drawn by mutual negotiation and they often require compromise. Thus, a woman who has a deep-seated distrust of men, or who has been brought up in purdah, may find it very difficult to agree to a vaginal examination by a male doctor. Similarly, it may be hard for a person who feels in danger from physical illness to leave the safe haven of home in order to enter the territory of the doctors and nurses who run a hospital.

Social influence and control

At every level of social organization, some form of control can be observed. This is as apparent when observing a couple, a family, a factory, a nation, or a summit conference of nations. Crucial to a secure place in the world is a reasonable degree of control over our means of survival. This arises, as we have seen, partly from self-trust, faith in our own ability to attain our ends, and partly from other-trust, trust in our ability to obtain the support of others by authority, by charm, or by transferring our resources to them. In human society, money is a more convenient resource to transfer than territory, but both increase security by increasing our ability to control the world in which we live. So, too, does a high place in the status hierarchy, but this also requires the exercise of roles and responsibilities which may themselves tax our competence.

Both within the family and in the outside world, individuals attempt to find a place in which this worth is recognized and their contribution rewarded. Out of interaction with others, they learn a view of themselves which enables them to adapt and conform to the needs of others. What emerges is a continually shifting field of interaction, the stability of which arises from the mutual rewards which each member of the social unit obtains. Homeostatic mechanisms emerge to ensure that members of the group agree on most important issues, that leaders can lead, and that conflicts are regulated. These mechanisms often take the form of shared assumptions which nobody challenges. Thus, the family myth that 'father is strong and unbeatable' and that 'mother, though stupid, is so beautiful that father will always worship her', may be a source of reassurance to the entire family.

In addition to mechanisms which facilitate conformity, there are mechanisms for controlling individuals or groups who attempt to challenge shared assumptions and patterns of behaviour. These include specific punishments meted out by parents and schools, rejection and exclusion from peer groups, and the sentences imposed by courts of law.

The mentally ill, because of their assumed lack of self-control, or unacceptable behaviour (i.e. shared assumptions) have been subjected to the current means of social control during all periods in history. They have been controlled by the forces of religion in the punishment of witches, by the forces of law in imprisonment, and by the forces of medicine by hospitalization. Such controls may benefit the patient, or society, or both. Sadly there are times when they benefit neither. This may result from misperceptions of danger which often lead to intolerance of social deviants, or from the rigid application of social rules which, though benign in intention, do not fit particular cases. Thus, the rule of thumb that anyone with a hallucination should be admitted to a mental hospital may be appropriate in some cases but quite inappropriate in others. Likewise, the uncritical assumption that people who attempt suicide, take off their clothes in public, or oppose the government are mentally ill and in need of segregation under compulsion can lead to injustice.

Change in social units

From time to time the homeostatic mechanisms which maintain the stability of a family or larger social group are thrown off balance by some major change. This may arise from changes in individuals within the group or threats from outside. Father may suffer a serious illness or have an affair with his wife's best friend. Mother may stop pretending to be stupid and demand respect rather than worship. There is much evidence that life events not only affect individuals' own health but that of those around them (see Section 1.3 for further discussion). Such events give rise to anxiety throughout the social unit and normal group functions may be suspended. Those who are in crisis tend to cry for help and to cling to those whose reserves of strength are assumed to be equal to the occasion. Feelings of sadness, rage, or guilt need to be shared, and the situation 'talked through' in an attempt to review the interlocking assumptions which are challenged by the change. Preparation for some life events, such as, for instance, the birth of the first child, can help both individuals and the social unit of which they are a part to cope.

Rituals

Society has its own way of helping, and the rituals, customs, and rights around the life changes which occur at times of sickness, birth, adolescence, marriage, retirement, death, etc. are helpful to many. At such times the succession of social rituals which Van Gennep[1] termed 'rites of passage' may be initiated.

Typically there is a ritual of induction, a transitional period, and a ritual of termination. The rituals of induction identify those people who are entering transitional status and draw in social support for them. They include funerals, introductory courses, retirement parties, or attending a doctor's surgery to obtain a sickness certificate. During the transitional period which follows, people become 'marginal'. They are given special sympathy and consideration, aggression and competition are inhibited, and peers provide protection. It is rightly assumed that people are particularly vulnerable and that they are entitled to ask for help and to depend upon others in ways which would not be tolerated normally. In some cases they are placed under 'taboo'. They are excluded from responsibilities and decision-making and their activities may be severely restricted. After a limited period, which may be fixed, for example the 40 days '*Quarantina*' during which Italian widows were expected to withdraw, or flexible, as when a sickness certificate is renewable, a second ritual of passage takes place, after which the person is expected to take a new place in society or to return to the old. In some societies it is believed that the spirits of the dead remain Earth-bound until the second ritual, when they go to their final resting place and the bereaved are relieved of their obligation to mourn them. In like manner the spirit of sickness may linger until a doctor finally registers a patient as disabled or certifies fitness to work. The clergyman, the doctor, the social worker, and the undertaker are all ritual specialists in our society.

The group response to threat

In the world in which most of man's evolution took place, social groups were surrounded by enemies. These included not only predators, but members of the same and other species who were in competition for food and other resources. Similar situations exist today. Alliances are made for mutual protection, and selection procedures determine who is admitted to an in-group and who must remain without. Only those with a surplus of resources can afford to be generous to 'marginal' groups (e.g. the old, the handicapped, and those of lowest status). Strangers and others who deviate from familiar norms are regarded with suspicion and even hostility. Conversely, friends and allies draw together in the face of threat.

Western people in their affluence, like to think that they can rise above the brutal facts of Malthusian life. But civilization has not changed their nature. In the jungle of committee and boardroom, battles rage and the weak go to the wall. Social security provides a safety net, but in so doing creates a new kind of transitional status for those who lose out. Increasing numbers are now finding that there may be no end to the transition. They have become marginal people.

Even within the family unit threats emerge. Pressures to change the familiar status quo commonly arise as a result of maturation in the younger generation or deterioration in the old. Each tries to defend the assumptions they are making and to discredit or overrule those of their opponents. Alliances are made which split the family into camps, scapegoats are identified and extruded, lines are drawn, dependants forced to confirm or change their commitment to a particular view of reality (the family myth), ritual battles are fought, the 'family script' is re-enacted.

Health professionals as agents of change

When changes are coming about and there is nobody within the social unit who is seen as able and willing to cope, it is usual for people to seek help from outside. Doctors are often seen as trusted members of the community, but their role requires persons to define themselves as 'sick' to be entitled to help. Thus, family or group problems may present in the guise of individuals who are asking for 'treatment' of 'symptoms'. It is important for doctors to interpret the situation correctly if they are to give the help that is needed to enable the change to take place smoothly.

Alcohol and other drugs are popular ways of coping with anxiety in the face of change and doctors may be involved in authorizing, monitoring, or limiting their use. This is only possible if doctors have a clear idea of the circumstances in which drugs are being taken and of the dangers of abuse. On the whole, alcohol and drugs are a poor substitute for emotional support and counselling; there are few doctors who have not regretted the injudicious prescription of drugs at a time of family crisis.

Doctors also have the power to sanction absence from work and to authorize, and even demand, that their patients relinquish a variety of roles and responsibilities. Their credibility in society is such that people often prefer to 'go sick' rather than to ask for permission to interrupt accustomed roles on compassionate grounds'. When family conflicts take place, doctors are in an ambiguous position. We like to think that we are impartial and detached from such conflicts, our role being to patch up the casualties and, in our small way, to undo some of the injustice which can result from being sick or handicapped. But we are also governed by our own myths; we are members of various 'in-groups' and perceived by others as allies of these groups. Thus we may be asked to take sides in a family conflict in which one side is denigrating the behaviour of the other as 'sick' or 'mad'. On the whole, we are more often called by middle-aged adults to control or 'cure' their children, or their elderly relatives, than we are by the children or elderly to control or 'cure' the family leaders. The process of medical or psychiatric 'labelling' is a subtle one because it is claimed to be done for the patient's benefit. Moreover, the diagnostic labels used in psychiatry are so broad that we may find it quite difficult to decide whether a particular act fits the label or not.

A 15-year-old boy brought along by his father because he stayed out until 10 o'clock at night, smoked with his friends, and occasionally stole money at home, could have been labelled as 'disturbed', until viewed in the context of the boy's need to achieve independence and of his father's authoritarian behaviour at home. The son was expected to do all the washing up and gardening, was given very little pocket money, and had that 'docked' if he didn't do the house jobs properly. The father and son both expected the doctor to identify with the father.

Clearly, in cases like this, it is more helpful to perceive the 'symptoms' as the reflection of the problems of a family faced with the need to change than as a mental illness, but this does not mean that we should go to the other extreme of denying the reality of all psychiatric illness and regarding psychiatric diagnosis as a conspiracy by the establishment to control dissidents.

Sadly, this paranoid view is often held by people who need our help. Hence, young people may fail to seek the help of a doctor who is 'old enough to be my father' and elderly people have been known to commit suicide rather than confide in a 'young fool who thinks he knows everything'.

To be effective caregivers we must have a clear picture of the social attributions that are being made about us and we may need to make special efforts to discuss and redefine these with the patient when we feel that they are hampering our work. At times we may need to draw in others whose social identity is more acceptable than ours to the people who need help. For instance, in the above example the enlisting of help in the form of a young female social worker was beneficial for all concerned, including the mother caught between the two strong-willed males in the household. Other members of the primary health-care team will be appropriate on other occasions.

Social circumstances

In understanding the experience and behaviour of individuals in society, it is important to consider the social circumstances in which they live. Such variables appear in most studies in the form of social class indicators such as income, housing, and education, and are relevant in matters of health. So, too, are the support systems of family, friends and neighbours.

The Black report[2] highlighted the differences in morbidity and mortality between rich and poor. Although this report focused mainly on organic disease and lower social class, residence in inner city areas and poverty are also known to be associated with increased morbidity, including mental illness.[3] Geographical mobility is known to be associated with increased incidence of coronary heart disease, as is moving from the country to factory work.[4] Being poor and having three or more children under the age of 11 is known to be a factor in depression.[5] Unemployment has proved a difficult area to research, but, on balance, it seems likely that it contributes to increased morbidity and mortality, including suicide. There is much argument whether people become poor or unemployed because they are already harbouring illness or whether the social circumstances cause the illness; in our view both are usually true.

A critical feature in people's social environment is the amount of social support available to them. Confiding relationships are protective against many illnesses, of which depression[5] and angina[6] have been particularly well researched. A large study in the USA found the following protective in decreasing order: marital relationships, contact with friends and relations, church membership, formal and, least, informal group associations.[7] For example, army wives who had been involved in many house moves had fewer complications of pregnancy when they had had good social support than when they felt unsupported.[8]

It seems that most of us need both a confiding relationship which supplies our daily needs, and also an extended network of friends who may be needed occasionally, but who can also be called upon in times of crisis. It is of interest that the Church of England in its recent report on the inner cities *Faith in the City*[9] emphasizes that what is amiss in the inner cities is that social networks have broken down and somehow need to be restored. Readers might find fascinating the description of the effects of the breakdown of social networks which occurred when London Eastenders moved to the new towns in the 1950s.[10] Recent research in the USA has shown that asking the simple question 'How many people do you have near you that you can readily count on for real help in times of trouble or difficulty, for instance watch over the children or pets, give a lift to the hospital or store, or help if you are sick?' was predictive of increased sickness in women. An answer of 'none' or 'only one' predicted a statistically significant excess of illness over the succeeding 6 months compared to those with more available assistance.[11]

The role of the extended primary health-care team

The team of general practitioners, social workers, health visitors, and perhaps voluntary co-ordinators is particularly well placed to foster community networks of, for instance, meetings for antenatal women and young mothers, pre-retirement courses, old people's clubs, and good neighbour's associations. New patients registering with a practice can be helped by being given a leaflet about the organizations and activities available in the community. In one practice, the children of service families who were billeted in a block of flats on the periphery of the practice and geographically distant from the fathers' work and the mess, presented more frequently to the practice with coughs and colds, and their mothers with depression, than those who lived closer to the service community. As a result of a meeting between the Warrant Officer in charge of the families and the social workers and health visitors, all new arrivals were invited to crèches, coffee mornings, and clubs. A dramatic fall in surgery attendances followed. In another practice, a lady who had lived in the area for some time presented with symptoms of depression. It was easy to elicit that her marriage, though stable, was unrewarding. There was little sharing of confidences, and she was lonely. Introducing her to the local dramatic society changed her life and relieved her depression.

'No man is an island.' It is of fundamental importance for those working in health care in the community to bear in mind the interaction between the individual and society. The primary care team is in a key position not only to use, but also to create, a community. This will be a theme to which we shall return in forthcoming pages.

References

1. Van Gennep, A. (1960). *Rites of passage.* Routledge and Kegan Paul, London.
2. Townsend, P. and Davidson, N. (1982). *Inequalities in health: The Black Report.* Penguin, Harmondsworth.
3. Marsh, G. N. and Channing, D. M. (1986). Deprivation and health in one general practice. *Br. Med. J.* **292**, 1173–6.
4. Cassell, J. (1976). The contribution of the social environment to host resistance. *Am. J. Epidem.* **104**, 107–23.
5. Brown, G. W., Bhrolchain, M. N., and Harris, T. (1975). Social class and psychiatric disturbance among women in an urban population. *Sociology* **9**, 225–54.
6. Medalie, J. H., Snyder, M., Groen, J. J., Neufeld, H. N., Goldbourt, U., and Riss, E. (1973). Angina pectoris among 10,000 men: 5 year incidence and univariate analysis. *Am. J. Med.* **55**, 583–94.
7. Berkman, L. F. and Syme, S. L. (1979). Social networks, host resistance, and mortality: a 9 year follow-up study of Alameda County residents. *Am. J. Epidem.* **109**, (2), 186–203.
8. Nuckolls, K. B., Cassel, J., and Kaplan, B. H. (1972). Psychosocial assets, life crisis and the prognosis of pregnancy. *Am. J. Epidem.* **95**, 431–41.
9. *Faith in the city.* A call for action by Church and Nation. The Report of the Archbishop of Canterbury's Mission on Urban Priority Areas (1987).
10. Wilmot, P and Young, M. (1960). *Family and kinship in East London.* Routledge and Kegan Paul, London.
11. Blake, R. L. Jr. and McKay, D. A. (1986). A single-item measure of social supports as a predictor of morbidity. *J. Fam. Pract.* **22**, 82–4.

2 The prevalence of psychological problems in general practice and the organization of care

2.1 INTRODUCTION

When looking at the literature on the epidemiology of psychological problems in general practice, one is immediately struck by the wide variations in their reported prevalence and incidence. Shepherd and Clare[1] reproduced the figures given in Table 2.1, showing a variation in psychological morbidity rates from 3.7 to 65 per cent (although it is important to realize that these figures relate to different time-spans). Other more recent workers have shown similar widely scattered figures. As it is highly unlikely that these are true variations between different populations, one must immediately ask the question—how do different authors define psychological disease? Are they talking about psychiatric diagnoses of the kind seen in mental hospitals, or are they taking into account the minor problems or feelings of dis-ease that patients frequently present to doctors in primary care? Although an extensive review of nomenclature and classification is out of place here, these variations in reported morbidity require us to gain insight into the presentation of psychological problems in general practice.

In countries without a primary care 'gate-keeper' system of the type we have in the UK, patients refer themselves to psychiatric or other health workers direct and therefore become, by definition, psychiatric (or other) 'cases'. The concept of what constitutes a 'case' depends, in essence, on whether the health worker and the patient between them consider professional help to be required. This will vary with the doctor's or other health worker's own concept of disease, the patient's perception of their own well-being, and what is accepted by society as health and disease.

Questionnaires

In recent years, standardized questionnaires have been devised which aim to overcome some of the inconsistencies of definition of psychological disease mentioned above. Of these, the most widely used is the General Health Questionnaire (GHQ) of Goldberg.[2,3] These questionnaires pick up the commonest symptoms of psychological problems—anxiety, irritability,

Table 2.1. *Psychiatric morbidity rates reported from a number of general practice surveys*

Surveys of patients registered	Number at risk	Period of survey	Conditions specified	Percentage of patients at risk
Ryle (1959)	2400	one year	neuroses	4.1
Logan (1953)	27 000	one year	mental and psychoneurotic disorders	4.7
Logan and Cushion (1958)	380 000	one year	mental and psychoneurotic disorders	5.0
Martin et al. (1957)	3700	one year	mental and psychoneurotic disorders	5.6
McGregor (1950)	2500	one year	anxiety states and hysteria	6.8
Kessel (1960)	900	one year	'conspicuous psychiatric morbidity'	9.4
Primrose (1962)	1700	one year	psychiatric morbidity	13.2

Surveys of patients consulting	Number consulting	Period of survey	Conditions specified	Percentage of patients consulting
Davies (1958)	2700	one year	psychoneuroses	6.4
Fry (1957)	4000	five years	psychoneuroses	8.5
Hopkins (1955)	650	six months	psychiatric illness	11.1
			stress disorders	31.7
Hewetson et al. (1963)	650	one month	psychiatric disorders	23.2
Paulett (1956)	—	five years	neuroses	65.0

Surveys of illnesses	Number of complaints or episodes	Period of survey	Conditions specified	Percentage of complaints or episodes
Handfield-Jones (1959)	2700	one year	mental and psychoneurotic disorders	3.7
Davies (1958)	3400	one year	psychoneuroses	5.2
Pemberton (1949)	4800	two weeks	mental and psychological ill health	6.5
Perth (1957)	150	one month	'non-organic'	53.7

Surveys of consultations	Number of consultations	Period of survey	Conditions specified	Percentage of consultations
Logan and Cushion (1958)	1 400 000	one year	mental and psychoneurotic disorders	5.0
Horder and Horder (1954)	2000	consecutive series	psychiatric disorder	7.7
Finlay *et al.* (1954)	—	four months	stress disorders	20.0
Pougher (1955)	500	consecutive series	neurosis	47.6

Reprinted from Shepherd and Clare (1981)

depression, fatigue, and sleeplessness, but do not necessarily identify people with major psychotic problems or those with personality disorders.

Although these questionnaires provide a more consistent and reproducible estimate of the prevalence of psychological abnormality in the community, it must be stressed that the cut-off point between 'normal' and 'abnormal' is arbitrary and derives from society's and the health worker's concept of what is disease. Also, screening questionnaires like the GHQ are designed to have a low false negative rate to ensure that all positives are identified. Therefore, the false positive rate is high and the questionnaires can give a misleadingly high figure if used to assess prevalence, unless appropriate corrections are applied. The whole matter has given rise to much research over recent years, to which the disciplines of sociology and psychology have contributed.

References

1. Shepherd, M. and Clare, A. (1981). *Psychiatric illness in general practice* (2nd edn). Oxford University Press.
2. Goldberg, D. (1972). *The detection of psychiatric illness by questionnaire*. Maudsley Monograph, No. 21. Oxford University Press.
3. Goldberg, D. (1978). *Manual of the General Health Questionnaire*. National Foundation for Educational Research, Slough.

2.2 PRESENTATION OF MENTAL ILLNESS IN THE COMMUNITY

If it is accepted that standardized questionnaires give a consistent estimate of the incidence of psychological problems in the community, and one which can be used to look more objectively at differences between various communities, we are in a better position to look at what happens to those who are identified by the questionnaires, and what problems they have.

In order to interpret a table such as Table 2.2 (modified from Goldberg and Huxley)[1] a number of definitions of terms need to be clarified. *Incidence rate* (annual inception rate) refers to the number of individuals with a new episode of a given disease each year, per 1000 population. *Prevalence* (point prevalence) refers to the number of people with a given disease in the population at any point in time, expressed per 1000 population. *One-year period prevalence* (e.g. annual patient consulting rate) refers to the number of people who suffer from a given disorder during the course of a year on at least one occasion, per 1000 population. Table 2.2 seems to indicate that at any time between 5 per cent and 11 per cent of British men and 12–23 per cent of British women are likely to be suffering from a psychiatric illness as measured by these questionnaires.

Table 2.2. *Prevalence rates per 1000 population at risk for random samples of the general population for all psychiatric illness: results from recent surveys*
(GHQ = General Health Questionnaire; CMI = Cornell Medical Inventory; SADS = Schedule for Affective Disorders and Schizophrenia; RDC = Research Diagnostic Criteria; PSE = Present State Examination; ID = Index of Definition; CIS = Clinical Interview Schedule)

Type of rate	Investigators	Location	Case-finding method	Size of sample	All psychiatric illness rates per 1000 population		
					Males	Females	Total
Rates calculated from psychiatric screening questionnaire	Goldberg, Kay, and Thompson (1974)	South Manchester, UK	GHQ	213	114	233	184
	Finlay-Jones and Burvill (1977)	Perth, Australia	GHQ	2342	89	150	120
Point prevalence	Ingham, Rawnsley, and Hughes (1972)	Industrial Wales (Rhondda)	modified CMI	300	120	230	175
		rural Wales (Vale of Glamorgan)		581	50	155	203
Clinical assessments	Dilling (1979)	Bavaria, W. Germany	CIS	1231	160	218	193
Point prevalence	Weissman, Myers, and Harding	New Haven, USA	SADS-RDC	511	164	189	178
Clinical assessments	Wing (1979)	Camberwell, London		800	59	119	90
	Orley and Wing (1979)	Ugandan villages, Africa	PSE-ID	191	194	291	241
One-month period prevalence	Duncan-Jones and Henderson (1980)	Canberra, Australia	GHQ/PSE/ID	756	70	110	90
Clinical assessments	Brown and Harris (1978)	Camberwell, London	PSE	458	—	170	—
One-year period prevalence	Brown et al. (1977)	North Uist, Outer Hebrides	PSE	154	—	120	—

Reprinted from Goldberg and Huxley (1980) by permission of the authors and publishers.

Incidence and prevalence rates for morbidity may be obtained from population questionnaires, presentation to (or identification by) primary physicians, attendance at psychiatric out-patient departments, and admission to hospital beds. These various 'stages' along the pathways to psychiatric care have been considered by Goldberg and Huxley in their concept of 'levels' and 'filters'. This is summarized in Table 2.3.

Level 1 represents the total detectable psychiatric morbidity in the community, determined by population screening questionnaires. As mentioned above, the decision by individuals to present themselves to the doctor depends on their own and their family's concept of what is an illness, and on the accessibility of the doctor, both in terms of time, and in some countries, money. This is the first filter.

Having passed through the first filter an individual becomes a 'patient' at level 2, which expresses the total morbidity in primary care. The figure shown here is the prevalence of psychiatric illness as measured by questionnaires in random samples of GP attenders. Only a proportion of these patients will be diagnosed by the doctor as having psychiatric morbidity (they may, for instance, come to the doctor with physical symptoms and be managed only on a physical basis), thus introducing a further filter before entering level 3, the 'conspicuous' or overt psychiatric morbidity of primary care. The figures are the rates of psychiatric illness diagnosed by GPs. The chain from here involves further filters — referral to the psychiatric service to enter level 4 and admission to in-patient care to enter level 5.

It will be seen that levels 1–3 are applicable to self and primary care, and levels 4 onwards are in the province of psychiatrists — at least in normal practice in the UK. In countries where psychiatrists are the doctors of first contact a different progression may be followed.

The levels and filters applicable to primary care are illustrated in a Venn diagram (Fig. 2.1). The square includes all patients registered with a practice, of whom the approximately 66 per cent who consult in any one year are included in Circle A. The eccentric design of the diagram draws attention to the fact that some patients pass through filters they should not have done, and vice versa.

When examining Table 2.3 it is interesting to note the close similarity in numbers between level 1 and level 2.[2] This suggests that most patients suffering from psychological problems do visit their doctors, though only just over half have psychological problems labelled as psychiatric illness.

In one study by Goldberg,[1] GPs were asked to categorize 262 patients who had been diagnosed as having psychiatric problems (i.e. were at level 3). Of these, 31 per cent were said to be suffering from anxiety states, 25 per cent from depression, and a further 31 per cent from a mixture of anxiety and depression. Eight per cent suffered from phobias, 0.8 per cent from schizophrenia and 4.2 per cent from miscellaneous other conditions. The vast majority therefore suffered from anxiety, depression, or a mixture of the two, and the whole represented 20 per cent of all attenders (262 out of 1310).

	The community	Primary medical care		Specialist psychiatric services	
	Level 1	Level 2	Level 3	Level 4	Level 5
	morbidity in random community samples	total psychiatric morbidity, primary care	conspicuous psychiatric morbidity	total psychiatric patients	psychiatric in-patients only
One-year period prevalence, median estimates	250 →	230 →	140 →	17 →	6 (per 1000 at risk per year)
	First filter	Second filter	Third filter	Fourth filter	
Characteristics of the four filters / Key individual	illness behaviour / the patient	detection of disorder / primary care physician	referral to psychiatrists / primary care physician	admission to psychiatric beds / psychiatrist	
Factors operating on key individual	severity and type of symptoms / psycho-social stress / learned patterns of illness behaviour	interview techniques / personality factors / training and attitudes	confidence in own ability to manage / availability and quality of psychiatric services / attitudes towards psychiatrists	availability of beds / availability of adequate community psychiatric services	
Other factors	attitudes of relatives / availability of medical services / ability to pay for treatment	presenting symptom pattern / socio-demographic characteristics of patient	symptom pattern of patient / attitudes of patient and family	symptom pattern of patient, risk to self or others / attitudes of patient and family / delay in social worker arriving	

Reprinted from Goldberg and Huxley (1980) by permission of the authors and the publishers.

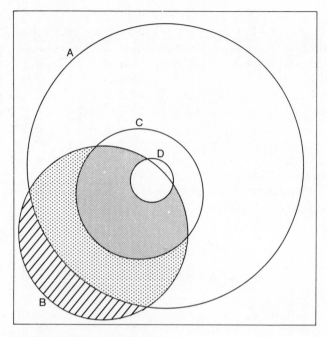

A=Consult their doctor during year
B=Psychiatrically ill during year (level 1)
C=Identified by their doctor as psychiatrically ill (level 2)
D=Referred to a psychiatrist (level 3)

▨ Do not pass 1st filter (ill but do not consult)

▨ Do not pass 2nd filter (illness unrecognized by doctor)

▨ Do not pass 3rd filter (not referred to a psychiatrist)

Fig. 2.1. Venn diagram showing the relationship between the first three levels (reprinted from Goldberg and Huxley 1980,[4] by permission of the authors and publishers).

Of those who do have such problems detected, only 17/140 (12 per cent) are referred onwards for formal psychiatric opinions and treatment. This emphasizes again the high proportion of psychiatric morbidity which is managed in the primary care setting and prompts the question—can general practitioners be trained to pick up a higher proportion of the morbidity that patients present—and would that alter the outcome? Johnstone and Goldberg[3] showed that if the patient's doctor is made aware of these hidden problems, the patients are likely to accept help and to have fewer symptoms at follow-up after a year. Studies by Marks *et al.*[4] and Goldberg[3] have demonstrated some of the determinants which correlate with GPs' ability to detect psychiatric morbidity, and which are amenable to improvement by training (see p. 52).

A further possibility would be to screen the community by distributing questionnaires, thus identifying those with psychiatric morbidity. This would bring to notice not only those who do not attend the doctor, but also those who do attend but are not recognized as having psychological problems— for instance, those suffering from Somatoform disorders (see Section 6.3). The use of questionnaires has been found very effective in identifying patients with alcohol problems (see Chapter 8)—there is scope for using them in other areas.

It is good for GPs to become aware of the psychological problems of their patients, but this does not necessarily mean that we should be too keen to make psychiatric diagnoses or even to think of people with these problems as 'sick'. It is often possible to give due weight to psychological issues without labelling a person as psychiatrically ill.

References

1. Goldberg, D. and Huxley, P. (1980). *Mental illness in the community*. Tavistock Publications, London.
2. Goldberg, D., Kay, C., and Thompson, L. (1976). Psychiatric morbidity in general practice and the community. *Psychol. Med.* **6**, 565-9.
3. Johnstone, A. and Goldberg, D. (1976). Psychiatric screening in general practice. *Lancet* **1**, 605-8.
4. Marks, J., Goldberg, D. P., and Hillier, V. F. (1979). Determinants of the ability of general practitioners to detect psychiatric illness. *Psychol. Med.* **9**, 337-53.
5. Goldberg, D. (1982). In *Psychiatry and general practice* (eds A. W. Clare and M. Lader), pp. 35-41. Academic Press, London.

2.3 FACTORS ASSOCIATED WITH PSYCHIATRIC ILLNESS IN GENERAL PRACTICE

Social

Much information has become available in recent years concerning the relationship between psychiatric morbidity and social factors, which may affect the onset, course, and outcome of both physical and psychological problems.[1]

Long-term factors

A study in Chicago[2] showed that first admissions for schizophrenia were more prevalent in poor, socially disorganized central areas of the city, while those for manic-depressive psychosis were distributed at random across the city. In considering findings of this kind, the question always has to be asked whether schizophrenics drift to poor neighbourhoods after developing the condition, or does the neighbourhood induce the condition to develop. Evidence suggests that both factors contribute.[3]

Much interesting work has come from Brown *et al.*[4] These workers have studied the prevalence of depressive illness in women in Camberwell and found that some factors increase vulnerability to the depressive effect of major life events. Such factors include the loss of a mother before the age of 11, absence of an intimate, confiding relationship, unemployment, and the presence of several young children at home.

The effect of social factors is further confirmed by studies such as those of Tischler *et al.*[5] in Connecticut, USA. Their study, based on patients who have passed the first filter and attended primary care services, showed that the groups which made most use of services were the unmarried, unemployed, those who live alone, and those without religious commitment.

Anyone working in the community is aware of the difference in the strength of the supportive networks available to different people — not only in number but in intimacy. It has been found[6,7] that old people in the community who are mentally ill have restricted social contacts when compared with those who are well. Intimate relationships perceived as inadequate are associated with the presence of neurosis.[8] The studies by Brown and others in Camberwell (quoted above), also relate to this subject, but one is frequently left with a chicken and egg question 'Which came first?' — the absence of social support or the development of a condition which rejected intimacy. Again, it seems likely that both factors play a part.

Short-term factors — life events

The above factors constitute the soil in which psychological problems can grow. They persist for long periods of time and their influence is undramatic and chronic. They seldom constitute a main cause of the disorders with which they are associated, but they increase vulnerability and need to be considered in conjunction with other causes.

More obvious are the major life changes and threats of change which have been lumped together under the general term 'Life events'. These have been the subject of much study in recent years, notably by Rahe[9] and his colleagues in the USA, and by Brown and others in Britain (e.g. as quoted above). Rahe used a check-list to measure the frequency of commonly occurring events. He found that patients with a variety of psychiatric and somatic disorders reported more life events during the weeks preceding the onset of the illness than controls. He also showed that life events affecting a family were often followed by 'illness clusters', episodes of sickness arising in more than one member of a family and taking a variety of forms.

Rahe's work has been criticized on the grounds that many of the events included in his check-list may have resulted from the behaviour of the person who subsequently presented with psychiatric problems. Thus, the break-up of a relationship may cause depression or may be caused by depression. Brown's significant work successfully answer this and other criticisms of life event' studies. By separating 'dependent' and 'independent' events, he was able to demonstrate that even those events that are independent of the patient's behaviour are increased in frequency before the onset of a depressive illness. He also showed that life events can bring forward or precipitate the onset of schizophrenia.

The least satisfactory aspect of 'life events' studies is the catch-all character of the events in question (a problem which they share with the similar concept of 'stress'). Paykel[10] has looked more closely at the types of events which carry the highest risk, and has concluded that events whose influence is transient, or which are classed as 'positive' in quality, seldom constitute a threat to mental health. On the other hand, events which are lasting in their effects and 'negative' in quality, i.e. they are classed as losses rather than gains, contribute significantly to the psychological disorders which follow them.

Losses have been regarded as potential causes of mental illness since biblical days, but it is only in recent times that they have been subjected to scientific scrutiny. Bereavement by death is the classic example and has been widely studied (see Section 5.11 for details) but there are many types of loss which remain to be investigated. In general, unexpected losses and those with prolonged effects are most stressful.

Physical morbidity associated with psychiatric illness in the community

This subject will be dealt with in greater detail in Chapter 6 but it must be mentioned when considering the ways in which mental illness presents in the community. General practitioners are familiar with the presentation of physical illness when the major problem is psychological — for instance, when a patient with depression presents with generalized aches and pains. This may be due to the belief held by patients that physical problems are a more acceptable way into the 'busy' doctor's consulting room, carrying less of a stigma than psychiatric problems, or it may reflect real ignorance. But there is also evidence for a real association between many physical and psychiatric illness. In a careful study[11] of a sample of 1500 patients in London, it was found that individuals with psychiatric disorders had a significant excess of ischaemic heart disease over controls. This could not have been due to worry about the disease, because most patients were not aware that they had ischaemic heart disease. This psychiatric group also had a general increase in other physical disorders over the control group, and the authors suggested that some individuals have a generalized vulnerability to disease, physical and psychological.

References

1. Cassel, J. (1974). An epidemiological perspective of psychosocial factors in disease aetiology. *Am. J. Publ. Hlth* **64**, 1040–45.
2. Faris, R. E. L. and Dunham, H. W. (1939). *Mental disorders in urban areas. An ecological study of schizophrenia and other psychoses.* University of Chicago Press, Chicago.
3. Goldberg, E. M. and Morrison, S. L. (1963). Schizophrenia and social class. *Br. J. Psychiat.* **109**, 785–802.
4. Brown, G. W. S. and Harris, T. (1978). *Social origin of depression: A study of psychiatric disorder in women.* Tavistock, London.
5. Tischler, G. L., Henisz, J. E., Myers, J. K., and Boswell, P. C. (1975). Utilisation of mental health services. *Archs Gen. Psychiat.* **32**, 411–15 and **32**, 416–18.
6. Nielsen, J. (1962). Geronto-psychiatric period prevalence in a geographically delineated population. *Acta psychiat. Scand.* **38**, 307–10.
7. Kay, K. D. W., Beamish, P., and Roth, M. (1964). Old age mental disorders in Newcastle upon Tyne. Part II: A study of possible social and medical causes. *Br. J. Psychiat.* **110**, 668–82.
8. Henderson, S., Byrne, D. G., Duncan Jones, P., Scott, R., and Adcock, S. (1980). Social relationships, adversity and neurosis: A study of associations in a general practice population sample. *Br. J. Psychiat.* **136**, 574–83.
9. Rahe, R. H. (1979). Life change events and mental illness: an overview. *J. Human Stress* **5**, (3), 2–10.
10. Paykel, E. S. (1974). Life stress and psychiatric disorder: application of the clinical approach. In *Stressful life events: their nature and effects* (eds B. S. Dohrenwendt and B. P. Dohrenwendt), Chapter 8. Wiley, New York.
11. Eastwood, M. R. and Trevelyan, M. H. (1972). Relationships between physical and psychiatric disorder. *Psychol. Med.* **2**, 363–72.

2.4 PRACTICAL PROBLEMS OF PROVIDING ADEQUATE PSYCHIATRIC SERVICES IN THE COMMUNITY

It is evident from looking at the Goldberg 'levels' (Table 2.3) and the work of Shepherd and Clare[1] that, whatever definition of psychiatric disease is used, a large number of psychological problems are brought to the general practitioner. The proportion dealt with by the GP—either by general support or attempts at solution—depends on factors within the GP, the patient, and their past relationship. When the patient feels confident that the GP understands and cares, the simple sharing of distress may be enough to alleviate the problem. More complex problems will require expertise which the GP may not have. Between these extremes will be situations with which this book will hopefully help the GP to cope. Overall, the large majority of psychological problems in general practice are dealt with by the GP alone.

The traditional way of coping with patients who need specialist care is by providing hospital facilities to which individuals may be referred. Looking t the distribution of main psychiatric diagnoses, Shepherd found that only bout 4 per cent of patients attended GPs for the treatment of major sychiatric conditions, the rest constituted 'neuroses', personality disorders, nd other less serious conditions.

Formal referrals have a place in the scheme of things as they concentrate oth the GPs' and consultants' minds on making an assessment of the resenting problem and working out some form of management plan. There s, however, very little advantage for GPs in the sense that they are unlikely to e helped to increase their own skills by the process of referral. In addition the onsultant is unlikely to learn a great deal about the commoner psychological roblems found in general practice, and the patient is stigmatized by being sent o a mental hospital. Hospital-based teaching of psychiatry to medical students oes not prepare young doctors for the types of problems they are going to face n general practice and, although some attempt to remedy this deficiency is nade in most vocational training schemes, those trainees who are attached o psychiatric units often find themselves confined to an in-patient setting.

The need for help in coping with this load—both in management and in ersonal support—is obvious. Michael Balint[2] drew attention to this need or support, and mention of his contribution and methods will be made later n the book. However, in recent years a trend has appeared, almost without notice, towards much closer liaison between general practice and hospital sychiatry.

Three different methods are possible by which GPs can get help for their atients' psychological problems from members of the secondary care team, uch as psychiatrists, clinical psychologists, and counsellors.

The 'replacement' method

This is based on the American type of system where patients with psychiatric roblems go directly to psychiatrists, or others, either in hospital or ommunity settings. This is at variance with the British concept of a generalist rimary care doctor, and, of course, presupposes that patients can always ecide in which specialist area their problems lie. The patient with backache nd a masked depression would be more likely to end up with an orthopaedic urgeon than with a psychiatrist.

The 'referral' method

This method is more traditional in Britain. In theory this might enable GPs o deal with any increased workload by passing it on to the secondary services. Of course these services may then deal with their increased workload by assing it back to the primary care team. Hence this could become an increased throughput' situation. It is interesting to note that, in spite of a 8 per cent increase in the number of psychiatrists in the UK between 1970 and 1975, there was no increase in the number of patients referred[3], so the number of new patients seen by each psychiatrist fell. It appears, therefore, that not only is this 'increased throughput' not occurring, but if it did, it would have important consequences — firstly in requiring a large number of extra psychiatrists, and secondly in the effect it would have in stigmatizing patients with a psychiatric label.

Studies of the outcome of traditional referral patterns to psychiatrist suggest that almost a third of new patients do not keep their appointment at all, and that the majority of those seen are discharged, or lapse from treatment, after a few consultations. Johnson[4] concluded that 'although the expertise of the consultant psychiatrist may be required for diagnosis and advice on treatment or management, in a substantial proportion of out-patients the hospital does not offer any form of treatment that is not available in the setting of general practice'. It is also likely that compliance with appointments made is higher in general practice than in hospital, though there is no firm evidence on this point.

Shepherd[1] concluded some years ago, and his assessment still remains true today: 'Administration and medical logic alike suggest that the cardinal requirement for the improvement of the mental health services in this country is not a large scale expansion and proliferation of psychiatric agencies, but rather a strengthening of the family doctor in his therapeutic role.' This leads to:

The 'liaison-attachment' method (see also Section 4.8)

This pattern involves movement of the psychiatrist, psychologist, and others out of the hospital to operate alongside the primary care team within their premises. It is only recently[5] that the extent and implication of this type of service has been documented as regards psychiatrists. A study at the General Practice Unit of the Institute of Psychiatry, based on postal questionnaires to all the psychiatrists in England and Wales, showed that one in five psychiatrists or their junior staff spent at least one session a week working in a general practice setting. Three types of working pattern emerged.

(1) Twenty-eight per cent adopt a 'consultation' pattern — a consultant psychiatrist spends time with GPs in group settings, discussing doctor-patient relationships and patient management problems with reference to patients the GPs are looking after themselves.

(2) Sixty-four per cent adopt a 'shifted out-patient' type of approach. Here the psychiatrist holds formal out-patient clinics from the GPs' premises, but even with this, a different spectrum of patients is seen, and closer collaboration with GPs in management is quoted as an advantage.

(3) The remaining small number of psychiatrists institute training links with the whole primary health-care team — health visitors, social workers,

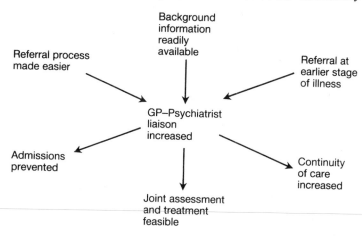

Fig. 2.2. Perceived advantages of clinical care provision in GP psychiatric liaison-attachment schemes.

community nurses, and psychologists attached to the practice, and reduce their own direct involvement in patient care to a minimum — a 'transfer of skills' approach.

The advantages of the liaison models as perceived by psychiatrists are shown in Fig. 2.2. GPs feel that they not only gain confidence in managing psychological problems but receive valuable support with some of the frustrations provoked by patients whom they find it difficult to cope with.[5,6]

Disadvantages quoted by the psychiatrists are the time involved in travelling to general practice premises and the difficulties some of them find in readjusting their attitude to the differences in professional roles in general practice. They miss the hierarchical model of hospital care within which they feel more secure.[7]

The evolution of liaison schemes of this kind, applicable not only to psychiatrists but to clinical psychologists, and other community psychiatric workers, and the assumption that the majority of psychological problems in general practice should continue to be cared for by the primary health-care team, has implications for communication within the practice, for the referral process (see Chapter 4(g)), and for the training of GPs and the other professional groups.

Training

Many GP trainees comment on the inappropriateness of their hospital-based psychiatric training to prepare them for the psychological problems they encounter in general practice. To a certain extent this can be compensated

Table 2.4.   *Medical behaviours which relate to accuracy of psychological assessment and which can be significantly improved by training*

Start of the interview:

- Making eye contact with the patient
- Clarification of the presenting complaint

Form of the 'problem-solving' questions:

- Proportion directive (rather than closed)
- Use of directive questions when dealing with physical symptoms
- Focusing on the present rather than the past

Some special techniques:

- Sensitivity to verbal cues relating to psychological distress
- Sensitivity to non-verbal cues indicating distress
- Ability to deal with over-talkative patients

Adapted from Goldberg (see ref. 5, p. 45).

Closed questions are ones which can be answered only by 'yes' or 'no', for instance 'Doe the pain get worse after meals?', or 'Do you wake early?'

Directive questions are ones which direct towards a certain symptom but are phrased to allov the patient to describe the symptoms, e.g. 'Tell me about the pain in your arm.'

Open questions allow the patient to choose the area of reply, e.g. 'How are you?', 'I've go a pain in my foot', or 'I'm having problems with my teenage son.'

for during the general practice year of vocational training (see table 2.4) but liaison attachments open up a form of continuing training adapted to the personality and experience of the GP in practice. In addition, traine hospital psychiatrists and other professionals could, perhaps by taking par in assessment meetings in general practice, learn to adapt their technique to the conditions, including time constraints, under which GPs work in the area of psychological medicine. As Lesser[8] has commented 'if a successfu partnership is to occur, not only must the psychiatrist come equipped witl the knowledge-base and eclectic experience suitable for general practice and its patients, but general practice must be prepared to identify and treat the problems of . . . their patients who are emotionally disturbed.' Simila considerations apply to the integration of clinical psychologists and counsellors into general practice.

References

1. Shepherd, M. and Clare A. (1981). *Psychiatric illness in general practice* (2nd edn) Oxford University Press.

2. Balint, M. (1964). *The doctor, his patient and the illness* (2nd edn). Pitman Medical, London.
3. Williams, P. and Clare, A. (1981). Changing patterns of psychiatric care. *Br. Med. J.* **282**, 375–77.
4. Johnson, D. A. (1973). An analysis of out-patient services. *Br. J. Psychiat.* **122**, 301–6 and **123**, 185–91.
5. Strathdee, G. and Williams, P. (in press). Patterns of collaboration. In *Mental health illness in the primary care setting* (eds. M. Shepherd, G. Wilkinson, and P. Williams). Tavistock, London.
6. Strathdee, G. and Williams, P. (1984). A survey of psychiatrists in primary care. *J. R. Coll. Gen. Pract.* **34**, 615–18.
7. Wilson, S. and Wilson, K. (1985). Close encounters in general practice: experience of a psychotherapy liaison team. *Br. J. Psychiat.* **146**, 277–81.
8. Lesser, A. L. (1983). Is training in psychiatry relevant for general practice? *J. R. Coll. Gen. Pract.* **39**, 617–18.

3 Models of prevention and therapy

3.1 INTRODUCTION

You can cure anything if you believe in it: you can cure neuroses with hypnotism, or with a walking stick, if that is what you believe in. Freud was kind to people and gave them his interest, that was what cured—the human contact. What you believe in is what cures.[1]
Sensitivity and a willingness to offer assistance are necessary but not always sufficient. We need knowledge, skills, attitudes and self-knowledge. (source unknown)

There will never be unanimity regarding the importance of the various factors which contribute to successful therapy, but it is reasonable to suppose that the ones referred to in the quotations above—love, belief in what is being done, kindness, genuine interest, sensitivity, willingness to help, and, of course, knowledge, skills, and self-understanding—are all necessary. However, unless some structure is imposed and some aims set, it is easy to lose direction. Forms of therapy range from counselling—which involves, through the use of a reflective technique, helping people to express their feelings, clarify their thoughts, and consider the consequences of possible actions—to psychotherapy—which aims to help people to come to terms with experiences which have damaged them, by intensive exploration aimed at uncovering the relationship between current assumptions and past experience. For all therapy, a model is helpful. In the introduction to this book we discussed the use of models as ways of understanding psychological mechanisms, and we emphasized that models are only maps; they are not the territory and must not be accorded the precision and fixity of reality. Some maps will be useful to some doctors and some patients, others will need different models. We intend to describe some maps which have been helpful to us and to others, and to provide some indication of when they may be most applicable.

Therapists can be seen as attempting to remove symptoms, and to change perspectives. They seek to alter responses in behaviour, thought, and feeling to the difficulties which either create or maintain problems—in other words, to help people to change. The therapist works to clarify goals, to discover in what ways patients are perpetuating the problems they define, or preventing themselves from reaching their goals, and to help them to change their approach so that, where possible, the problems are solved and the goals achieved.

Beliefs and theories held by general practitioners may strongly influence not only their technique, but also the length and outcome of treatment. Thus the doctor's expectations may affect the patient's behaviour and recovery.

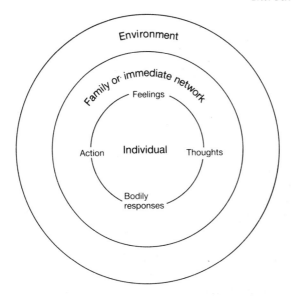

Fig. 3.1. The individual as part of a system

Psychoanalysts may expect to see patients in 50-minute sessions for five days a week for several years, while some family therapists and general practitioners expect improvement in one session. Although the goals may be very different, expectations may be fulfilled in either case.

Systems as a model

The framework shown in Fig. 3.1 introduces the idea of systems. The person is a system. No one part can be changed without changing other parts and consequently the whole person. If I have *thoughts* that someone has deceived me, I may *feel* angry, my pulse rate may increase and I may *go* and have a row. If I wake up with a hangover and *feelings* of depression, I may make myself *think* that I am not needed at work today and *choose* to stay at home.

In the centre is the self, the essential 'I' which can make choices and become aware of it's own thoughts and behaviour. This self is part of the body, it observes the body and controls it from within. Many models of therapy recognize that people's intentions, their desire to get better, and their self-healing abilities need to be acknowledged. Many systems are homeostatic. They operate to maintain the person unchanged.

People may find themselves in predicaments or with problems that in some sense seem the only solution to their situations. Mr A avoids crowds because to do so is less distressing than to face them. Mrs B consumes too much alcohol because if she did not do so the pressures of life would be intolerable.

These examples are grossly simplified and caricatured, but it is easy to forget that while people may wish to lose their symptoms, the cost to the whole person may be too great. However, with a little help, individuals may be as capable of solving predicaments as they are of making problems of them.

Surrounding the person is the family or the immediate network. The family may also be considered as a system of which the individual is a part. One person in a family may not be able to change or act without affecting the other members of the family. If, therefore, we are considering helping the individual to change, it may be necessary to consider the family or at least the marital pair. Mrs C remains inadequate because if she were competent she would rival her husband who might then leave her. Master D gets abdominal pain to defuse his parent's marital conflict and reduce the chance of one of them moving out.

The family's immediate circle and close friends also live in communities and thus belong to other circles which again may be termed systems. If the factory goes bankrupt and father loses his job, this will in turn affect the family and the individuals in the family.

Most of the general practitioner's work is, or seems to be, with individuals, yet we often need to consider the family in order to be in a position to help.[2,3] Inevitably, the influence of the larger system, the environment, and the community will also have to be considered.[3]

The goals in therapy may be to treat disease, relieve symptoms, or to increase the patients' autonomy to live their own life as they would choose it. This may be broadly rephrased as increasing the range of choices people have in different and difficult circumstances, and helping them to have some control over these choices. Choices include not only decisions about actions and behaviour, but also about thoughts and moods. Most people would prefer not to have thoughts about being worthless or feelings of depression, but they see no way out. Therapy may be about exploring alternatives.

Much good therapy consists in helping people to step outside themselves and look at their lives from a different viewpoint. Taking a history is the first step, and there are many people for whom the act of explaining themselves to a doctor is all the therapy that is needed, though in most cases the therapist will need to go further. There are various tactics for this. The therapist can reflect and restate the problem in different terms. Patients can keep a diary to develop perspective, or can be asked to list the positive and negative aspects of their situation. Patients may be invited to behave in a different manner, thus altering not only their viewpoint but also the response of their environment. It must be remembered that change in the consulting room is useless if it is not reflected by change in the outside world. However, valid the interpretation, reframing of the problem, or suggested task, these are only effective if they stimulate different behaviour elsewhere.

Throughout this chapter there will be descriptions of ways in which patients, couples, or families can be encouraged to take a new look at themselves, hear things differently and possibly experience altered feelings. One task of the therapist is to develop skills which help the patient to see another side of the problem. The empty nest provides opportunities for new hobbies and growth, and even the death of a spouse, while involving the loss of the old world, may allow new opportunities to arise.

General practitioners often feel powerless to alter people's distress without resort to pills. This chapter will suggest alternative ways to help people to gain some control over their thoughts, feelings, behaviour, and bodies. The ability of GPs to accept, tolerate, and affirm patients may in itself be helping, if not healing, and may facilitate other more specific techniques.

One of the difficulties in treatment is the fine line between caring for people and making them dependent, between helping people to make choices and taking responsibility away from them, between being outside the system and becoming engulfed, between objectivity and subjectivity. Doctors need to remember that they do not cure people — people cure themselves. If general practitioners become too involved in attempting to cure, they may become lost in the patient's system and will lose their effectiveness.

References

1. Jung, C. G. (1976). *Letters* Vol. 2 *(1951–1961)*. Routledge and Kegan Paul, London.
2. Fosson, A., Elam, C. L., and Broaddus, D. (1982). Family therapy in family practice. A solution to psychological problems. *J. Fam. Pract.* **15**, (3), 461–65.
3. Galazua, S. S. and Echert, J. H. (1986). Clinically applied anthropology. Concepts for the family physician. *J. Fam. Pract.* **22**, (2), 159–65.

3.2 PREVENTION

There can be a few aspects of psychiatry that have given rise to more controversy than prevention. Attitudes vary from enthusiasm to scepticism. Some utopian schemes, religious faiths, and political systems have promised to abolish mental illness, but most psychiatrists remain sceptical, and scientific justification for such global solutions to our problems are lacking. Even so, there are some communities with low rates of mental illness. For instance, Eaton and Weil[1] found a surprisingly low prevalence of schizophrenia and psychopathy among the Hutterites of North America. This fundamentalist sect have cut themselves off from many of the 'advantages' of Western society and form communities in which social pressures and social supports provide closed networks which concern themselves with nearly every aspect of life. Giving and withholding of approval and love are the principal and very effective means of maintaining conformity. All important decisions are made by the elders of the community and many of the sources of information and pleasure which others take for granted, such as television, music, and dancing, are disapproved of.

The lesson that the Hutterites have to teach us would seem to be that our much prized freedom of individual action and thought is a mixed blessing, and that, in rejecting traditional beliefs and rigid social structures, we may leave people without support systems and guidance which they need. Certainly, there is no chance of persuading our patients to become Hutterites even if we wanted to do so. We have to live with the society we have got. What then can be done to reduce the incidence of mental ill health?

As in other types of preventive medicine, three approaches are possible. These have been termed primary, secondary, and tertiary prevention.

Primary prevention

Primary prevention sets out to reduce the incidence of a disorder by identifying its causes and intervening to prevent them from taking effect. Examples from the general medical field are the prevention of tuberculosis by means of pasteurization of milk and the prevention of diphtheria by immunization. The causes of mental illness are seldom as clear-cut as that of tuberculosis or diphtheria but there is, as we have seen, no shortage of known causes; in fact one is often faced with a multiplicity of causal factors, many of which are potentially modifiable. *Genetic factors* can sometimes be identified before birth (e.g. by amniocentesis) and the mother may then choose to terminate the pregnancy where the fetus is diagnosed to have a condition which would result in severe mental handicap. *Early childhood influences* are a common cause of later difficulties. Measures which seek to prevent and ameliorate the effects of mother–child separations, or which will support mothers who are depressed or under stress, may well reduce the risk of damage to the child. So, too, will any activities which foster the development of secure bonding between parents and children, and reduce the risk of physical or mental abuse of children. The members of the primary care team are in a position to monitor and advise parents and children throughout these crucial years.

Later in life, the support of people who face a psychosocial transition (see Section 3.3), i.e. people who are about to reach a major turning point in their lives (*anticipatory guidance*) or who are already in transition (*situational crisis counselling*) may ensure a healthy rather than an unhealthy adjustment to change. The identification of such turning points, be they associated with growing up or other life events, is quite practical for the GP, since many of these changes arise from medical illness or death, and others cause people to seek help from their doctors.

Of course, not all harmful influences occur at times of change. Some go on for years, sapping the reserves and undermining the support systems of those who suffer them. Lasting malnutrition is rare in our society, but other forms of deprivation may starve people of social contact, physical affection, or space, place them in danger, restrict their freedom to defend themselves, undermine their trust in themselves and others, or block their capacity to reach their most basic goals.

There is great individual variation in vulnerability to such things as overcrowding, aircraft noise, social isolation, alienation, and threat. This does not mean that measures to mitigate these stresses should be ignored, though it does make the investigation of their effects more difficult. Housing conditions can have measurable effects upon the mental health of the people who live in them and local authorities are becoming aware that the tower block is far from the ideal solution to problems of urban relocation.[2]

We shall be examining many of these issues in more detail elsewhere in this book, but we do not imply that it is a major responsibility of the general practitioner to 'put the world to rights'. Even so, there are many occasions when GPs are involved either directly, as when a patient asks for support in an application for rehousing, or indirectly, as when the GP asks a social worker to call on an unsupported mother who may be having difficulties in coping. Clearly, GPs need to understand the risks to mental health which result from events or circumstances which come to their notice, and they need to know what can be done about them.

Many GPs, and especially those who live in the small communities which they serve, may choose to involve themselves in such local activities as adult education, local government, and voluntary bodies. Taking part, if they have the talent, in activities such as music and the arts may help to improve the social supports within a community and enable them to contribute to its mental health.

Secondary prevention

Secondary prevention involves the identification of incipient or hidden cases of a disorder in order to take prompt action to prevent the condition developing into a full-blown illness. In the area of cardiovascular disease, taking regular blood pressures is an example. In the mental health field it includes any activity which enables people to get help quickly and easily for problems that do not yet justify the designation of mental illness but which may well lead to one if they are ignored. It includes a variety of drop-in services, telephone 'hot-lines' (such as the Samaritans), and general crisis services. General practitioners are often in a position to recognize symptoms which are indicators of distress rather than illness. They can educate patients to recognize that they can come for help with problems which are primarily emotional and not just physical.

Appropriate action by counselling (q.v.) crisis intervention (q.v.) or other means to be described in later chapters, may well prevent further escalation of problems.

Tertiary prevention

In the mental health field, tertiary prevention involves the prevention of recurrence in people who have now recovered from an episode of illness. In the example of tuberculosis it includes the six-monthly X-ray and sputum tests which ensure that the treated patient remains free of infection. In the case of mental illness we can cite regular follow-up of people who have been discharged from a mental hospital following a psychotic illness and special measures to ensure that those who are vulnerable to recurrent disorders continue to receive support and to take any medication which may be necessary to prevent relapse (e.g. lithium carbonate for the prevention of recurrence in cases of cyclical mania).

General practitioners are often the only people available to provide this kind of care. When community psychiatric nurses or other professionals are available the GP needs to liaise closely with them, agree on where 'the buck stops', and organize satisfactory follow-up systems.

In conclusion, GPs have important roles to play in the primary, secondary, and tertiary prevention of mental ill health. However, they will easily become overwhelmed with all the 'slings and arrows of outrageous fortune' unless they adopt a clear and realistic approach to this difficult subject and make use of all the ancillary sources of support, both statutory and voluntary, which exist in, or can be introduced to, the community. It may be a more effective use of their time to lobby for the appointment of a community psychiatric nurse, or to foster the inception of a self-help group, than to provide preventive care themselves.

A report by a sub-committee of The Royal College of General Practitioners summarized the logistic implications of GP involvement in prevention:

> . . . rather than more consultations there is a need for a change in attitude towards the consultations already taking place. Rather than increase the time taken for each consultation, there is a need to re-examine how the time is currently spent. Rather than increase the number of members of the primary care team, there is a need for the present members to learn to work together in new and different ways. Rather than increase the number of psychiatrists, psychologists and social workers, there is a need to increase their knowledge of first-line care by encouraging their attachment to general practice.[3]

It is one of the purposes of this book to show how this can be done and to spell out the scientific justification for these measures.

References

1. Eaton, J. W. and Weil, R. J. (1956). Mental health and the Hutterites. In *Mental health and mental disorder* (ed. A. M. Rose). Routledge, London.
2. Fanning, D. M. (1967). Families in flats. *Br. Med. J.* 4, 382.
3. Royal College of General Practitioners (1981). *Prevention of psychiatric disorders in general practice.* Report from General Practice, No. 20. R. Coll. Gen. Pract., London.

3.3 CRISIS THEORY AND PSYCHOSOCIAL TRANSITIONS

Crisis theory

The words 'stress' and 'crisis' are broad and imprecise in meaning and are best defined in terms of their effects — thus a stressor is stressful if it produces distress or a crisis is critical if it upsets people (see also Section 3.4). It then becomes a tautology to say that psychological disturbances are caused by stress. Another way of saying the same thing is to indicate that in crises the demands of a situation exceed a person's ability to cope. At such times normal homeostatic mechanisms are thrown out of balance; anxiety or its physio-logical accompaniments become pronounced, and may themselves give rise to more problems. Gerald Caplan, who has played a major part in the development of 'Crisis Theory', points out that at times of crisis, people are both more vulnerable and more amenable; they need help and are more willing to accept it than at other times in their lives. He suggests that crises are often turning points at which the course of life may be reset for good or ill. A little help can go a long way towards turning the experience into one of growth and encourage the development of increased competence rather than defeat and illness.[1]

Situational and emotional crises

Caplan's model is helpful as far as it goes, but needs to be elaborated. A further subdivision into situational crises and emotional crises is sometimes made. This allows for two kinds of response — situational crisis services aimed at particular life situations (e.g. bereavement, major surgery, disaster relief) and emotional crisis services open to anybody in distress (e.g. 'open doors' and 'hot-lines'). In either case the idea is to provide prompt, effective help to individuals or groups who are at special risk.

The advantage of situational crisis services is that, by defining the special situation which they cover, they enable people with special knowledge of the situation to provide help that is 'tailor-made'. By contrast, emotional crisis

services have to cope with a wide range of life situations and they may b
tempted to use methods of intervention which focus on reducing distress rathe
than influencing its causes. Their value arises from the fact that there are man
life crises that do not fall neatly into a particular situational category and man
episodes of distress the cause of which is not evident. Clearly, both kinds o
service are needed and both are, in fact, provided by the primary care team

As described in Chapter 2, analysis of the life events associated with th
onset of depressive illnesses shows that they tend to have three characteristics

(1)   they are lasting in their effects (rather than transient threats);

(2)   they are undesirable, negative rather than desirable, positive events; and

(3)   they involve 'exits' from the person's environment rather tha
'entrances'.[2]

In other words they are life changes which involve major losses rather tha
gains.

Of course not all life changes can be easily categorized into losses and gain
many involve both, and some are so ambiguous that the attribution of 'los
or 'gain' can only be made with hindsight. But they all require a person i
some degree to give up one set of assumptions about the world and to develo
another. This has been termed the 'Psychosocial Transition Model' and
enables us to take the analysis of the psychosocial reaction to life event
beyond that of losses and gains.[3,4]

Psychosocial transitions

Psychosocial transitions occur whenever situations arise in which people'
existing world models prove to be at variance with what they meet. T
understand these we need to know something of their world models as we
as something about the emerging situations. Thus, the birth of a baby ma
be completely consonant with the parents' plans and expectations or it ma
be disastrously at variance with them. How a person reacts to a life ever
cannot, therefore, be understood if our knowledge is limited to the life ever
alone. Even something as unambiguous as the death of a husband or wi
may be anticipated and prepared for in such a way that very little chang
in the survivor's model of the world is needed, or it may leave a perso
bewildered and unable to cope.

Information

As mentioned in Section 3.4 under 'Information giving', patients who ent
any psychosocial transition with some knowledge of what it is going to invol

are better able to cope. Thus, giving information before a surgical operation reduces post-operative pain, and warning of a coming death and a description of what normal grieving is like helps individuals cope when a death occurs — so-called anticipatory guidance.

Perhaps one of the reasons for the pathogenic effects of events involving losses as opposed to gains arises from the fact that people don't really anticipate or 'look forward' to the things they don't look forward to! This is most notable when a person's basic assumptions need to change. If these include, for example, the notion that 'I am a weak and helpless person but I shall always be looked after by an adoring parent or parent-substitute', then that person may cope well with disablement but badly with the death of their mother. If, on the other hand, security derives from the fact that 'I can stand on my own feet even though nobody else can be trusted to care for me', that person may cope well with the loss of a person but badly with the loss of a limb.

The world model or 'assumptive world' contains all that we take for granted, all facts we assume to be true on the basis of our previous experience, and it includes our view of the past and future as well as the present world. Hence, it is quite possible for us to grieve for something we have never had. Medical students work for many years to acquire a model of the world of the doctor, which will eventually enable them to make the transition from student to doctor relatively smoothly. If, however, they fail completely the final examinations, they will grieve the loss of a future and be forced to rebuild their assumptive world. Assumptions are, of course, held with various degrees of conviction, and it is worth making a distinction between 'expectations' and 'contingency plans'. Contingency plans have a provisional quality which makes it easier to give them up. 'If the operation is a success, then I shall return to work; if not, I shall have to remain at home.' The coexistence of two alternative models of the world may make it easier for a person to cope with either outcome.

The theory of 'psychosocial transitions' makes it easier to understand why education and anticipatory guidance are important. General practitioners are often in a position to help people to prepare for the changes that are likely to come about. But we also need to understand why people often find it very difficult to change. They disbelieve our prognoses, misinterpret our explanations, and forget or ignore what they have been told. Only if we understand enough of their internal world to appreciate the impact of our attempts at communication, will we appreciate the true nature of the problem and act appropriately (see Section 4.2, Beliefs).

When we ask someone to explain to us how they see their situation, we not only add to our own understanding; we also help them to stand aside from their view of the world and to treat their assumptive world as itself a part of their life space, an area to be explored or assessed. In explaining themselves to us they may begin to question assumptions which, up to then, had been taken for granted. Hence, the great therapeutic value of case-history taking. Patients often improve as a result of history-taking only, before any attempt at formal counselling or therapy is made.

Of course, some assumptions are more 'open to question' than others. Self-examination can be a painful process because of the danger of internal chaos if basic assumptions should be found to be wrong. 'If I can no longer trust the accuracy of my view of the world, what can I trust?'

People are unlikely to share with us their basic assumptions unless they know that they can trust us to treat them with respect. Doctors who enjoy scoring points off their patients, or who feel that they have not done their job unless they point out the inconsistencies in their patients' assumptions, will soon find that the door is barred and bolted. Psychotherapy exists to make change easier and this is only possible if the therapist adopts a permissive, non-judgmental attitude in which the patient feels safe to talk about the things that are unsafe. Hence the importance of rapport in the therapeutic relationship.

It takes time to revise a complex model of the world, and we must allow for this in any situation when we are attempting to ease a major transition. Doctors are sometimes annoyed when patients refuse to agree to major operations which are obviously necessary. We tend to put pressure on patients by warning them of the dire consequences of refusal. Such pressures may only serve to increase fear and, with it, resistance to our arguments. If, on the other hand, we encourage the patient to take time and to 'talk things over with your family', we usually find that a sensible decision will be made.

Ideal or hoped-for models of the world seldom qualify as assumptions any more than do worst-outcome or dreaded models. They have a function in providing an extreme model against which our perceptions of reality can be tested. Discrepancies between the assumptive and the ideal world constitute gaps to be filled, and any change which reduces such a gap will be construed as a gain. The fact that the person may well have rehearsed in their mind behaviour and assumptions appropriate to this new, more ideal world, may enable the transition to take place more smoothly. Likewise, the person who has worried about a possible dreaded event may cope better with the event than one who has refused to consider the possibility.

People who cling to unrealistic ideal models and hopes as if they were justifiable assumptions are usually defending themselves against their fear of the opposite. Thus, patients may insist on endowing their doctor with magical and god-like powers in order to remain secure in a world which has begun to terrify them. If the doctor fails to live up to these unreasonable expectations, he or she may come to be seen as the opposite, a malevolent monster who can no longer be trusted. It is often the role of the helper to enable people to feel safe enough to give up extreme models of the world be they positive or negative.

Life events may give rise to changes in personal relationships, familiar environment, possessions, physical or mental capacities, roles, status, plans, and expectations. Some events will change one of these fields, others will change several of them. Thus, an illness may not only alter physical and mental functions, it may lead to the break-up of relationships. loss of status, unemployment, poverty, and the ruin of cherished expectations. Each of these changes must be examined and its implications faced if a person is to find a new place in the world which is now being entered.

Support systems

One of the most important functions of a family is to provide support to its members at times of change, and doctors (with the patients' consent) can sometimes help them to do this by keeping them informed of the situation and making them aware of their need for help. As we saw in the last chapter, the normal attachment behaviours which mediate this support do not always function as they should. Far from being supportive, family members may cling for support to those who themselves need support, or they may withdraw their help when it is most needed, misguidedly blocking emotional expression or telling lies when truth is sought. At such times the members of the primary care team must be prepared to support family members as well as patients.

Further attention will be given to the practical aspects of crisis intervention and the management of psychosocial transitions in Chapter 4. In helping people through these turning points in their lives we become agents of change, catalysts, whose presence can make the difference between defeat and mastery of the situation.

References

1. Caplan, G. (1961). *An approach to community mental health*. Tavistock, London.
2. Paykel, E. S. (1974). Life stress and psychiatric disorder. In *Stressful life events: their nature and effects* (eds B. S. Dohrenwendt and B. P. Dohrenwendt). Wiley, New York.
3. Parkes, C. M. (1971). Psycho-social transitions: a field for study. *Soc. Sci. Med.* 5, 101–15.
4. Parkes, C. M. (1988). *Prescription for change: psycho-social transitions and health care*. (In preparation.)

3.4 COGNITIVE AND BEHAVIOUR THERAPIES

All therapy attempts to produce change with the aim of solving patients' problems or helping them to tolerate those that are insoluble. The change may be in how the individual thinks, feels, or behaves; it may be in the external physical and social environment; or it may be in the physical state of the patient, and be achieved by pharmacological or psychological means.

Some changes take place without therapy or in spite of it — when these are improvements it is easy to interpret them as benefits of therapy, but this may be misleading. When patients consult a doctor seeking help for psychological problems, a number of 'non-specific' factors will contribute to their improvement. First, patients are likely to consult when a problem has reached some kind of peak; if it is a problem which tends to fluctuate spontaneously, then it is very likely to show improvement soon after consulting the doctor as part of the normal fluctuation. Secondly, patients consult when they have decided to do something about the problem; there may be an intention to change, or other attempts at problem-solving which lead to improvement. Sometimes patients will only appear to have improved, describing the problem as less intense at later consultations, although no change has in fact occurred. This is known as the 'hallo-goodbye' effect, as patients give a very full account to engage therapeutic help, and then minimize the problem after therapy in appreciation of the help they have been given, perhaps because they are embarrassed by what they have revealed.

Placebo/expectancy

All therapies are helped, to some extent, by the placebo effect — improvement in the patient's condition which is not due to what is thought to be the active component of treatment. This is true of drug treatment, including that with psychotropics and analgesics, it is true of surgical intervention, and it is also true for psychological treatment. The suggestion that the procedures are therapeutic is important; for example, experimental studies of audio analgesia to minimize dental pain showed that playing the music did not achieve analgesic effects unless it was suggested to the patients that the music would reduce their pain. Some individuals are more susceptible to placebo effects than others.

The patient's expectations are highly predictive of success in any psychotherapeutic treatment. Two types of expectation are important, the expectation that the treatment will have the desired outcome and the expectation that he or she can fulfil the treatment requirements: patients holding such expectations are much more likely to have successful outcomes than those with pessimistic views.[1,2]

Clearly, it is necessary to take advantage of these important therapeutic opportunities. In order to maximize the placebo effect, it is therefore wise not only to introduce the suggestion of therapeutic effect, but also to ensure that patients share the expectation that the treatment will be effective and have confidence in their ability to carry it out. These expectations are not necessarily fixed, and it may be necessary to give further information, or to work on inaccurate information and beliefs, during treatment, though always respecting the patient's viewpoint.

Information-giving: predictability and control

Experimental studies with humans and animals show that the ability to cope with threatening events is increased if the events are predictable and controllable. Information-giving can increase this ability, and patients have had better outcomes in a variety of clinical procedures, e.g. endoscopy and surgery, if given additional information in advance.[3]

These improved outcomes may involve less distress, greater ability to co-operate in treatment, less need for medication (for pain relief, anxiety reduction, and sleep), faster recovery, and less requirement of expensive medical care, including hospitalization. There is now a very large body of research on surgical patients, showing that information about procedures, techniques, and sensations experienced all improve outcomes, but that information about the sensations the patient will experience may be the most effective, (see also Section 4.3). Even more effective may be approaches that enable the patient to use better cognitive strategies[3] (see later in this chapter).

Patients frequently complain that they are given too little information or that they are given conflicting information; on the other hand, doctors are wary of giving information that may cause distress. This is particularly true when the doctor is in a position to give bad news about a patient's condition. Furthermore, patients may reject what they are not ready or able to hear. A group of patients with cancer were informed that they had 'cancer', but six months later 17 per cent denied that they ever had a diagnosis of cancer made.[4] People differ in their personal style of coping with stressful situations. Some prefer to seek out all possible information about a threatening event, while others take avoiding action. The information-seeking style tends to be associated with high levels of anxiety and distress. Those who adopt an information avoidance style may cope better with short-term stresses, especially if there is nothing that they can do to avert the dangers, but in the long term they may show more signs of physical and psychological illness. These findings also have parallels in animal studies where those subjected to chronic stress with no available method of active coping have shown high levels of disease and death.

Desensitization/exposure

Some of the most successful therapeutic approaches developed over the past 20 years have depended on desensitization or gradual exposure. These are particularly applicable where the patient needs to overcome some fear or develop some skill. Systematic desensitization was originally introduced for patients with phobic disorders, and was based on conditioning theory (see Section 1.2). The treatment is analogous to the desensitization treatment of asthma, patients being exposed to graded examples of the frightening stimulus. Patients are first trained to relax and then asked to imagine the feared situation (or objects) while maintaining a state of relaxation. A start is made with items that are only mildly feared, progressing up a hierarchy until they can imagine the most feared item without distress. It is then possible to expose the patient to the feared situation in a similarly graded manner. This treatment was more successful and more efficient than other procedures available when first introduced. Subsequent research has confirmed the success of systematic desensitization but has not confirmed the theoretical basis—it works, but we do not know how. Simple conditioning theory no longer offers an adequate explanation, and cognitive factors, such as expectancy, or the development of new coping strategies, are included in most of the current attempts at explanation.[5]

It has now been shown that this type of treatment can be radically modified and still be effective. It is not necessary to climb a hierarchy gradually, as treatments such as 'flooding' and 'implosion', which subject the patient to very frightening stimuli in the initial stages, can be equally effective. In flooding, patients are asked to face the most frightening event in the hierarchy that they can tolerate, while in implosion they are exposed to frightening images, e.g. pictures, thought to be associated with the unconscious meaning of the stimuli. The essential components appear to be:

(1) an explanation which gives the patient confidence to participate; and

(2) the exposure of the patient, in imagination and eventually in reality, to the phobic stimulus.

In spite of other methods being effective, the favoured approach is still the gradual one, as this is generally less unpleasant for the patient and therapist alike. Patients' spouses can be trained to act as therapists and have been very successful in the treatment of agoraphobia. A manual has been published which guides practitioners, health visitors, or relatives working with these patients.[6]

These treatments can now be conducted with a minimum input of professional time and are compatible with the time constraints of general practice. A typical example is a patient who was asked to keep a record of her outings and to return, after a week, with her husband. The record showed that she was not going anywhere alone. She and her husband were given the 'client's' and the 'helper's' manuals and instructed on how to practise going out alone in the streets and to the shops near home. When she returned after one month, she reported being able to go where she wished on her own. She had found the booklet helpful both in explaining her problem and in guiding her in the gradual exposure programme.

Exposure treatments are also successful in dealing with obsessional disorders. Treatment may be conducted in imagination: in *habituation* the patient is encouraged to think and maintain an obsessional thought; in *response prevention* the patient is exposed to conditions where they wish to perform a compulsive act, but are prevented from doing so. For example, a patient with an obsession about dirt and contamination might be instructed to think and maintain the thought 'If I use the toilet, I will contract a disease' or might be asked to use the toilet and not permitted to wash her hands immediately. Both methods have been shown to be useful in treating patients and, although the methods may be difficult to translate directly into general practice, they suggest possible strategies.

These behavioural treatments of phobias and obsessional disorders attempt to modify symptoms by modifying the immediate causes that maintain the problem, rather than exploring the historical reasons for it's existence. The original cause of the fear may be long past, but the symptoms have become self-perpetuating; the patient may have come to dread the fear rather than it's original source. Experimental studies show that these treatments usually work; that is to say, they are effective in relieving symptoms and are often both more effective and more efficient than treatment by psychotherapy.[6,7]

Desensitization or exposure programmes inevitably involve a shared understanding of the nature of the problem in order for the patient to be able to co-operate. The patient's understanding of the problem and the sharing of that understanding may both be therapeutic.

Skill development

While work on the development of skills has had the greatest application in industrial and educational fields, it has also proved relevant in solving some of the problems referred to medical practitioners. The best-known examples are in social skills training (including assertiveness training) and in basic self-care skills for mentally handicapped children, although the latter is likely to be carried out in collaboration with educational services. All skills training involves certain basic components: division of the task into its component parts, rehearsal of the parts, feedback on performance, and assembling the total performance.

Social skills training has been undertaken with a number of clinical groups, including schizophrenics, social phobics, patients complaining of extreme shyness or difficulties in social situations, and others whose complaint is caused or exacerbated by their lack of skill in making and maintaining relationships. The training starts with the identification of skill deficits, a procedure which depends on previous research defining the components of normal social interaction. These consist of verbal behaviours and also non-verbal ones, such as eye-contact, gestures, listening, style of dress, and interpersonal distance. This analysis may depend on the patient's own report, 'I just can't look at people', the clinician's direct observations, or the use of video recordings in selected social encounters. When deficits have been identified, the therapist may use modelling, role-play, or real-life rehearsal, with or without video feedback, to develop the relevant skills. So, for example, someone who complains that they cannot cope with ordinary social encounters might be filmed while simulating going into a shop and making a purchase. This might reveal a lack of eye-contact, which accompanies the feeling of being unable to cope and feeling very exposed. After watching the video together with the patient, the therapist might simulate the same behaviour and observe the patient attempt an improved performance. Later, the therapist encourages the patient to perform some real-life tasks, such as going to buy a box of matches or a newspaper, with an instruction which encourages eye-contact, such as 'Note the colour of the shop assistant's eyes.' Obviously, the task must be well chosen and within the individual's capacity. The procedures are very similar to those used in many training schemes to teach general practitioners to learn a very specific set of social skills, those used in the consultation.

In all skill training the task is divided into parts that the learner can achieve. Success is rewarded and this motivates further effort. Defining relevant manageable targets and providing feedback on performance are the critical features of this approach. Some simple aspects of this approach can easily be incorporated into ordinary general practice consultations. For example, a shy young woman described having difficulty in ordinary social situations and the feeling that people were looking at her. In the consultation it was observed, and this did not require complex video procedures, that she made little eye-contact with the doctor. Her poor social skills prevented her from seeing how other people behaved. She was set the task of noting whether anyone else who attended the same bingo club as she did looked uneasy or nervous. This task achieved two objectives: first, she discovered that other people were not looking at her; and secondly, she found that there were always several people who looked nervous and that it was, therefore, not such an unusual experience as she had previously thought.

Reward and punishment (operant methods)

Behaviours that are rewarded are likely to increase in frequency, while those that are punished decrease in frequency. It seems reasonable to suggest, therefore, that a problem behaviour occurs because it is rewarded or that a desirable one is absent either because it is not rewarded or because it is punished. It may then be possible to design a programme to change behaviour by changing the schedule of rewards and punishments. These approaches offer both an explanation and a therapeutic approach.

These *operant* methods derive from Skinner's original work with pigeons, but subsequent workers applied these basic findings to human behaviour. They found these approaches successful in the modification of a wide variety of problem behaviours, such as children's behaviour in the classroom, delinquency, overeating, anorexia nervosa, schizophrenic behaviour, marital problems, and chronic disability arising from (minor) impairments. This is probably the most researched approach to therapy, as it rests on a major body of fundamental research. Those applying the methods to clinical practice have evolved research designs, the 'single-case study designs', which allow controlled studies of the methods within an individual subject.[8]

Rewards and punishments are defined for the individual; for example, children from deprived backgrounds may find attention rewarding, regardless of whether it is friendly or hostile. In such cases scolding would increase the frequency of the scolded behaviour but turning away might decrease it. For ethical and practical reasons, reward is the main method used in practice. It is usually possible to get rid of an undesirable behaviour by rewarding an alternative, desirable behaviour. For example, a child who screams when put to bed at night can be rewarded for settling down quietly rather than punished for screaming.

The general practitioner is frequently in a position to choose between reward and punishment. When the patient who was told to give up smoking returns saying 'I've cut down from 20 a day to five', the GP can say 'Well done, you'll soon succeed in giving up altogether', or 'That is not good enough, you must give up completely.' The former is likely to be more effective both in reducing smoking and in encouraging the patient to return to the GP for further help with the problem.

Rewards can be part of a self-control programme or part of a contract between two individuals. For example, an obese patient on a self-control programme to reduce food intake might reward herself with new clothes, or a trip to the theatre, if, and only if, she lost weight; a couple in marital therapy might agree a contract whereby the husband arriving home from work at the specified time would be rewarded by a glass of sherry, and the wife having meals ready on time for five nights in a row would be rewarded by a meal in a restaurant. In each case the agreed behaviours must be precisely specified in advance, the rewards well defined and given if, and only if, the behaviour occurs.

Operant methods may be applied inadvertently in the consultation. It has been shown that the symptoms reported can be influenced by selectively rewarding some rather than others simply by the doctor saying 'yes', 'mmhmm', and nodding after some symptoms. For some patients the doctor's attention may be particularly rewarding and, since the doctor is likely to be interested in symptoms, illness behaviour may be encouraged. Many case-study reports have now been published which show that excess symptomatology may be reduced by rewarding, i.e. by paying more attention to, healthy behaviour.[9]

Cognitive therapies

In the 1970s a number of therapeutic approaches were developed which attempted to change particular beliefs or styles of thinking. The best known of these is Beck's cognitive therapy[10] for depression, which has recently been adapted for use with anxious patients.

Beck postulates that the depressed individual has negative thoughts about the self, the world, and the future, and that these negative thoughts lead to the depressed mood. This, in turn, leads to selective attention to, and recall of, negative information, and the depressed person is said to operate negative schemata. This theory gains support both from experimental studies of normal and of depressed individuals, showing that a change in thinking leads to changes in mood and vice versa. For example, in the study by Bower[11] quoted on p. 22, two important findings emerged: first, recall is better if the subjects are in the same mood as when they learned the material; and secondly, recall is better for material which matches the recall mood.

This type of finding is easily replicated and may help to explain why depressed patients can produce so many negative thoughts. It can be puzzling to try to understand why depressed persons who paint gloomy pictures of their abilities, their home, their spouse, and their job can, when the depression lifts, describe in glowing terms the same abilities, home, spouse, and job.

In cognitive therapy, these negative beliefs are challenged, both by working on them in the clinical setting and by setting patients homework assignments to test out their beliefs. A woman who asserts that she is a bad mother might be asked what good and bad mothers do, before being asked to compare her own behaviour with these standards. A man who says that he is an uninteresting person and that no one could like him, might be asked to make a list of the friends he has, and to note whether it was he or the friend who initiated the last contact. Beck asserts that depressed individuals distort the data in various ways. The above examples illustrate 'generalization', the woman generalizing from one occasion on which she could not comfort her crying infant, and the man from one occasion on which he had to take his coffee break alone. The therapy aims to teach individuals to identify and reverse the distortions in their thinking.

Other approaches to depression also focus on the individual's thinking. In the original theory of learned helplessness, depression was said to be caused by experiencing uncontrollable unpleasant events; the modified theory suggests that the critical factor is the individual's explanations for the negative events. If they are thought to be caused by internal, stable, and global factors, depression is more likely than if they are attributed to external, unstable, and specific factors. For example, according to this theory, a man who attributes a broken leg to his own carelessness (internal, stable, global) is more likely to become depressed than if he attributes it either to a failure to notice the step he fell down (internal, unstable, specific) or to the dog that ran in front of him (external). In therapy, therefore, patients are trained to identify occasions when they inappropriately attribute blame to themselves rather than to others or to bad luck; when they attribute blame to a constant, unchanging factor rather than a transient state of affairs; and when they attribute blame to a general feature of themselves or their environment rather than something that was only relevant in this particular situation.

Cognitive therapy is newer and less researched than operant therapy, but there are controlled trials showing that in experienced hands it can be as effective as imipramine in the treatment of depression (see Sections 4.7 and 8.5). The use of this model to treat anxiety or anger is still exploratory. The main reservation about its wider application is that it is very labour intensive, each patient requiring many hours of treatment, and each therapist requiring extensive specialized training to become competent in the techniques. In the general practice setting, its importance may lie in the attention which needs to be paid to identifying patients' explanations of unpleasant events that contribute to depressed thinking.

Cognitive approaches have also proved useful in the treatment of pain. It is widely recognized that distraction may help to reduce pain and this can be used systematically. It has also been shown that systematically focusing on the pain can reduce it. Both techniques are cognitive, controlling what the individual thinks about, and both work by interfering with the generation of worrying thoughts about the pain.

Relaxation/meditation/hypnosis/biofeedback

Emotions are accompanied by physiological changes which may themselves evoke distress and become self-perpetuating. Minimizing or controlling these changes can sometimes break this vicious circle and reduce or eliminate the distress. This section deals with techniques designed to reduce physiological arousal.

Relaxation training attempts to achieve changes by verbal instruction. Various forms of instruction have been used including Jacobson's progressive relaxation, autogenic training and yogic relaxation.[8]

Progressive relaxation

This produces the most reliable bodily changes, using instructions which ask the patient to tense and then relax muscle groups, working systematically over the body.

Autogenic training

Autogenic training describes sensations associated with relaxation and ask the subject to imagine these feelings in their body; for example, 'You fee your hands becoming warmer and as they become warmer your arms begin to feel heavy.'

Yogic relaxation

In yogic relaxation the subject is asked to work systematically over the body allowing each part in turn to become as relaxed as possible; it is incorporated in the practice of yoga. Most forms of training will involve some element of all three approaches.

Meditation training

Meditation training may also seek a similar objective, but does so by training the individual to focus attention on a limited word ('mantra'), sound, or idea In the simplest form patients may be asked to think 'one' on each exhalation

Hypnosis

Hypnosis is a form of collaboration between hypnotist and client in which the client voluntarily allows the hypnotist to induce a state of focused attention and increased suggestion (hypnotic trance). By reducing distractions to a minimum and making repeated emphatic suggestions, the hypnotist can evoke moods, thoughts, sensations, and even behaviour which replace the moods, thoughts, sensations, and behaviour which are troubling the patient.

Unfortunately, not all people are sufficiently suggestible to become hypnotized, and in most people the effects soon wear off. Hence, they may either give up hypnosis or become unduly dependent on the hypnotist.

To some degree the effects of hypnosis can be prolonged by auto-hypnosis. This technique enables the client to re-induce the hypnotic trance and to repeat and reinforce the suggestion made by the hypnotist.

Like most forms of therapy, hypnosis is most effective when both the patient (or client) and the practitioner have faith in its efficacy.

Biofeedback

Biofeedback involves the amplification of normal biological signals. On receipt of these signals, the subject can attempt to control them. The signals may be from EMG (electromyograph from the frontalis, corrugator, or other relevant muscle group), EEG, peripheral temperature (an index of peripheral blood flow), skin conductance (an index of sweat-gland activity), heart rate, or some other relevant measure. Some biofeedback is designed to have a specific effect, as when frontalis EMG feedback is given for the control of tension headache, or anal sphincter dilation feedback is given for the control of faecal incontinence. Other forms of biofeedback are designed to give the patient more generalized control of physiological arousal, either to reduce the pathophysiological changes associated with stress or to reduce the distress experienced.

All of these techniques encourage learners to practice regularly on their own, except where complex, non-portable biofeedback equipment is involved. There has been some experimentation with audio-cassette instruction for relaxation training, and some cassettes are available commercially. While these are useful, there is evidence that suggests that a greater degree of relaxation is achieved with live instruction.[12]

There is little doubt that these approaches can be effective in the treatment of physical conditions which have a psychological trigger, such as tension headache or essential hypertension.[13] However, it is not clear that they are effective in the treatment of emotional disorders, such as anxiety, unless they are incorporated in a more complex treatment package involving cognitive techniques or more general stress-management approaches.

Stress management

People experience stress when they perceive threats, or demands, that either tax or exceed their coping capacity. This can happen when they are subject to major life changes, such as a new job, losing a spouse, or moving house. It can also happen with the accumulation of ordinary day-to-day hassles, such as getting up late, spilling a pint of milk, arriving late at work, or having a colicky baby that requires a lot of attention during the day and interrupts one's sleep at night. The over-anxious person will see threats where they do not exist. Stress may be experienced when objectively there are no demands which are not met; people frequently perceive their spouses, children, parents, employers, friends, etc. to be dissatisfied when, in reality, they are not. The effects of stress can be seen in the individual's mood or in physiological changes which may present as symptoms. These may range from palpitations or pains caused by muscle tension, to disorders such as peptic ulcers or essential hypertension (see Chapter 6).

Stress management involves the following components:

(1) *Identification of the stressors*—the situations which make the individual feel taxed or threatened.

(2) *Assessment of the stressors*. Is it reasonable to feel stressed in these situations? If not, can cognitive technique help in reaching a more realistic assessment?

(3) *Reduction of the stressor.* Can the dangers be averted or avoided? It may be possible by using problem-solving techniques to prevent the threat arising without losing anything, but one must be wary of strategies that lead to the avoidance of useful parts of life; it does not help an agoraphobic to avoid going out in order to avoid feeling frightened. The stress may be reduced by increasing the patient's ability to deal with the situation, for instance by increasing social skills.

(4) *Redefinition of the stressor.* Given that there is an unavoidable stress, some of the effects may be reduced by restructuring or reframing the situation. For example, a woman who reported being continuously upset by the repeated criticisms of her by her mother-in-law, might be more able to deal with the situation if she saw this as the behaviour of a rather unhappy older woman than if she saw it as a true reflection of her own competence as a wife.

(5) *Reduction of the effects of the stressor.* It may also be necessary to reduce some of the unpleasant physical effects of stress by training the patient to gain control using biofeedback or relaxation techniques. These skills then need to be used when exposure to any of the triggering situations occurs.

These techniques have been used successfully with patients facing stressful medical procedures, such as surgery,[3] and also with patients suffering from stress-related physical symptoms, such as tension headache. They have also been used in the management of irritable bowel syndrome, essential hypertension, and even myocardial infarction.[13] They obviously draw heavily on the cognitive, skills, exposure, biofeedback, and relaxation techniques described above, and it would be quite possible to use the stress-management framework for working with a large number of psychological problems presenting in general practice. The techniques are likely to be most useful in working with patients who present with symptoms of anxiety, either physical or psychological.

Marital and family applications (see Chapter 4)

Older models of therapy viewed such problems as existing within the individual and independent of the social environment. The therapists therefore worked with the presenting patient. Many of the more recent models see the problem, or the solution to the problem, as embedded in the patient's family situation, and therefore the problem needs to be solved in a family context. Any of the above models can be applied in such a context: indeed, operant therapies frequently depend on family members who deliver rewards; and exposure, stress management, and cognitive therapies may involve spouses as therapists.

References

1. Bandura, A. (1977). *Social learning theory*. Prentice-Hall, Englewood Cliffs, NJ.
2. Lick, J. and Bootzin, R. (1975). Expectancy factors in the treatment of fear: methodological and theoretical issues. *Psychol. Bull.* **82**, 917–31.
3. Mathews, A. and Ridgeway, V. (1984). Psychological preparation for surgery. (eds A. Steptoe and A. Mathews). In *Health care and human behaviour*, Academic Press, London.
4. France, R. and Robson, M. (1986). *Behaviour therapy in primary care; a practical guide*. Croom Helm, London.
5. Rimm, D. C. and Masters, J. C. (1974). *Behavior therapy: techniques and empirical findings*. Wiley, New York.
6. Mathews, A. M., Gelder, M. G., and Johnston, D. W. (1981). *Agoraphobia: nature and treatment*. Guildford, London.
7. Marks, I. and Horder, J. (1987). Phobias and their management. *Br. med. J.* **295**, 589–92.
8. Gambrill, E. (1977). *Behaviour modification: handbook of assessment, intervention and evaluation*. Jossey-Bass, London.
9. Fordyce, W. E. (1976). *Behavioral methods for chronic pain and illness*. C. V. Mosby, St Louis.
10. Beck, A. T. (1976). *Cognitive therapy and the emotional disorders*. International University Press, New York.
11. Bower, G. H. (1981). Mood and memory. *Am. Psychol.* **36**, 129–48.
12. Borkovec, T. D. and Sides, J. K. (1979). Critical procedural variables related to the physiological effects of progressive relaxation. *Behav. Res. Therapy* **17**, 119–25.
13. Johnston, D. W. (1982). Behavioural treatment in the reduction of coronary risk factors; Type A behaviour and blood pressure. *Br. J. clin Psychol.* **21**, 281–94.

Further reading

France, R. and Robson, M. (1986). *Behaviour therapy in primary care; a practical guide*. Croom Helm, London.
Gambrill, E. (1977). *Behaviour modification: handbook of assessment, intervention and evaluation*. Jossey-Bass, London.
Mathews, A. M., Gelder, M. G., and Johnston, D. W. (1981). *Agoraphobia: nature and treatment*. Guildford, London.
Rimm, D. C. and Masters, J. C. (1974). *Behaviour therapy: techniques and empirical findings*. Wiley, New York.

3.5 UNCOVERING THERAPIES

Nasrudin was sent by the King to investigate the lore of various kinds of Eastern mystical teachers. They all recounted to him tales of the miracles and the sayings of the founders and great teachers, all long dead, and of their schools.

When he returned home he submitted his report which contained the single wor 'Carrots'.

He was called upon to explain himself. Nasrudin told the King: 'The best part is burie Few except the Farmers know, by the green, that there is orange underground; if yc don't work for it, it will deteriorate; there are a great many donkeys associated with it.

So much has been written about the distinction between the 'conscious' an the 'unconscious' minds that one is tempted to forget that by far the large part of the mind lies between the two. Many mental processes take plac outside of consciousness but are accessible to introspection and they belong therefore, to the subconscious rather than to the unconscious. Everythin which previous experience causes us to take for granted, all habits of thoug and action, belong to this great realm. Thus, many of the irrational and se defeating behaviours which are seen as psychiatric disorders are the resul of habits of thought whose roots are quite open to inspection, if only w turn our attention in their direction.

If we accept that our internal model of the world contains assumption based on our previous experience, it is very likely that many behaviou resulting from these assumptions, which may have been appropriate or lif saving in the past environment in which they were learned, do not apply t the current world. A woman who learned to escape her father's drunken wrat by adopting a subservient attitude to men may find herself quite unable t cope when placed in a position of authority later in life. Freud, in his writing on psychoanalysis, has described ways in which the pain of anger, sorrow or anxiety attached to damaging events may be repressed and avoide Perhaps his greatest contribution to psychology and psychotherapy may b simplified into the concept that trauma in childhood may create discomfort disorders, and distortions of perception in the present. Whatever the theor behind these explanations of disordered perceptions, their occurrence obvious in our everyday life.

These processes, which are often called the psychological defenc mechanisms, and are considered below, operate at various levels of consciou ness, so that some may be easy for the patient to verbalize, understand, an perhaps change, while others may be very deeply buried. It would be wron to assume that all defences are pathological. We must ignore one proble if we are to deal with another. We would find life difficult, if not unlivabl if we did not modify and forget some of our pain.

Defence mechanisms

Repression

It would be intolerable to be aware of all our problems all the time. We ofte forget and ignore unpleasant experiences, sometimes deliberately, though the

emain accessible in our minds. Repression of memories shades into denial,
hen access to the memories becomes more difficult.

Denial

Mr A on his return from hospital was asked about his future. He had been told that
e had an inoperable cancer with not long to live. The following week he was planning
n active summer holiday 'when I am better'.

In a way, denial is similar to repression but refers more to the denial of our
wn fears, unacceptable wishes, and thoughts. The denial of these may often
nderlie current thoughts and behaviours which seem illogical, inexplicable,
nd sometimes painful and damaging. Denial is often an unstable defence
which may not last long, but it is usually a mistake to challenge it outright,
s it may be vital for adapting to life.

Displacement

t must be a common occurrence to witness or experience the phenomenon
f venting spleen on the door, the dog, or the daughter. It may relieve tension
f we punch the cushion or the golfball, when the true object of our rage
may be absent. Many people are unable to assert themselves directly or show
their anger openly to close contacts. It may be damaging to all concerned
o displace anger which should be directed, say, against an employee, onto
ne's spouse. Much therapy is concerned with attempting to achieve honest
nd open communication between members of a family and others.

Projection

ome emotions and qualities are too painful to own but may be attributed
o other people instead. 'My wife is very sad about John's death', may be
 true statement but may also avoid acknowledgement of one's own sorrow.
Even more common, and dangerous, is a tendency to attribute hostility to
eople who frustrate us or happen to get in the way. Doctors often get blamed
or the effects of an illness.

Introjection

t is normal for developing children to model themselves on their parents
nd to incorporate their behaviour, thoughts, and feelings into their own
epertoire of responses. It may be inappropriate for an adult to identify with
another person in such a way as to acquire their characteristics. For example,
 woman who had wished her husband dead, felt deeply guilty after that
vent. In the course of the next year she attended her general practitioner

for treatment of each of the symptoms from which he had suffered befo⟩ he died.

Regression

It has been the experience of every doctor to witness sick people who beha⟩ in a childish way. The child who is ill may revert to bed-wetting. It will ⟩ a strong adult who does not become a little demanding and dependent if p⟩ to bed in strange surroundings and treated as a child.

Rationalization

Some people do not acknowledge that they experience painful thoughts ar⟩ feelings. They deny their emotions by intellectualizing and theorizing. 'The⟩ is no point in getting upset,' they say, 'that won't solve anything.' Suc⟩ patients create difficulties for doctors who realize that the talk is a scre⟩ which seems logical and irrefutable, but which prevents emotional problen⟩ from being reviewed. This may obstruct, for instance, the work of grievin⟩ Such patients often present with 'inexplicable' physical symptoms.

Uncovering therapies help people to acknowledge memories, thoughts, ar⟩ feelings. The mere recovery of these, or the acquisition of insight, may n⟩ in itself be helpful. What matters is their integration into a more appropria⟩ model of the current world. Uncovering interpretations will only be possib⟩ if the patient feels safe. This depends upon the development of a trustin⟩ relationship between therapist and patient.

Freud used the techniques of free association and interpretation to uncov⟩ memories of traumatic events in order to free patients from the continuin⟩ power of such events to obtrude into current life and create symptoms an⟩ other problems. By 'free association' he meant allowing the patient to follo⟩ one thought with another, on the assumption that, sooner or later, patien⟩ would be drawn towards the emotionally meaningful memories that la⟩ behind their current problems. By 'interpretation' the therapist drew attentio⟩ to the psychological defences of the patient and clarified the underlyin⟩ assumptions and memories which lay hidden in the patient's unconsciou⟩ mind. Much use was made of the interpretation of dreams, which were see⟩ by Freud as 'the royal road to the unconscious'.

As time passed, Freud's 'talking cure' changed its focus from recent traum⟩ to uncovering earlier and earlier memories in the patient's childhood. Th⟩ tendency reached its logical extreme in the work of some of his followe⟩ (e.g. Otto Rank) who came to see the trauma of birth as the primal stre⟩ from which all else developed, and who would not accept that therapy cou⟩ be complete unless memories of this experience had been 'recovered'.

Although Freud did not adopt this extreme position, and himself becam⟩ sceptical of the veracity of many of the 'screen memories' which his patient⟩

eported, the form of therapy which he developed (psychoanalysis) became, and remains, very expensive and time-consuming, often involving daily sessions of an hour's duration for 2–3 years. Consequently, it is beyond the pocket of all but the wealthiest patients and is never likely to be provided by the National Health Service.

There are psychotherapists today who see the uncovering of early childhood memories as a main object of therapy, and some fewer who set out to demolish the 'defences' of their patients, though most now see this type of uncovering' as akin to rape. But the practice of psychoanalysis did provide therapists with a source of ideas, many of which have been taken up and used in other forms of psychotherapy. These include the recognition that behind many symptoms there lie problems which stem from attitudes and assumptions that may have been quite appropriate in the past but which are now inappropriate and harmful. The 'uncovering' and clarifying of these assumptions can free people to review them and to discover new ways of coping with current challenges.

Transference and counter-transference

One type of interpretation, which often results in successful therapy, is the drawing of parallels between the way in which the therapists are being perceived and treated and the way in which the patients perceived and treated their own parents—the interpretation of 'transference'.

Freud noticed that in the course of therapy patients began to see and treat him as though he were a significant person from their past lives, perhaps as though he was their mother, their father, or a sibling. He used this behaviour by pointing it out to patients, encouraging them to remember episodes relevant to these relationships. This, in simple form, is the essence of transference. But there is more to it than this. By allowing the patient to transfer onto the therapist assumptions which properly belong to an earlier relationship, the patient is helped to re-learn that relationship. By accepting his projected material without criticism, the therapist shows, for example, that not all mothers denigrate their sons, that not all fathers sexually assault their daughters, and that the patient is worthy of attention, whatever the behaviour.

Because we are all open to the influence of suggestion, therapists also tend to react to the patients' transference as if they were the significance persons patients makes them out to be, or they may react towards patients as they would to significant persons in their own families. To ensure that therapy does not confirm the patients' worst fears, therapists need to be aware of their own reactions to patients; this is termed '*counter-transference*'. In other words, the therapist has to remain self-aware without becoming too detached, even when being treated as someone with attitudes that may be quite alien. It is for this reason that analysts claim the need to be analysed before they

can become effective. Few general practitioners will want to have an analysis
but it is helpful for all GPs to be aware of the more obvious problems o
transference and counter-transference because they occur in many day-to-da
consultations and form the basis of many therapeutic problems.

Mrs G had had an unhappy childhood and what seemed, to her male GP, to be an
unusual marriage. After the death of her husband in his late forties, she presente
with a series of inexplicable symptoms in a rather childish and flirtatious manner
which irritated the GP. With difficulty, he managed to talk to her about the manne
of her presentation, which seemed to reflect the way she had interacted with her father
After this, the patient became able to express her feelings of being unloved, and he
need to be loved, and the general practitioner began not only to tolerate, but als
to like her. This did not solve all her problems, but she gradually presented fewe
inexplicable symptoms.

   Balint's[2] gift was his ability to interpret ideas derived from psychoanalysi
in a manner which made them accessible and useful to general practitioners
The groups he founded encouraged doctors to become aware of their ow
feelings which may reflect or mirror the patient's feelings toward someone
else in their life. Doctors, by using insight into their own feelings, may thu
be able to help patients explore their own emotional life.

Insight

An important test of progress in therapy is the grasp of insight or 'flash' —
'Ah, now I understand' — when a person suddenly comes to comprehend th
true nature of the problem. Perhaps a behaviour which seems inappropriate
or illogical, suddenly makes sense, assumptions which had been taken fo
granted are seen as inappropriate, a new way of viewing a problem spring
to mind; such insights are important milestones in therapy, but they ar
seldom sufficient in themselves to solve the main problems. It is not enoug
for a mother to realize that she is battering her child because of the resentmen
which built up inside her when she was battered by her own mother — sh
needs to find some other way of expressing that rage.
   Insight is, therefore, a part of the process of re-learning which ca
eventually liberate people from the shackles of the past and enable them t
fulfil their true potential.

Abreactive techniques

Sometimes the recall of traumatic events is accompanied by intense emotio
and an experience as if the person was re-living the event in question. Thi
is termed 'abreaction'. Abreaction usually leads to an immediate reductio
in levels of anxiety and tension and sometimes to improvement in othe
symptoms. It will occasionally occur spontaneously when a person is talkin

about an event of this kind but it can also be induced by means of drugs, hypnosis, or strong suggestion. A clue to the presence of relevant traumatic memories that are being repressed may come from the observation that the emotional reaction to a current situation is inappropriate and inexplicable. One approach is to ask the patient to experience the reaction more deeply, to verbalize it repeatedly in louder and louder tones, and to exaggerate the non-verbal behaviour that accompanies it (the twisted foot, the clenched fist, or the rigid posture). In the hands of experienced therapists, and given enough support and trust, the patient may then re-live or 'abreact' a traumatic event from the past, speaking in the present tense as though to the relevant person, parent, sibling, etc. who was involved in their earlier memories. After such abreaction there is usually a time of profound relief and relaxation.

Mr X had been talking about his eight-year-old son, John, who was truanting from school, and explaining how angry John made him. The therapist noticed that he seemed restless, a bit flushed, was breathing more quickly, and was drumming the chair with his right hand. Empathy, reflection, and silence did not help the patient to express the thoughts, which were perhaps not fully accessible to him. The therapist leaned forward and suggested that Mr X exaggerate the drumming and repeat more loudly his last statement 'John makes me so angry'. Encouraged to continue drumming more violently and to repeat the sentence more loudly, the behaviour eventually reached a climax. At this point, it was suggested to the patient that he state what the drumming hand was really saying. The patient crumpled, and in a childish voice, using the first person and the present tense, described his terror of his own father who used to thrash him, and his repressed anger towards him. When, after a few minutes, Mr X seemed to have said all that was needed, it was suggested he might relax and breathe deeply. He drifted into a light sleep and on waking, after another few minutes, he remembered what had happened but felt calm and relaxed. He was encouraged to integrate the abreactive experience that he had had into his handling of the current problems with his son, and found this helpful.

The unconscious

Freud's work was carried out before the days of sexual liberation and at a time when repression of sexual feelings was endemic throughout (mid-European) society. 'Uncovering' therapies seem to be particularly useful in the treatment of hysteria (conversion disorder) and other conditions in which repression plays a large part. Today, hysteria is a rare condition, at least in the gross forms reported by Freud and his contemporaries, and the uncovering therapies less often provide us with a solution for patients' psychological problems.

Some of the phenomena which Freud attributed to fantasies of incest and sexual abuse are now revealed as literally true, as these forms of behaviour

are much commoner than they were once thought to be. The climate of th
age often makes it possible for patients to share their feelings about suc
events, instead of diverting their emotional energy to repressing then
Somehow 'the unconscious' seems to be less unconscious than it was mad
out to be, and our patients, with support and encouragement, find less tha
is unthinkable, unspeakable, or unchangeable.

One of Freud's great contributions to helping patients was the concept tha
the unconscious can be made accessible and understandable within
framework of care and support. It is again important to remember that hi
is only a model, and other models have arisen out of his work which ma
be more easily used by some doctors with some patients. Jung, Adler, an
Klein, to mention only a few, developed differing theories of huma
development, but all accepted the idea of unconscious processes.

The ideas of uncovering therapies are usable in general practice and, indeed
awareness of defence mechanisms, transference, and the skills of helpin
patients to unburden their easily accessible thoughts need to be part of ever
consultation.

Evaluation

The scientific evaluation of any method of treatment as complex as psycho
analysis is obviously difficult. It is not easy to persuade patients to accep
random assignment to therapy or no therapy at all, and in those few studie
in which this had been done, results have been disappointing. Other type
of psychotherapy derived from psychoanalysis are too numerous and to
varied to make it possible for us to make broad generalizations about th
success of psychotherapy as a whole. Numerous comparative studies do
however, enable us to point to some of the factors which seem to predispos
to successful psychotherapy; but none of these has much to do wit
'uncovering'. They have been summarized by Frank[3] as follows:

- the establishment of a confiding relationship with a person seen to b
  a professional;

- holding the sessions in a setting identified as secure;

- having a therapeutic rationale which the patient finds meaningful i
  explaining symptoms;

- prescription of a course of action to relieve symptoms which involve
  active participation by both patient and therapist.

These principles apply not only to 'uncovering' therapies but also to th
behavioural treatments considered in Section 3.4.

References

1. Idries Shah (1986). *The exploits of the incomparable Mulla Nasrudin*. The Camelot Press, Southampton.
2. Balint, M. (1957). *The doctor, his patient and the illness*. Pitman Medical, London.
3. Frank, J. D. (1986). Psychotherapy—the transformation of meanings; discussion paper. *J. R. Soc. Med.* **79**, 341–5.

Further reading

Bandler, R. and Grinder, J. (1979). *Frogs into princes*. Real People Press, Utah.
Bendix, T. (1982). *The anxious patient* (ed. H. J. Wright). Churchill Livingstone, London.
Berne, E. (1974). *What do you say after you say hello?* Andre Deutsch, California.
Fisch, R., Weakland, J. H., and Segal, L. (1985). *The tactics of change. Doing therapy briefly*. Jossey-Bass, London.
Lankton, S. (1980). *Practical magic*. Meta Publications, California.
Pincus, L. and Dare, C. (1978). *Secrets in the family*. Faber and Faber, London.

Part II Methods

4 Practical management by the primary care team

4.1 INTRODUCTION

n Chapter 2, attention was drawn to the high prevalence of psychological problems in the population and the fact that the majority of these have, of necessity, to be managed within the primary care team (PCT). In this chapter we discuss the various aspects of this management, and convert some of the theory of Chapter 3 into practice.

It is becoming increasingly clear that patients are not always best served by the prescription of drugs. Tranquillizers seldom provide cures, and may mask the expression and working-through of emotional problems. They soon lose their effectiveness, and are habit forming. Antidepressants can be literally life saving in severely depressed people, but have serious side-effects and most of them can easily kill people in overdose. They need to be used judiciously. Major tranquillizers should be reserved for major, usually psychotic, illnesses. In this chapter we consider the indications and practicalities for the use of drugs but also put forward some of the alternatives available.

We believe that members of the primary care team, by virtue of their long-term involvement in the community, have, if for no other reason than to contain their own work-load, a vested interest in the early discovery and treatment of health problems — not only mental. Half of the GP's work is generated by 15 per cent of the patients on his or her list.[1] Most of these patients have psychological problems. If a few of these could be made less dependent, the total work-load would be reduced and most patients made happier. Some of those patients have somatic symptoms and no organic illness (see Chapter 6); if these can be diagnosed at an early stage, and effectively treated, they need not become chronic.

For all these reasons we see prevention, primary and secondary, as crucial to the management of psychological problems in the community. At the heart of management lies the consultation, within which a trusting relationship between doctor and patient, or health professional and client, is built up. There will be few consultations, whether for physical or psychological problems, which do not require counselling skills, and the dividing line between these and psycho-therapeutic skills is blurred. Neither need be lengthy. Both are examined here.

While not many GPs become involved in group therapy for patients, we need to know how this operates, so as to be able to identify those patients who might benefit.

Lastly, few doctors in primary care now work in isolation. Most work closely with other members of the team, not only with nurses and health visitors, but with a wider team within which are clinical psychologists, social workers, community psychiatric nurses, counsellors, and psychiatrists. The benefits and problems of team work are examined in Section 4.8.

Reference

1. Wamoscher, Z. (1966). The returning patient. *J. R. Coll. Gen. Pract.* **11**, 166–72

Further reading

Balint, E. and Norell, J. S. (1973). *Six minutes for the patient: interactions in general practice consultation*. Tavistock, London.
Balint, M. (1957). *The doctor, his patient and the illness*. Pitman Medical, London

4.2   THE CONSULTATION

Background

In order to understand the consultation it is helpful to remember what both parties, the doctor and the patient, bring to it in terms of their personalities, memories, experiences, hopes, fears, and expectations.

Symptoms

Most illnesses start with a symptom or a cluster of symptoms which may or may not be familiar to the person. Whether this is dismissed or taken seriously depends on its meaning, implication, and effects. Hoarseness in an opera singer requires a different response than it would if it happened to a farmer. Bleeding piles will be viewed differently if a friend has died of carcinoma of the rectum than it will if a near relative has had piles all their life

Symptoms are likely to be seen as significant if they:

● interfere with normal activities, e.g. phobias;

● are obvious to others, e.g. twitches;

● are regarded as serious by others, e.g. hearing 'voices';

● occur concurrently with an unrelated personal crisis;

● exceed the individual's threshold of tolerance (pain is tolerated differently in different cultures);

- are unfamiliar, e.g. feeling 'far away';

- are thought to be due to serious illness;

- are thought to lead to incapacity or death, e.g. forgetfulness or severe headaches;

- persist after self-medication.

The course of action taken depends on how the patient interprets the meaning of the illness. If it is thought of as a weakness, it may be denied; if as a punishment, suffered; if as a threat, challenged; if as a loss, grieved; if as a relief from a stressful situation, grasped. At opposite ends of a spectrum people either attribute the illness to outside events, which may give rise to anger or even paranoia, or to themselves, when they are more likely to become depressed. People who attribute externally (i.e. have an external 'locus of control', see Section 1.2) are often best helped in a more formal manner than the internal attributers, who need their self-esteem boosting.

Life may, or may not, be made easier for doctors by the fact that almost all patients consult their family, friends, or both, before seeing their doctor, and will have decided whether their symptoms imply a serious illness, whether it should be self-medicated, to whom it should be referred, and how it should be presented.

Mrs Smith had a funny feeling in her chest after dinner (probably extra systoles resulting from several cups of tea). She remembered that her mother's angina and death seemed to have started like this, and as she did, so her discomfort increased and she overbreathed a little and developed a rapid heart beat. She mentioned this casually to her daughter who, used to her mother's panics, suggested some Alka Seltzer. Mrs Smith was not happy with this. She recalled how angry she had been with her husband the night before, and decided that this must have affected her heart. She had been to the doctor before with other discomforts and, after barium meals and endoscopies, had been told there was nothing wrong with her. She was reluctant to go again.

As it happened she met a friend on her way back from the chemist. They discussed her 'pain' and her friend said she should make an emergency appointment at the doctor's, as only the day before, in *Woman's Own*, the importance of early treatment of heart attacks had been explained. So Mrs Smith went to the doctor, but found a new one, and felt frightened because he spoke with an upper-class accent. She said she had this pain in her chest and could it be indigestion? (She was frightened that it might be her heart but didn't want to say so.) The doctor was very thorough and took a careful history of the pain. 'What was it like and where did it radiate to?' (What does radiate mean?) He examined her and said all seemed well, but he would get his nurse to do an ECG 'just in case'. By the time the nurse had done the ECG the doctor was running late and saw her in the treatment room, assuring her that all was well. He prescribed a few diazepams. She felt confused and still didn't understand her sensations. Her friend said she didn't think she ought to take tranquillizers ''cos they are addictive like drugs'.

Later that week she saw another partner. By now she thought that it was probabl' 'the nerves' but felt that to be a sign of weakness and didn't like to ask if it coul< be, so she described the funny breathing that accompanied the chest feeling. The docto' was again thorough, examined her and arranged a chest X-ray. She left feeling mor' frightened than ever and her anxiety was confirmed by the family, who reminde< her that her sister had died of cancer of the lung. When she heard that the chest X ray was normal she was still not convinced that she was not ill.

A more satisfactory outcome might have occurred if the doctor had bee> able to elicit what was frightening her at the first consultation.

Beliefs

The Health Belief Model elaborated by Becker[1] provides a structure fo' understanding why patients do or do not follow advice, based on their ow> perception of their susceptibility to a disease, its seriousness, and the influenc' of various modifying factors. These modifying factors may relate to age sex, race or ethnicity, or to media or friend's advice. Considered together if the perceived benefits outweigh the perceived barriers, the patient wil comply. These considerations can be applied to advice given during an' consultation. It is important to explore the patient's beliefs if an outcom satisfactory to both doctor and patient is to ensue.

Illness, culture, and religion

The doctor and the patient will bring different beliefs to the consultation An oriental patient may not accept a 'hot' food for a cold illness: poorl' informed patients will avoid acid fruit if they think they have 'acidity' o' ulcers; patients may not see their depression as an illness if they think it i due to sinful action.

Many men and women are convinced that there is a divine power of som' sort operating in human affairs, but they are not sure what it is, nor do the' know how to bring this divine presence into their daily experience. It ma seem outside the doctor's province to talk about religion but questions suc' as 'Do you have any religious belief?', or 'Is it in any way a religiou problem?' may produce surprising answers. Having elicited that there ar' indeed ethical or religious problems, most health professionals will prefe to listen and then attempt to find a suitable priest or cleric. For such a referra the patient may be eternally grateful! Possession of a strong faith may enabl patients to overcome many hurdles, though a rigid one may limit the abilit' to change, and may be associated with illness. There is evidence that churcl membership is protective against illness.[2]

The doctor's contribution to the consultation

Doctors also bring a series of thoughts and beliefs to the consultation an< it is salutary to remember that these beliefs may be as ephemeral and changin:

s the patient's. Is diverticulitis treated with a low- or high-fibre diet? Is omosexuality an illness to be treated, or the predominant orientation of minority of normal people?

Doctors also vary in their beliefs or are inconsistent, even if they, like atients, attempt to disguise them; adultery is a sin; a variety of sexual xperience is valuable.

Much of this book describes a set of thoughts and beliefs about psychological problems, but individual members of the helping team need o acquire their own set of thoughts and beliefs based on good scientific vidence where this is possible. It will help if all members of the team nderstand each other's ideas. While models of therapy and interpersonal kills are important, the personal attributes of the therapist may be even nore so.

Attributes

Research[3] has suggested that in addition to general rapport, the ingredients f accurate empathy, non-possessive warmth, and genuineness are essential o therapy whatever the model used, and these attributes are discussed in he next few pages. To some extent, all health professionals have to accept hemselves as they are, but there is evidence that some change is possible. ruax and Carkuff[4] describe an improvement in genuineness, non-possessive varmth, and accurate empathy after the use of videotapes and group work o improve self-awareness. Balint[5] describes a limited change in doctors' ersonality that may result from attendance of seminars focusing on this issue, nd changes in personal attributes after completion of GP vocational training chemes have been evaluated.[6]

Everyone has different sets of behaviours which are used in different ettings (compare a doctor's behaviour at a party and at an FPC hearing), nd, therefore, the capacity to adapt without having to change fundamentally s already there.

Rapport

Good rapport is essential for good consulting. It seems that some people chieve this with little effort and some find it more difficult. Observation f doctors establishing good rapport shows, above all, that they listen, but lso that they are shrewd observers of their patients and use these bservations, either consciously or subconsciously, to good effect. The art f rapport can be learnt. It is important to greet patients and make eye-contact s soon as they enter the room. Some doctors will shake hands, some only n the first meeting, and some never, but a positive greeting, both verbally nd non-verbally, perhaps by change of posture or by standing up, is mportant. Once patients are seated, it is important to note their posture, one of voice, speed of talking, and need for eye-contact.

It is helpful, in some measure, to mirror the patient. If a courting coup(e) are observed in a restaurant, it will be seen that they both lean forwar(d) together and lean back together; they both rest their chins in their hand(s) they both smile; they are on the same wavelength. Doctors need to be o(n) the same wavelength as their patients; this helps non-verbal communicatio(n) which seems emotionally more powerful than words. If the patient is ale(rt) and upright, the doctor should avoid leaning back, because this suggests lac(k) of interest. If the patient's tone is low and sad, it is unwise to be brusq(ue) and humorous. For the most part, this kind of adjustment happens natural(ly) and automatically, but if it does not, it needs to be done consciously, so (as) to put patients at their ease. This may, at first, seem artificial but it soo(n) becomes second nature and is not seen as mimicry by the patient. Videotapin(g) confirms that it looks natural. Once contact has been established we ma(y) change these rules on the assumption that the patient will imitate us; th(us) a doctor may deliberately lean back in his chair or make a joke in order (to) relieve tension and help the patient to relax. Leaning forward, to indica(te) interest and support, and leaning back, to indicate relaxation and to tak(e) a break from intense involvement, become part of the warp and weft (of) therapeutic interaction.

While non-verbal language is in some ways more powerful, or basic, tha(n) the verbal, it also helps to use similar language; for instance, to reflect on(e)-syllable words with one-syllable words. Most people have a preferred wa(y) of expressing themselves and predominantly use visual, auditory, (or) kinaesthetic words. If a patient tells me that the future looks *black* and h(e) can't *see* the *light* at the end of the tunnel, and I reply in terms suggestin(g) that I find it *hard* to get the *feel* of the situation but have some ideas abo(ut) *lifting* the *load* from his shoulders, he may not, at an important level (of) consciousness, understand what is being said.

Patients come to all consultations, and particularly to those in which the(y) seek help of a psychological nature, with their own expectations. They ma(y) wonder if they will be lying on a couch and confessing all, or imagine th(e) doctor as an important professional in a big chair who will make decisio(ns) about their lives. These expectations need to be sensed.

Doctors can legitimately touch people when examining them. Don(e) sensitively and with awareness, this can create trust and rapport. The us(e) of touch may be appropriate during, and at the end of, a consultation. Mo(st) patients will welcome the reassuring touch on the arm or the supporting ar(m) around the shoulder. Shoulders to cry on can sometimes be more tha(n) metaphorical, and holding hands often seems appropriate in a situation (of) acute loss, such as with the recently bereaved, or the dying.

Accurate empathy

A simple definition of empathy is understanding the other person's assumpti(ve) world. In attempting to understand patients and their problems, all th(e) doctor's skills of rapport are needed, especially the ability to give full attention. Close observation may enable the doctor to follow the patient's feelings — the minimal pallor of anger, the dilated pupil of fear, and the flush of embarrassment can be vital clues, as can the tremulous lip and the moist eye.

Doctors live in their own assumptive world and it is natural for them to expect to understand other people's thoughts and experiences in terms of their own. However, this accurate empathy is not tantamount to complete identification with a patient. A doctor who makes claim to the latter could easily arouse a patient's resentment. It is not usually helpful or true to say 'I understand, I have felt the same', but it may be helpful to say 'Yes, I too have experienced the loss of a mother.' This does not imply having had the same emotional response.

In the course of everyday life, and especially in the practice of medicine, doctors will have acquired a fair knowledge of different lifestyles and some insight into how different people think. However, no one can experience all the ills of life (for a start, no one knows what it is like to be a member of the opposite sex) and some doctors may have led rather restricted lives — the race-track of school, university, medical school, house jobs, and vocational training may have left little time for the wider world. For instance, a heterosexual doctor might find it hard to empathize with the beauty and difficulties of a gay relationship. The discipline of understanding a patient's world and interpreting their words in terms of that world can be helped by discussion with colleagues.

Sometimes it may help to understand the patient by referring to textbooks of sociology, psychology, or anthropology, but it is also possible to extend life experience through novels and biography, or theatre, television, and art. Freud once said 'Creative writers are valuable allies and their evidence is to be highly prized, for they are apt to know a whole host of things between heaven and earth of which our philosophy has not yet let us dream. In this knowledge of the mind they are far in advance of us everyday people, for they draw upon sources which we have not yet opened up for science.'

Non-possessive warmth

Fry[7] defines a therapeutic relationship in the following terms. 'A culturally sanctioned relationship between doctor and patient in which care and concern, and sometimes love, produce a feeling of safety for the patient, subsequently allowing the development of understanding and change which may also involve the application of technical procedures and therapeutic agents.' A person suffering from psychological problems will need caring warmth to be shown by the doctor. Only then can the ambience be created in which a patient feels they can trust the doctor with their feelings. This gives the doctor a better chance of identifying and helping with the problem. Moreover, this support may temporarily assuage the patient's feelings of fear, loss, or uncertainty. The patient might, for instance, come to the doctor with a embarrassing or self-revealing problem, or one that is felt likely to provok criticism from others. If any sign of hostility or lack of interest were to b shown, that patient would certainly be discouraged and without some positiv warmth and encouragement might find it hard ever again to speak abou the problem.

Inevitably, this kind of doctor–patient relationship involves the danger tha the patient becomes emotionally dependent on the doctor—the very fact tha the doctor provides psychological support could, in some cases, make a degre of dependence inescapable. In the case of a patient who has experience personal loss, that patient may project the image of their own lost perso or someone else in their life onto the doctor, and with it their desire to becom dependent. For the doctor the relationship may invoke subconscious need to be loved and wanted. It is important that care and warmth are showr but there is a vital distinction between the warmth shown in such a situatio by a doctor and the warmth of friendship. Compared to the warmth of friendship, the doctor's warmth must be non-possessive and unconditiona. In other words, professionals must avoid seeking their own emotiona satisfaction from the relationship and should not allow the patient more tha a limited emotional dependence, though in every practice there are a fev isolated people who have only the doctor to turn to. Support is most usefu when offered steadily in a clearly controlled, unambiguous way, regardles of whether or not treatment appears to be successful. It helps to be warm open, and available, not to create dependency, and not to imperil our ow lives and health by giving in to all demands. Limits must be set about tim and privacy.

It is a paradox that people towards whom doctors do not immediately fee warm, or whom they may even dislike, may be the people who can benefi most from help. It is probable that if the doctor finds these people difficul or bristly, so does much of the rest of the world. If enough time and effor is spent on understanding their isolation and feelings of rejection, they ma become not only tolerable but lovable, though one needs to beware of pity For them to know that they are at least tolerated can be a great boost to their self-esteem. An important extension of non-possessive warmth i availability and commitment. The doctor must have the ability 'to stay wit the patient' and be able to tolerate their distress and anger and not shy of into questions or reassurance. Being there can be more important than doin things.

There are occasions when things seem to be going badly. It is then necessar to distinguish between a true breakdown in the relationship, when referra to a partner or other professional may be desirable, and the situation in whic the patient is transferring feelings from other relationships in their life o to the doctor, when it is therapeutic to stay with the patient. If this distinctio is in doubt, and it is important to get it right because rejection of the patien will reinforce their self-distrust, discussion with a colleague can be helpful. The demands of psychological counselling involve a delicate balancing act between, on the one hand, non-possessiveness and a certain emotional reserve and, on the other hand, personal warmth and 'genuiness' (see below). To preserve this balance, the doctor needs to be aware of what is happening in the relationship with the patient, and be able to monitor his or her own involvement. This has been likened to being in the control tower of an airport. Once the doctor becomes totally part of the system, objectivity and effectiveness are lost. Doctors need this skill not only to prevent themselves becoming over-involved but also to plan tactics and strategies. Discussion with colleagues, group work, and audio- and videotape analysis of consultations are the best methods of learning this skill.

Genuineness

The *Shorter Oxford Dictionary* defines genuineness as 'natural, not acquired, not spurious, authentic'. Genuineness does not mean responding with unthinking honesty. However, patients may need to hear the truth and they may be helped by an honest appraisal of their problem. As with accurate empathy and non-possessive warmth, sensitivity is required in treading the path between extremes. Certainly there is a tendency amongst some doctors to avoid openness and truth in their dealings with patients; white coats, desks, and titles, particularly in hospitals, may have the effect of over-sheltering the doctor. Marinker[8] stated that 'one of the hidden agendas of the undergraduate curriculum is that it is profitable for doctors to distance themselves from their patients and to conceal, or even repress, their natural feelings'. Some distance may be necessary so as not to be overwhelmed by patients' pain, suffering, and demands. This in itself involves a genuine recognition of the doctor's own needs. It is appropriate that personal friendships and love are kept separate from professional lives, but there are occasions when it is right to tell someone they have done well, that they possess kindness and warmth, that they are worthwhile and have enhanced the doctor's own life. It may also occasionally be appropriate to confront patients with the difficulties they have created for the doctor. People depend on others to affirm and confirm their identities and this can be an important part of the counselling role.

The above attributes are important, but in addition, whatever the situation, doctors need to retain a positive expectation of their patients. This is not to say that they must display unjustified optimism, or false hope, but at a deeper level they must believe in the possibility of positive change. Goethe said 'If we take people as they are, we make them worse. If we treat them as if they were what they ought to be, we help them to become what they are capable of becoming.'

Although authoritarianism is not normally helpful, it is sometimes necessary to speak with authority in psychological treatment. For instance it may need to be pointed out that problems with families may persist if some secrets are retained, that continued avoidance of the feared situation will maintain a phobia, that the denial of grief is often productive of adverse symptoms, that marital problems are more difficult to overcome if both partners do not accept help, that children may be damaged by divorce if evil is spoken of the absent spouse, and that death in the family should be discussed honestly, sensitively, and appropriately to the age of children, who should be allowed to express their feelings. Doctors can speak with authority without being authoritarian.

Support for the carers

Doctors and others need to be warm, genuine, and empathetic to help patients in distress, but this can be emotionally draining. It is said that a problem shared is a problem halved. Sometimes the therapist can be left with a very painful half. Therapists react in different ways to their own stress and to the demands of patients. Some will deny the usefulness and validity of psychological help for themselves, even though they offer such a service to their patients. Some will be cold, remote, and defensive, some will struggle but will sacrifice their own families or health. Some will displace their anger, sadness, or helplessness onto others — staff, friends, or families — and some will resort to alcohol or drugs, or become workaholics. Some will cope, help, survive, and grow.

More than the rest of the population doctors die from suicide, alcohol, and drugs. They also suffer from 'burn out', the phenomenon of disenchantment after initial enthusiasm. The apparent need to be competent, infallible, and strong in order to support patients makes it difficult to admit to weakness and sadness. This denial may be an inappropriate defence and one which is both damaging to physical and mental health and prevents growth as an individual and as a professional person.

> Men, said the Devil,
> are good to their brothers
> They don't want to mend
> their own ways, but each other's.[9]

Jonathan Gathorne Hardy[10] in his book *Doctors* writes eloquently about the fact that some, perhaps many, doctors, join the profession in part to cure themselves and to satisfy subconscious needs. This is not to deny or invalidate more conscious motives of altruism or desire for security and status. Such factors have to be accepted and make it important that facilities are available for doctors who need help — partners in a group practice may be the most readily available resource. Within a team, people need to be aware

of signs of stress in each other and be able to respond. 'Burn ou
in any member of the team, but is less likely to occur where the
sympathetic working relationships. If it does, families and fri
of invaluable help, but there are dangers inherent in these opt
helping agencies are available, such as groups run by the Br...
Postgraduate Federation. Sometimes an attached counsellor or psychotherapist may be able to offer individual advice, though this can be difficult
if there is to be a continuing professional working relationship. Outside help
may then be required.

The setting

Before considering the structure of the consultation, it may be helpful to
examine the effect of the setting on its outcome. There are advantages in
consulting in the home, particularly in crises, and with families (see Sections
3.3 and 3.4). The doctor has a chance to observe the lifestyle and scenario
of the patient's problem. Moreover, it is the patient's or family's territory
and they may be less inhibited within it than in a consulting room. But doctors
have to have the confidence to leave their own territory.

However, most consultations, for logistic reasons if no other, take place
in the territory of the primary care team.

The consultation does not start at the door of the consulting room. The
reception and waiting rooms are the doctor's responsibility. If there have
been problems, or undue delays, it may be helpful to discuss these briefly,
allowing emotions to be expressed and put into perspective to clear the way
for a better consultation.

The physical layout of the premises, in particular of the consulting rooms,
also has an effect on the patient. If the rooms are kept neutral, and free from
personal belongings, an impersonal style is implied. On the other hand, too
many family photographs may be intrusive. If bibles or crucifixes are too
much in evidence, atheists may be alienated.

Similarly, very formal clothes may encourage respect, appealing to the
middle-class and middle-aged, but alienating some younger patients. Relaxed
clothes may help to diminish the status gap between the poor or the young
and the professional, while others may see it as unprofessional for a doctor
not to wear a tie.

A desk placed directly between the doctor and the patient tends to make
it difficult for both to be open and may lead to confrontation and discord.
If there is no desk and only chairs, the patient may feel exposed. Most prefer
the corner of a desk between themselves and their doctors.

People have an invisible boundary around them of about 18 inches, so
that a comfortable distance between a couple conversing is abou 3–5 feet.
Most consultations will be comfortable at this distance, but occasionally,
in order to 'get close' to people, it may be helpful to encroach on this

boundary. Similarly, moving further away will distance the patient. Ideally the notes, or computer, should be consulted before the patient arrives and not referred to again until the consultation has been completed.

By choosing to consult in their own territory doctors enhance any difference in status between them and their patients; this may be due to knowledge and class but will probably involve power. There is evidence that doctors talk less, explain less, and listen to fewer problems when seeing patients of lower social class than themselves.[11] It is also customary to exclude the patient's friends and often relatives from the consultation, yet research suggests that doctors are more polite, and distance themselves less, when an ally of the patient is present. This knowledge may help counteract unnecessary barriers.

The ritual

The consultation does more than provide a prescription or management. It may turn a symptom into a disease. This has implication for patients about their perception of themselves — 'I have diabetes and will never be healthy again.' It may turn a reading of a continuous variable into a disease — 'I have hypertension.' It may turn a behaviour into a disease — 'The doctor sees me as an alcoholic.' It may turn a problem into a disease — 'I was worried about my mother and now I have an anxiety state and am on diazepam.'

The ritual of the consultation fulfils functions in addition to diagnosing, managing, and prognosing. It may be a gateway for benefits. It is also a gateway to the sick role. Not only may the illness become labelled as a disease, but may be confirmed as a sickness.

It may bring with it certain rights and duties. A sick person may need cherishing, need not work, but must try to get better and do what the doctor and family say. When better, a ritual to escape from sickness is needed — 'I can't go back to work until I have been back to the hospital.'

The structure of the consultation

The framework of the consultation, as described by Byrne and Long,[12] may be applied to consultations about psychological as well as physical problems (assuming the two can ever be separated):

● greeting;

● discovering the problem;

● making an assessment or a diagnosis;

● agreeing the nature of the problem;

● agreeing a possible solution;

● ending the consultation.

Greeting

Having made the non-verbal gesture with which the doctor feels most comfortable, an open-ended question such as 'What can I do for you?' or 'How can I help you?' is usually appropriate. Sometimes one can just wait for the patient to open the conversation.

Discovering the problem

The high prevalence of psychological problems in the population and the failure of diagnosis of these problems in general practice, together with the value of recognition, have been referred to in Chapter 2.

All consultations have a psychological component but not always a problem. Any illness or distress, or change, will have some meaning to the patient — 'Why should I get this illness?', and some implication — 'How will this affect my relationship with my husband?', and some effect on self-esteem — 'It is good that I have got over this so well' or 'Why haven't I got over this better?' A few patients will present, openly, problems of a psychological nature — their anxiety, depression, their marriage, or shop-lifting. In others, the predominately psychological nature will be obvious — 'the radio told me that I must accept God and cut off my penis.' Others will present a minor physical problem, as a ticket of admission, to sound out the sensitivity and willingness of the doctor to listen.

The role of the doctor will be to help people present the problems that they want to present. This is complicated because initially there may be some areas about which the patient is ambivalent and other areas which the patient had not thought relevant, but which become important in the course of the conversation. It is possible to lead patients to disclosures which they feel delighted to have shared or which they regret having made. Some of the techniques described can be powerful, and doctors must beware of being intrusive and pursuing solutions alien to the patient (see empathy, p. 94). In its extreme forms this amounts to raping the patient's mind. Sometimes a doctor's kind, mild manner can be deceptive and insidious; the patient may be subtly pressurized without knowing how to resist.

Sensitivity, for example asking patients if they want to discuss difficult subjects, is a safeguard. However, if patients do disclose information which they regret, it may be possible to turn this to advantage by discussing their fears and continuing to show that we affirm and respect them.

Discovering the patient's problem uses the skills of listening (see p. 109) aided by asking open questions — 'Tell me more', 'Anything else?' A statement such as 'I am worried about my cough' may elicit several responses which may determine the course of the rest of the consultation. 'How long have you had it?' 'Do you bring up any phlegm?' (closed question) may end in a prescription for an antibiotic. 'Tell me more about it?' (a directive but open question) or 'You say you are worried' (a directive, open statement) may end up in a discussion about a relative's death from cancer of the lung or about an anxiety state.

If the doctor is to ascertain the presence of psychological problems, as well as physical, all clues must be attended to, for instance:

- If there is a suggestion of reticence or something hidden and eye-contact is avoided, it may be helpful for the doctor to ask 'What is it that you had decided not to say when you came in?'

- Non-verbal communication of distress, agitation, depression: 'I notice the trembling of your hand, would you like to tell me what this means?'

- The non-verbal communication of schizophrenia is as revealing as the verbal content (see Section 8.6).

- Incongruence between verbal content and non-verbal communication: 'I hear you say that you have no worries but I notice your white knuckles.'

- The physical appearance — extreme neatness or dishevelment, or alcohol on the breath.

- The incongruence of symptoms, or the absence of physical signs.

- The presence of depression, poor health, or alcohol abuse in someone else in the family.

As well as discovering the nature of the problem, it is necessary to elicit what the patient feels is the cause of their being unwell, so that appropriate information and reassurance can be given. 'You must have given some thought to the problem. I wonder what your explanation is? Do you have any other?'

Sometimes it helps to elicit the patient's expectations of the doctor and of treatment. If the consultation seems difficult and meandering, the questions 'What did you hope I would do for you today?' or 'What did you expect of today's consultation?' may simplify the situation. 'Oh, I just wanted to tell somebody, I don't want you to *do* anything.' 'I just wanted a certificate.' 'I just wanted you to know, that's all.' Doctors often think they are expected to do something, whereas patients have different expectations. Alternatively, 'I wanted tablets like my sister had' offers a basis for negotiation.

Making an assessment or a diagnosis

The detailed psychiatric history as taught in medical schools was developed for use in hospital practice with patients who have already been assessed by the primary care team. It is very time-consuming and can be intrusive. As a teaching tool it has great value in helping medical students to discover the main factors underlying mental illness but, even in hospital practice, the busy consultant psychiatrist soon learns to drop most of the questions which he asked as a medical student, and the general practitioner who must, of necessity, operate on a different time-scale and with different types of psychological problems, would do well to take a different approach in most instances. With psychological problems, as with physical, assessments are reached by formulating hypotheses about the possible causes, and checking these by further discussion, examination, or investigation. During this process some hypotheses will be discarded and new ones will be created. 'Good' doctors create more, and more accurate, hypotheses, usually because of previous experience, and are prepared to discard invalidated hypotheses and take account of negative information.

What does this mean in practice? Mrs X presents a problem about her son's behaviour and you notice tears in her eyes. Possible hypotheses are depression, sadness, hayfever, or epiphora. 'I notice tears in your eyes, would you like to tell me about them?' Mr Y describes palpitations and anxieties. Hypotheses which need to be tested include thyrotoxicosis, panic attacks, and hyperventilation. If the history and findings do not confirm any of these, further hypotheses may be made about phobias, depression, paroxysmal arrhythmias, and so on.

On occasion all hypotheses seem unrewarding and it them becomes necessary to resort to the standard method of taking a history — family, past, social, geographical, psychiatric, etc. It is often helpful to draw up a genogram (see Section 4.4).

As well as searching for clues about the origin of distress, it is important to enquire about the solutions that have been tried and what other agencies have been involved.

Patients are sometimes embarrassed, ashamed, or perhaps unconscious of the relevance of symptoms. Phobias, compulsions, obsessions and feelings of depersonalization, and some thought disorders may need to be positively, but sensitively, enquired about. Behaviour, such as the excessive use of alcohol, trouble with the law, or sexual deviations may also be hidden.

One will also need to remember that much physical illness is accompanied by depression,[13] and that much of this is not recognized.

Screening questionnaires administered either by the doctor or by a member of the team may be helpful (see p. 37). Some illnesses are presented as purely physical but seem to be a reaction of the whole person to past and present experiences. This is discussed under somatoform disorders (Section 6.3).

A vital part of assessment is ascertaining the severity of the illness, particularly the risk of suicide (see Section 4.6).

Almost by instinct, GPs will take into account the physical health of the patient and assess it's relevance to overall health. Most patients live within families who will have played a part in the aetiology and maintenance of the problem and who will be involved and affected by the management.

Of particular importance is the support available, within and outside the family, which may be crucial to the patient's management.

Agreeing the nature of the problem

In most consultations the process of assessing will have helped to define the problem in terms which are acceptable to both patient and doctor. However, it may be that restatement and clarification of the problem by the doctor is the trigger that enables the patient to consider new choices and the possibility of change. While delivering the summing-up, the doctor will remember the patient's theories and myths about their problem, as elicited earlier in the consultation, and will attempt to take these into account.

On occasions there will be a mismatch between the patient's and the doctor's beliefs, often about the psychological origins of physical symptoms. It may help to remind patients of accepted physical manifestations of emotion: the real tears of sadness, the rapid heart rate on witnessing an accident, or the looseness of the bowels or frequency of micturition before an interview. It may also help to recall such common metaphors as 'a pain in the neck', 'a load on my back', 'I can't swallow that', 'it breaks my heart', 'I feel all churned up'.

A framework for improving the consultation is to view it as a process of negotiation. It is a process which may need to be used in full, particularly with patients who present with somatic symptoms without a recognizable organic basis, or when the consultation is going badly. If doctor and patient have different explanatory models of the illness, the doctor needs to present his or her understanding in layman's terms and invite further questions. If the patient is genuinely able to accept this understanding and suggestion, there is no problem, but more often the patient is only able to take in a little information or accept only a part of the change that may be needed. This may enable the doctor to modify the interpretation and recommendations, so that they are compatible with the patient's view. If important differences remain, the doctor may agree on a compromise treatment, or involve the family and/or other members of the primary care team. If there is still no compromise, the best option may well be to offer another opinion, within or outside the primary care team.

Agreeing the treatment

At this stage the meaning and implication of the diagnosis and its management can also be discussed. The 'success' of the consultation will depend not only upon the accuracy of the diagnosis, the competence of the examination, and the expertise of the 'prescription' but on the hopes and expectations of the patient having been met by the doctor. The resolution of symptoms, in the short term, is highly related to the doctor and patient agreeing about the diagnosis.

If the nature of the problem has been agreed, there will be little difficulty in agreeing treatment. On most occasions the patient will desire the proposed management plan, but it is always important to clear its acceptability.

Ending the consultation

Some patients will wait until they are leaving the room before revealing some important piece of information. This may reflect the patient's realization that this is the last chance to pluck up enough encourage to 'spill the beans'. How we respond to such last minute bids is a matter for fine judgement. If the matter seems important, we should, at the least, indicate that we shall make a note to discuss this matter at the start of our next meeting with the patient. Certainly, patients should not leave any consultation without an agreement as to whether there is to be a follow-up consultation and if so, whether the appointment is to be made now or whether it should be left to the patient to make one. The doctor should not try to impose another appointment, but also should avoid being interpreted as rejecting the patient by not offering one.

References

1. Becker, M. M. and Maiman, L. A. (1975). Sociobehavioural determinants of compliance with health and medical care recommendations. *Medical Care* **13**, 10–24.
2. Hannay, D. R. (1980). Religion and health. *Soc. Sci. Med.* **14**, (A), 683–5.
3. Frank, J. (1974). *Persuasion and healing. A comparative study of psychotherapy.* Schocken Books, New York.
4. Truax, C. B. and Carkuff, R. R. (1967). *Towards effective counselling and psychotherapy.* Aldine, Chicago.
5. Balint, M. (1957). *The doctor, his patient and the illness.* Pitman Medical, London.
6. Freeman, J. and Byrne, P. S. (1976). *The assessment of post graduate training in general practice.* Society for Research into Higher Education Limited, Guildford.
7. Fry, A. (1984). The whole psychiatrist and the whole patient. *Br. J. Holistic Med.* **I**, 52–4.
8. Marinker, M. (1974). Medical education and human values. *J. R. Coll. Gen. Pract.* **24**, (144), 445–62.
9. Grooks, V. (1972). *Mist and moonshine* (ed. Piet Hein). Basil Blackwell, Oxford.
10. Gathorne Hardy, J. (1984). *Doctors.* Weidenfeld and Nicholson, London.
11. Cartwright, A. (1962). *Patients and their doctors—a study of general practice.* Routledge and Kegan Paul, London.

12. Byrne, P. S. and Long, B. E. L. (1984). *Doctors talking to patients*. R. Coll. Gen. Pract., Exeter.
13. Bridges, K. W. and Goldberg, D. P. (1987). *Somatic presentations of depressive illness in primary care*. R. Coll. Gen. Pract., Occasional Paper, No. 36, 9–11.

Further reading

Axline, V. M. (1971). *Dibs; in search of self*. Penguin Books, Harmondsworth.
Berger, M. M. (1977). *Working with people called patients*. Brummer Hazel, New York.
Neighbour, R. H. (1987). *The inner consultation*. MTP Press, Lancaster.
Pendleton, D., Schofield, T., Tate, P., and Havelock, P. (1984). *The consultation: an approach to learning and teaching*. Oxford University Press.
Satir, V. (1976). *Making contact*. Celestial Arts, California.

4.3 COUNSELLING AND INDIVIDUAL PSYCHOTHERAPY

In Section 3.1 counselling is defined as the process of helping patients to express their feelings, clarify their thoughts, to restate or reframe their problems, suggesting alternative understandings or potential solutions. So, armed with a wider range of choices, they are encouraged to make their own decisions. Psychotherapy aims to help people come to terms with past experiences which have damaged them, by intensive exploration which aims to uncover the relationship between current assumptions and past experience.

It is not really possible to make a distinction between counselling and the type of psychotherapy which it is appropriate to use in general practice. Both can be more or less structured, more or less goal-oriented, and more or less directive. They merge into each other.

The personality of the counsellor is a major factor in helping patients, and there is much to be said for allowing patients to have open access to the various members of the team, on the principle that they will then choose the most appropriate person (see Section 4.8). This is, unfortunately, not always possible, and patients may well need referral to someone with particular skills and more time. If the professional feels this is necessary, it is probably a good idea to refer early, before a therapeutic relationship has been built up. This avoids the feeling of rejection which many people suffer when referred elsewhere.

Most occasions necessitating counselling will evolve out of crises (see Section 4.6). 'I feel desperate, I have lost my job.' 'My wife died last week and I don't seem to be coping.' 'My son is glue-sniffing, what can I do?'

There are also situations in which it may be appropriate to offer counselling proactively, i.e. before the crisis occurs. For example, many people have difficulty in helping their children while in the throes of a divorce, or in discussing with their children a death in the family. There is evidence that counselling at such times may prevent future distress[1].

Goals

Counselling aims to help persons to get a new perspective on their current problems and emerge stronger and autonomous, or even enhanced, by the experience of conquering their problems. An important negative goal is the avoidance of dependence.

Having agreed with the patient that the problem is psychological, it is only too easy for the counsellor to become involved without any overall plan. When considering the goals it may be helpful to make a tentative agreement about:

- the extent of the problem to be tackled;

- whether any underlying illness is to be treated;

- the role of the counsellor.

If, for example, the patient says he wants to be less depressed, clarification of this may be made by some such question as 'How will you know that you are less depressed?' 'What is the minimum change that will tell you that you are improving?' 'How will I be able to tell that you are less anxious?' 'What would you like to do that you can't do now?' The answers to these questions form the basis of a target for the therapist and the patient, so that each has a clear idea of the commitment that has been made by the other and a reasonable hope of what the outcome may be.

It may be important to record this target in the notes, and perhaps remind the patient of it, though frequently, as treatment progresses, it has to be rewritten. This clarification of goals is important for both the therapist and the patient, because it can improve rapport between them and may also help patients to plan steps on their own.

Structure

If it is deemed necessary to set aside a session to counsel patients, it may be helpful to structure the session differently, and perhaps use a different room from that used for ordinary surgery sessions. Desks may be deserted and both patient and counsellor sit in similar easy chairs. This shift may make it easier for doctors to discard the prescriptive mantle. A time limit is also helpful not only because it concentrates the work, but because it safeguards other activities and family life.

Often one session will suffice, but if more are thought to be necessary it may be helpful to make a contract — 'Let's see if I can help you to resolve your problem in three sessions, if not, we can review the next move.'

It may also be wise to keep separate notes and to tell the patients that their secrets will not be available to anyone else, if that is their wish.

Principles

People have within them the potential to cope with most problems, but, to do this effectively, they need self-confidence, an ability to see choices, and the courage to make and implement decisions. The therapist's role is to facilitate these processes.

In Section 4.2, the value of rapport, accurate empathy, non-possessive warmth, and genuineness was discussed in relation to the consultation. In counselling, these factors are even more important, but informed self-awareness is needed as well. The counsellor needs to be aware of his or her own biases, prejudices, and ability to identify more with some people than with others. This latter will reflect the counsellor's personal position as wife, sister, father, employer, and so on. This is even more important in relation to those with whom it is difficult to empathize. Lastly, the skill to sort out one's knowledge of human affairs from one's value judgements is needed.

> This above all: to thine own self be true,
> And it must follow, as the night and day,
> Thou canst not then be false to any man[2]

Patients who come to the primary care team, whether with a physical complaint or a psychological problem, often have a low opinion of themselves. Part of therapy is to promote self-esteem. Perhaps the most important way in which we can do this is by an attitude of interest in, and respect for, the people we are treating. They may forestall possible criticism by criticizing themselves — 'I'm sorry to be so stupid', 'I didn't mean to cry', or 'I'm wasting your time.' Positive reassurance is needed. Those who have long-standing low self-esteem may need specific therapy to ameliorate the damages of past experiences, perhaps by uncovering and reframing the past, although most counselling will be focused on the here and now.

Unburdening is itself helpful in a secure setting and in a trusting relationship, and may be even more help if some of the distress can be reframed, or made sense of (see Chapter 3). Sometimes it may be helpful to ask the patient 'What do you *feel* about *feeling* angry, sad, etc.' This changes the patient's perspective and may give some control over emotions. All professionals will have had experience of enabling patients to share their sorrow, their burdens, their secrets, their guilts, and their worries. Sometimes one will not know what to do next. If one can just 'stay with the patient' and accept and affirm them as fellow human beings many will feel better, their self-esteem will be enhanced and they will be able to cope with the external world and their own thoughts and fears more adequately.

Much of what has been described as the attributes of good doctoring will help to raise peoples' self-esteem, but it may help to rephrase those principles. This may sound patronizing and trite, but is important to repeat: people are individuals, and unique, and we need to affirm them as such. They deserve full attention, skilled and practiced listening, affirmation, and acceptance, however sad, mad, or angry they may seem.

Methods

Traditionally, the GP is expected to educate, explain, and instruct patients, and we often possess the knowledge which will enable us to do this. However, there are many situations in which it is better for patients to figure out their own course of action and we do best to adapt the approaches pioneered by Carl Rogers under the title of 'non-directive counselling'. Having mastered these techniques, we soon discover when to use them and when they can safely be put aside in favour of more directive or 'proactive' approaches.

The simplest method of therapy is to listen and reflect patients' thoughts back to them without evaluation, comment, or criticism. Freud, particularly in his early days, encouraged patients to let their minds wander and to create associations freely to words of possible emotional significance. This method facilitates recall of events which are at the back of the mind, the subconscious, and not deeply buried.

Listening and reflecting is perhaps not as easy as it sounds. The general practitioner needs to be selective, so that the conversation is guided away from symptoms and into situations and events. Such guidance needs to be gentle and unobtrusive, using non-verbal cues wherever possible. By eye-contact we show interest, by looking away or frowning slightly we indicate lack of interest. Therapists who become aware of their own non-verbal communications soon learn what powerful effects these can have in blocking the endless repetition of symptoms or complaints about the behaviour of others ('It's all my wife's fault') and channelling the patient's thoughts into more profitable directions. If the patient 'dries up' or looks to the therapist for guidance, the simplest tactic is to repeat a significant word or phrase selected from the patient's last sentence. This sounds contrived, but is, in fact, less artificial than the staccato question-and-answer style of the normal clinical consultation; it is acceptable and unnoticed by most patients. If for some reason this technique seems inappropriate, the therapist can either make an empathic comment 'that sounds worrying' or sad, or whatever, or can remain silent. Silence may feel uncomfortable for both parties, but it is often helpful for patients to have time to make sense of their thoughts and to develop confidence to voice them. If the silence seems unbearable, the best intervention is to ask 'Could you tell me what you were thinking about?' Alternatively, one can try to draw attention to the feelings behind the patient's words by a phrase such as 'It seems that you are feeling angry/bewildered/ lost, etc.' This method of encouraging the patient to talk by using reflective statements, silence, and empathy may sound a little threatening, but it is easy to learn and is a useful approach. It has been well described by Bendix.[3] If we are to follow patients' thoughts and help them to explore their difficulties, asking questions can be distracting, as it is very unlikely that our questions will exactly match their thoughts. All we will get is answers to our questions. If the doctor is asked a question or is asked for advice, it is better not to provide the answer unless it is a matter of fact, but to summarize what has been heard so far as a statement and wait again.

Similarly, reassurance may be an anodyne that blocks thoughts. We are seldom in a position to give advice about people's lives. Towards the end of the consultation it can be helpful to summarize what has been heard or, better, to ask the patient to summarize it so that the pattern of the problem emerges.

With a few exceptions, which will be considered in the final part of this book, it is unhelpful to ponder about the diagnosis. There may be no diagnosis, only a situation. It is also unhelpful for therapists to worry about whether they are clever enough to conduct the interview properly. It is the patient who does the work. Many worry about the wisdom of encouraging patients to disgorge their thoughts and feelings 'Could it be unhelpful and how will I cope with the can of worms when it is opened?' Sharing patients' problems is unlikely to be harmful and almost certainly will be beneficial, not only through allowing the problems to be voiced, but also by changing perspectives. It is not we but the patients who have to decide whether they trust us enough to talk about the stressing 'can of worms'. If, however, they choose to do so we must be aware that it will take time for them to express their feelings and calm down to the point where they can reach some kind of natural end to the communication. If people are aware at the start of a consulting session of the amount of time available they will usually time their disclosures so that we can 'pick up the pieces'. Those who make such disclosures when there is no time left to deal with them may be making a bid for extra attention. Rather than following their lead we may do better to register our awareness of this need for attention, but postpone discussion of the issue raised. 'I can see that you are feeling very unhappy about the situation and I am sorry that we don't have enough time to continue our discussions now, but we can come back to these issues next time we meet.'

It is important that certain things are avoided, otherwise the healing process of change will be interfered with. If the patient's symptoms are physical ut thought to be related to psychological problems, further physical investigations should be avoided unless new evidence emerges to suggest these re necessary. Although it may, at times, seem prudent to offer one more est to reassure a patient that there is no physical cause for a problem, this undermines the agreement that this is a psychological problem (or at least n emotional one). Similarly, if tranquillizers or antidepressants are prescribed, there is the implication that patients can get better by having things done to them, and that there is no need for them to make the effort or go hrough the toils of change. Autonomy is infringed and a pattern of dependence is set for the future. This is in no way to decry the use of antidepressants in severe depressive illness.

In medicine in general, and in psychotherapy in particular, different methods are not necessarily right or wrong but more or less appropriate; the bility to be flexible and imaginative and to have a repertoire of responses s part of our skill.

Helping people to change

Most people know that they would be healthier if they did not smoke, drank ess alcohol, ate less, didn't gamble, and spent less on clothes and more on he family; but for varying reasons, conscious and subconscious, they do not follow their beliefs. People escape from this dilemma in various ways:

- They decide they are worthless and there is no point in attempting to change ('Don't waste your time on me, Doctor.'). They become depressed.

- They can say that it is too difficult to change and that they are helpless ('Nothing makes any difference'.).

- They can deny that there is a problem. Statistics are claimed to be unreliable and to be discounted ('It's all propaganda.').

- They can look for evidence to support the balance for maintaining the behaviour. ('Alcohol protects against cardiovascular illness and not everyone who drinks dies of cirrhosis.')

- They can blame other people ('She's the one who drives me to it.').

- They can change their behaviour.

The tasks of the doctor are to:

- bolster self-esteem;

- bolster feelings of self-efficacy;

- avoid confrontation and allow patients to verbalize their own decisions, and give a sense of internal attribution;

- increase dissonance by helping patients weight their own balances;
- give ideas and tactics for change;
- involve the family, if this is appropriate.

Self-esteem

This was mentioned in the previous section. It is helpful if the counsello reflects back the good aspects the patient has presented and emphasize strengths. 'I notice you were able to stop smoking last year.' 'You got ove losing your job.' Reflection can be used to change perspectives. 'I can't b an alcoholic because' may be reflected back as 'I imagine that that must b confusing for you. On the one hand you can see that there are seriou problems about your use of alcohol, but on the other hand the label alcoholi doesn't fit because things don't look that bad!' This task is the most importar and perhaps the most difficult for the doctor. It may entail uncovering reason for low self-esteem and giving people permission to change.

Individual responsibility and self-efficacy

Doctors do not need to take responsibility for the decisions individuals mak about their lives. The doctor's role is to elucidate, clarify, produce evidence and provide knowledge. It is for patients to decide if they have a problem and if they want to tackle that problem. The doctor then needs to provid a framework and support in which that decision can be implemented.

Internal attribution

Not only is it important that people make their own decisions, but it i important that they own their decisions. If for some reason a drinker decide to drink less, it improves their chances of keeping to it if they attribute th change to themselves. If they believe that the change is due to the increase tax, the doctors, the weather, or God, they are less likely to stick to it. Som people tend to see themselves as helpless because they attribute change t external agencies. One of the tasks of the doctor is to help the patient accep that they alone make the decision to accept that there is a problem with, fo example, drink or smoking, however helpful or unhelpful, forceful, or kin the external world is. The belief that an alcohol abuser or obese person i helpless is not founded upon evidence and is counterproductive to maintain

Labelling

Using these methods to help people change, it is not necessary and, in fac undesirable to apply labels. Many patients who would not accept the labe of obesity respond positively to treatment. Most people almost anywhere on the upper part of the continuum of alcohol consumption would agree that they have had a problem with alcohol at some time in their lives.

Avoiding confrontation

Confrontation tends to elicit denial. Thus, if in ordinary conversation, A tells B he is a coward (a pejorative statement), B's first reaction is to deny it. If the doctor tells Mrs J she is an alcoholic (interpreted as a pejorative statement), her first reaction will be to deny it. This is unfortunate, not only because it tends to drive people into a situation of conflict, but also because one tends to believe what one hears oneself say. The more one says one is not an alcoholic the more one will attempt to defend that position.

Eliciting self-motivating statements

The doctor's task is to change behaviour without challenging the patient, by helping the patient recognize that there is a problem, and to recognize the need for change. If patients can express the ideas themselves, they are more likely to believe in them and keep to them. Examples of questions are— 'What have you become aware of about your drinking that worries you?' or 'What else have you noticed?' 'What other things concern you about your obesity?' It will be noticed that not only do these questions create an opportunity for the patient to make a statement, but they also make the supposition that there is a problem. The answer to these questions can be acknowledged, but not used as a weapon by the doctor. Moving on to help the patient decide on action, a suitable question might be 'What makes you think you should do something about your eating?' This, again, contains an assumption about the patient's desire for change (and also gives internal attribution). If confronting the patient provokes denial, it may be helpful to side with the patient to invoke change. 'These ideas for change that we have discussed look difficult for you and, frankly, I am not sure if you really do want to change, and have enough motivation to do so.' This is a delicate strategy and some doctors will not feel comfortable with it.

Increasing dissonance

It is important that patients weight their own balances. What information we offer is best given objectively. This will vary according to the problem, but may come from research evidence about possible harms, from the results of examination or investigation, from filling-in of questionnaires or keeping of diaries. The more contrast there is between the evidence the patient believes, regarding, say, smoking, and their own behaviour, the likelier they are to change.

Tactics for change

Certain tactics aimed specifically to help people with alcohol and tobacco addiction will be considered in Chapter 8, although the tactics described there have wider application.

Family involvement

The above framework, while helpful, may still leave people with difficulties which necessitate looking at these in both a historical and current context. The pressures of family systems may be such as to necessitate their involvement (see Section 4.4).

References

1. Caplan, G. (1961). *An approach to community mental health.* Tavistock, London.
2. Shakespeare, *Hamlet*, I. iii. lines 78–80.
3. Bendix, T. (1982). *The anxious patient* (ed. H. J. Wright). Churchill Livingstone, London.

Further reading

Miller, W. R. (1983). Motivational interviewing with problem drinkers. *Behav. Psychoth.* **11**, 147–72.
Rogers, C. (1965). *Client centred therapy.* Houghton Mifflin, New York.

4.4 FAMILY AND COUPLE THERAPY

Family and couple therapy is based on the premise that couples and families are systems within which problems may persist or improve because of the behaviour of the members of the systems towards each other. Consequently solutions to the problems can be found by promoting change in the problem maintaining behaviour.[1] Instead of looking at the individuals in isolation as being sick, neurotic, or having a disordered personality, family and conjoint therapies look for the causes and cure of problems in the relationships between people.

In such a system, no one person is blamed or labelled as 'the problem'. A change in one part of the system (e.g. an illness, a behaviour or social dysfunction) creates change throughout the system. An example of this would be the death of a parent and its effect on the family system resulting in various physical, emotional, and social symptoms in other family members. In other words, when one family member is in trouble and experiencing pain, all are in trouble and experiencing pain. If the family is not functioning well as a support to its members, symptoms may develop in one or more of them.

Individuals may change because they have an enhanced understanding of their own interactional pattern or because they see available a more positive choice of behaviours, and the possibility of control over these behaviours. Alternatively, they may change because of the behavioural changes initiated by the therapist with little 'insight' by the family or couple. The limitations to the power of therapy should be recognized; even if complete solutions are found, the process of change can only be *initiated* in the consultation room—the bulk of the work is done outside, mainly in the home.

The same principles apply to helping a large system, such as the family, as to a small system, such as the parents, who may be called the 'parental subsystem'. Parents also have a task of cherishing each other, and may then be regarded as a 'marital subsystem'. In this chapter we hope to provide ideas which may be found useful for helping both families and couples, and also to look at ways in which the individual can be helped by using a family perspective.

Occasionally there may be a conflict between the interests of the family as a unit and the interests of an individual member. The question then arises 'Who is the patient?' Most of the time the interests of the individual will be seen as more important and ethically more acceptable in the context of Western society.

When dealing with couples, it must be made clear from the beginning that the therapist's job is to provide a framework in which the couple can come to the best possible solution for themselves and their family. This may entail splitting or staying together. We are not in the business of advocating either outcome, whatever our own private beliefs may be.

Family factors

The family affects the health of the individual in many ways.[2] The following examples begin to explore the interactional patterns that are of chief concern in this chapter. They also indicate the need for an awareness of family history in understanding individual patients.

The genetic predisposition

This contributes to the shaping of personality as well as predisposing to many psychiatric and physical disorders. The influence may be high in certain forms of mental handicap, moderate in schizophrenia, and low in most other psychiatric conditions.

Shared environment

People who live in small, overcrowded tenements have different expectations, and indeed different behaviours, from people who live in large manor houses.

Shared experiences

These can be important to health. A family which has been evicted will tend to have a common feeling towards landlords, while unemployment in the breadwinner may affect the health of the whole family.

Shared attitude

Children tend to accept or reject totally the views of parents on such things as drinking, smoking, race, class, and food preference. They also learn from parents what to fear: if parents see the world as dangerous, the children often do too. Families may bring different attitudes to discipline. A boy's encopresis can be a source of worry not only to him and his family, but its occcurrence may exacerbate the difference of opinion about child management that each parent brings from their family of origin. 'Should he be treated by reward or punishment?'

Problems also arise from the family's handling of everyday events by differences of approach.

Sixteen-year-old James stayed out until 2 a.m. one night, partly because he was embarrassed to disrupt the party and ask for a lift home, and partly because he wanted to be seen to be as free as his peers. His father's response was to demand that in future he returned at 9 p.m. instead of 11 p.m. His mother's response of crying and refusing to discuss the issue escalated the problem into repeated early morning returns and the use of alcohol to face his father's wrath.

Attitudes to illness often determine the nature of the problem the family develops.

Mrs X was feeling relatively helpless and hopeless by contrast with the competence of her kind husband. 'Depression is an illness. We should continue to shelter Mum (devalue her) and take her to the doctor for antidepressants (confirming a disease). We should also continue to cheer her up and deny her sadness.' The kinder, the more efficient, and the more solicitous they were, the more she felt devalued, condescended to, depressed, and ill. Treating Mrs X without helping the family to change might be almost impossible.

Shared responsibilities

It may be important to know who in a family bears the burden of responsibility and who wields power. First-born children often have a strong sense of responsibility, while younger children may be more dependent. Some families take all their problems to the doctor while others only do so *in extremis*.

Shared communication

The way in which a family behaves and communicates can have a profound effect on the health of the family. A family where people tend to speak for each other and share not only the same ideas but also emotions and bath towels, the 'enmeshed family', may find it harder to quarrel and express themselves as individuals; they have to repress a lot of thoughts and feelings and this leads subsequently to psychological problems, particularly psychosomatic disorders.

A family where people do not communicate or consider each other much of the time, but tend to act on their own, is prone to behavioural problems such as truanting, getting involved with the law, and perhaps alcohol abuse, as a consequence of the acting out of unrestrained impulses.

Taboos, secrets, denials

In some families taboos are in operation.

Mrs Q became depressed when her little boy was drowned in an accident. Straight after the accident her husband's solution was to distract his wife and not allow her to dwell on the tragedy. She never discussed with him her own feelings of guilt and her anger with him for being away on that particular day, but these feelings continued to emerge indirectly and to delay her recovery.

Secrets may be deliberate or inadvertent. The inadvertent will often unravel themselves in the course of discussion. The deliberate sometimes announce their existence to outsiders through the irregular behaviour that surrounds them. If the son's paternity is other than what is commonly believed, it may or may not be helpful to the son to know. Mishandling of this knowledge might be destructive of the spouses' relationship.

Unspoken family rules often contribute to health problems. Families have rules about what it is permissible to do or to talk about, but they are seldom discussed.

A girl aged 14, was dressing provocatively, to the annoyance of her parents, who banned the use of make-up. It was an unspoken rule that sex was not discussed. Before it could be, it was found helpful to ask where this rule came from and how such rules were made.

Family myths

Similarly, there are the basic assumptions and family myths that govern a family. The assumption that 'father is strong but unreliable' and that 'mother is weak but loving' may reflect wider assumptions that 'all men are dangerous' and 'women must stick together'. Children may be seen as sweet but fragile, or as monstrous tyrants who are set on destroying their parents. The outside world may be seen as a jungle or as a bag of goodies ready for picking. Because the list is endless, we may be tempted to disregard it. But there are major unifying principles in every family which are not difficult to recognize if we keep our eyes and ears open, and which reappear in succeeding generations. They may be difficult or impossible to change, but they always have to be taken into account if we are not to be faced by unexpected failures.

It will often be helpful to comment on these rules and myths so that the family gains a perspective of their effects.

Presentation

Families may present openly with relationship difficulties which may be marital, sexual, or between generations. Alternatively, an individual may come to the primary care team with a problem which later turns out to involve other members of the family. Often it is not a psychological but a somatic symptom which is presented—backache, a flare-up of colitis, or an exacerbation of headaches.

A child who is sick may often be an indicator of parental discord, and if a child is presented as 'the problem', it will be helpful at some stage to see anyone else who seems to play an important role in the family.

After seeing the family together, the parents can be seen alone—to discuss the marital situation or to strengthen the parental subsystem and to clarify the differences between the generations, perhaps by encouraging them to act cohesively with a definite framework of discipline.

Even when the couple present as the problem, it is occasionally helpful to include the children for one or two sessions. This may reveal unexpected alliances or antipathies across the generations, as well as helping us to understand the general dynamics of the situation.

Often it is difficult to recruit all the family, but it may help to see as many as will come. If only one person presents, and he or she does not wish anyone else to be involved, we need to continue to 'include' the absent family members. Occasionally, however, it may be necessary to insist on the presence of a key family member as a condition of therapy.

Therapy

A family may have asked for help, but this does not mean that they know that we can be trusted. In fact, they are likely to be extremely apprehensive at the very idea of being 'put on the spot' by a powerful person who can easily destroy their self-respect and make a bad situation worse. It follows that we are unlikely to get very far until we have shown ourselves to be friendly and genuinely interested in every person in the room. A good way to start is to shake hands all round, to explain how we came to be invited and what we already know about the situation. Of course, we may already have confidential information about a family and it may be advisable to seek permission to reveal this in advance of the meeting. This leaves us free to clear the way to open communication within the meeting. Thus, 'Mollie has told me that there have been arguments between her and George (her husband) recently and that on one occasion a blow was struck. I'm not concerned with judging the rights and wrongs of the situation, this isn't a court of law, but I imagine you are probably all worried about the situation, and it seemed to me that it would be a good idea if we all got together to try to understand everyone's point of view, in the hope that we may have some ideas about how things could be improved. Does that seem reasonable?'

By this time the family members will have an idea of what is going on, but they will be very uncertain of our ability to cope with the situation. Are we trying to put the blame on George? Do we really care what they think? Are we going to undermine the comforting myth that Mum and Dad love each other and that their tiffs should be disregarded? Who will keep the family safe if George's authority is undermined?

Defining the problem

At this point each member in turn may be invited to say what they see as the problem, or what they would like to see happen differently in the family. What difficulties do they have in living together? What would they like to do that they can't do now? This latter is a useful question as it also introduces the idea of treatment goals. If there are several problems, it is helpful to ask which is the most important.

In all probability their responses will include one or more of the following strategies:

Denial of facts and/or feelings, e.g. father's drinking is not a serious problem, mother could not care less if he goes out with other women, all children steal from their parents, the baby's bruises must be self-inflicted, etc.

Avoidance of important issues, e.g. by key members of the family failing to come to meetings, or by collusive keeping of secrets from the therapist and/or from each other.

Tunnel vision e.g. by ignoring or misinterpreting any statement or evidence that conflicts with their own comfortable view of the world ('What does it matter what he does as long as he loves his mother?'), evasion, talking past the point, and repetition of stereotyped viewpoints.

Projection of blame onto others, inside or outside the family. This may include the doctor ('If only you would give me something for my stomach, everything would be all right.').

   Scapegoats may be overt, as when parents blame all the problems in the family onto the bad behaviour of a particular child, or covert, as in the subtle labelling of a family member as 'sick', with consequent loss of status, power, and roles within the family.

Controlling of others by persuasion, alliance, or *force majeure*. This again may be overt ('You'll do what I say or it's out with you, young lady'), or covert ('Now I think we should all agree to do whatever the doctor says. You're so wise doctor. I'm sure that the doctor agrees with me that . . .').

Giving up on a problem may be easier than tackling it. One way of doing this is to set impossible goals ('We must just stop feeling angry with each other'), or blocking all suggestions for improvement with a 'Yes, but . . .' ('Yes, doctor, you're quite right, but it would never work because he's too stubborn').

   If marriage or relationships are in trouble there is a probability that at one level of consciousness, thoughts, feelings, and memories of parents are being projected by each partner onto the other, and it is also likely that similar thoughts will be projected onto the therapist. In these circumstances the therapist needs, at least, to avoid playing the role assigned to him or her as somebody's mother, father, of sibling and to help the couple understand the origin of these misplaced feelings and assumptions.

   The therapist may now need to summarize and clarify the findings by a review of the problems and perhaps by recalling the strengths of the family and the difficulties they have previously overcome. The assumption that they are all working in their own way for the common good will need to be encouraged.

Setting goals of treatment

It is helpful to agree goals which would indicate improvement in concrete behavioural terms, so that goals achieved may be compared with goal set. The goal can be a relatively small change, but one which is feasible. A suitable question could be: 'What small change would indicate to you that an improvement has been made?' For example, 'Mrs Jones will be able to shop in the corner shop'; 'Mr Green will take his tablets so that his blood pressure is acceptably lower'; 'James, aged 4, will only wake his parents once a night'.

Couples and families should be helped to define in positive terms how they would like themselves and things to be different. It is important not to accept negative goals. I want him to be less cold' could be rephrased into 'I would like him to express more affection', which is not only positive but is worded so that she can see whether there is any change. Goals may need changing and expanding as one gets to know the family better.

Changing perspective

The simplest form of intervention may be the redefining of statements, attitudes, or goals. The nagging wife may be described as expressing anxious interest. The husband who stays out late at work is avoiding the conflict of return. The kind, solicitous husband of the depressed patient is gently alluded to as being over-protective.

As in individual therapy, most change happens outside the consulting room. Whatever the theoretical models, the hope is to effect change by changing the participants' perspective of themselves and their relationships, to increase their choices of verbal and non-verbal behaviours, and to give them increased control over these behaviours.

The perspective may be changed in many ways—by keeping a diary, by noting the rules that govern behaviour, or by having a historical or analytical understanding of the current situation.

Communication

Relationship problems are often manifested by faulty communication. Teaching the couple or family to use direct and clear language may enable them to begin to change the relationship problems. 'Why is the toast always burnt?' needs clarifying into a direct and clear statement which might be something like 'I feel that you, Ann, let the toast burn because you don't care about me.' People should be encouraged to speak in the first person and not to use the impersonal, i.e. 'I am angered by you ignoring me' rather than 'People get upset if they are ignored.' Nor should they be allowed to speak for other people, 'We are all happy in this family.' Generalizations may need to be challenged, e.g. 'You never listen to me.'

A person's sense of helplessness might be seen in a phrase such as 'You make me angry' because the speaker acknowledges the other person's power over them. However provocative other people are, individuals can choose at some level how they will respond, and this possibility of choice can be pointed out to them.

The perspective may be broadened and choices increased by encouraging the participants to use their imagination, perhaps by a brain-storming session New ideas may be introduced by the therapist and the ability to use them may be enhanced by challenging assumptions. 'I'm damned if I'll say I am sorry', 'What would actually happen if you did say you were sorry?', or 'Can you imagine yourself saying you were sorry?'

In helping patients to establish greater control over their behaviour, the therapist may choose to insist on some simple rules of communication. If the conversation between a couple sounds as if it will escalate into a non-productive, repetitive argument, rules can be suggested which the couple can adopt when things get hot at home. Perhaps the simplest manoeuvre is to restrict each response to one sentence. This slows the pace and prevents it degenerating into a diatribe. Another way is to ask A to rephrase what he heard B say, before he makes his own statement. These tactics have the advantage of allowing therapists to limit themselves to commenting and reflecting on the process of communication between the couple, and to avoid getting bogged down in the content. This prevents being sucked into the conflict and being made to take sides.

Feelings

Confusion of thinking and feeling needs to be distinguished. 'How do you feel about our daughter's boyfriend?', 'I think he is in a poor job.' This response sidesteps any disclosure of emotion and personal involvement and the feeling aspect needs to be pursued. It may also be beneficial to understand and acknowledge each other's feelings. Encouraging the expression of loss and grief may be particularly important. 'If only I had known how much you missed your mother, I could have understood and helped you.'

Many couples seem locked into their own thoughts and have never learnt, or have forgotten, the act of empathy. Empathy may be enhanced by asking questions such as 'When, Ann, you say you feel fed up, what do you think John understands you to mean, and what thoughts do you think occur to him?'

An alternative to asking more questions is to ask the couple to reverse their roles. 'John, could you pretend you are Ann and, using the words she would use, answer your question?' It may be possible to encourage them to continue the discussion in reversed roles. This technique may sound difficult, but many couples rapidly understand the value of trying to understand their partner's thoughts and feelings. Brave therapists may risk appearing gimmicky by asking couples to change places, as this highlights the experience of trying to understand someone else's thoughts and feelings. A similar technique is to invoke the presence of an absent person. The family can often be 'brought into the room' by asking such questions as 'If your husband was here now, what would he say was causing you to be depressed?' or 'What would he say in response to that?'

A tactic for encouraging people to express their feelings is to ask them to talk to each other rather than through the therapist — but the latter must be prepared to comment on their communication. This technique has the advantage that it resembles the exchanges of everyday life, with the therapist as observer. 'I hear you saying that you find it difficult to listen to your mother-in-law criticizing your children, and I hear you, Peter, say that you do not realize that your mother did criticize the children. Could you two talk together and see if you could find a mutual understanding?'

Observing

Whenever the therapist sees two or more people together, observation of the patterns of communication will reveal facets of their relationship. Interactions between family members need to be watched closely. Who leads, who follows, who is nervous, who assured? What basic assumptions do they make about each other? What alliances exist and how are these viewed by others?

Communication embraces not merely the content of the sentence but the way it is expressed; the tone, the speed, and the hesitations. It also includes all the non-verbal communications of clothes, posture, gestures, and expressions. For instance, the doctor might detect a mismatch between what is said and what is expressed non-verbally. Much poor communication is based on misunderstanding of non-verbal communication. What A hopes will be interpreted as a conciliatory smile may be interpreted by B as a deceiving grimace. Clarification from both partners may be helpful: 'What did you think that smile meant?', 'Is that what you meant it to mean?'

Methods of therapy

Contract therapy

Contract therapy is a technique which helps people to understand each other. Once the therapist has established trust, and elicited the problem and the solutions to be aimed for by the patients, homework is suggested, acknowledging that it may be surprisingly difficult.

Week 1: Behaviours that the participants would like to change in each other are looked at, remembering to be firm about positive behaviours that can be observed, and not, at this stage, attempting to change thoughts or feelings.

Homework: Each partner to separately write

(1) three examples of their behaviour which they think the partner seeks to increase;

(2) three examples of their partner's behaviour which they seek to increase.

Week 2: The participants are asked to compare the examples and identify the items that they agree on. After discussion they are asked to agree to work on changing one item each in a contract: 'The reward for your effort is that your partner changes in this way.'

Homework: Each partner fulfils the contract.

Subsequent weeks: The contract is reviewed, revised, or added to.

Behavioural interventions

Sometimes apparently small, almost irrelevant changes can help behaviour, perhaps by showing that change is possible or by subtly changing dynamics. Many quarrels in marriage happen when a husband, exhausted by a day's work and the rush-hour traffic, arrives home. His wife, who has had a trying day with the children and with the broken vacuum cleaner, pounces on him and unloads her troubles. If she can give him ten minutes to unwind after he arrives home, the dynamics of the evening can change. Other suggestions such as swapping sides of the bed, or even accustomed places at the dinner table, can be dramatically helpful because it may give patients some control over their lives.

Mr and Mrs A were quarrelling regularly, and occasionally violently, but still wanted to stay together. The doctor acknowledged how difficult it would be for them to stop quarrelling, but suggested two changes of their normal routines. They should continue to quarrel verbally, but violence was forbidden, and they should anticipate their arguments by deliberately quarrelling at eight o'clock in the morning. The result was that they failed to get any steam up in the morning, and somehow did not quarrel during the rest of the day.

An easier suggestion for the therapist to give might be that whenever they felt like quarrelling they made sure they moved out into the hall to do it. These suggestions make people look at their behaviour from a different angle as well as offering some small chance of change.

Patients from families who seem resistant, and in a covert way to oppose all suggestions for change, may have their opposition articulated and utilized. The therapist may suggest that the patient is unlikely to resolve the problem and treatment can only attempt to help him to endure it, to which the 'Yes, but' answer is to challenge the therapist by getting better!

Two other methods are useful in eliciting patients' thoughts and feelings. Both of them, at first sight, appear to have more to do with events and situations than with thoughts and feelings, but the latter will emerge, often very profitably. While both of them may be thought of as ways of eliciting information from patients, they blend imperceptibly with therapy. They may be particularly useful when the family are using the defences of tunnel vision and projection. Both methods are based on the idea of the family as a sytem: all members of the family (or both members of a couple) are interdependent, so no one member can change without a corresponding change occurring in the rest of the family or other member of the couple.

Genograms

Genograms are a simple way of eliciting and recording information about a family. There are various ways in which information can be recorded on them. A standard format is shown in Fig. 4.1.

Genograms can be constructed with individuals, couples, or whole families but are particularly useful when only one family member is able to be present. The manner in which a genogram is taken is often as important as what is elicited or the technique of recording. Therapists need to be sincere, open-minded, interested, and non-judgmental, and even occasionally prepared to share vignettes of their own family. A favourite method is to use a flipchart

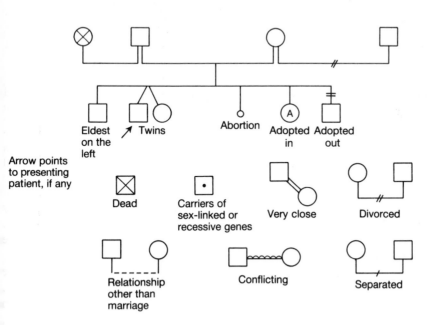

Fig. 4.1. Symbols used in genograms.

(32 × 24″) placed conveniently for the therapist and each member of the family. Thus the chart itself becomes a centre of interest and a focus for everyone's enthusiasm about its completeness, accuracy, and relevance. Surprising secrets are often revealed, such as abortions, stillbirths, liaisons, problems with alcohol, and even incest.

The first step is to create a family tree including the years of births, miscarriages, abortions, stillbirths, adoptions, marriages, separations, divorces, remarriages, and deaths. Careful recording of all years will enable everyone to see connections between events. Causes of deaths should also be recorded. When a three- or four-generational tree has thus been constructed, there may already be a clear, repetitive pattern which can be shared and explored with the family. The areas of discussion after the creation of the basic tree will depend upon the family and its problems.

Examples of useful questions are: 'Would it help us to know about any births, stillbirths, or miscarriages that we have forgotten?'; 'Have any important relationships been omitted?' (this can provide an opportunity for homosexuality to be discussed); 'Was there anyone to whom you were unusually close?', 'If so, why was that?'; 'Would you like to talk about the quality of your parents' marriage?'; 'To which brother or sister were you closest?'; 'Do you think your mother was as close to your grandmother as you are to your mother?'; 'Who else in the family has had pains like John?' Discussion of these areas can be helpful as patients begin to make sense of their own identity and the reasons why they have become as they are. Certain phraseology during questioning — 'Perhaps one of your parents taught you to worry?' — may trigger off constructive trains of thought in that patient, implying, for example, that learned behaviours can also be unlearned.

The completed genogram can be given to the individual or family at the end of the session so that it can be shared with the rest of the family and the therapeutic process can continue. A small-sized copy should also be made for the therapist to keep in the case notes. This will become an invaluable *aide-mémoire*.

Understanding and interpreting the genogram

Discussion of the complete genogram can offer alternatives to the family for their current behaviours, and a chance to escape from repetitive patterns. Furthermore, a genogram can make sense of hitherto unexplained fears and anxieties. In a family where emotions can be neither recognized nor displayed, distress may present as somatic symptoms. If, for example, strokes have been common in such a family, then headaches may be much more worrying.

The revelation of secrets, if handled with skill, is often therapeutic because of the anxiety, obtuseness, and deviousness which usually surround them. The sharing of previously denied emotion about death, miscarriages, or stillbirth is usually dramatically helpful. It is easy to elicit and display the event hemselves using a genogram, and not too difficult to assist people to come o terms with suppressed sorrow, guilt, and anger.

When relationships within the family are explored, alliances and behaviour :an be discussed and time can be spent on coaching individuals to strengthen more appropriate links (this is most usually within the marital subsystem). inappropriate alliances usually arise across generations, for example between mother and daughter, or between daughter and grandparent.

Where children are being used as a mechanism to defuse parental and marital quarrelling, the therapist can encourage parents to discuss problems directly, without allowing the children to interfere and without involving them as scapegoats.

'After-thoughts', children born after a stillbirth, a miscarriage, or a sibling who has died, are children at special risk, as are children born at the time of a grandparent's death, or those who have a handicap. Such children may be unduly susceptible to physical disease, mental distress, and behavioural problems.[3]

It is more important for the family itself to have an understanding of their own interactions than it is for the doctor to know this 'from the outside', so the family should be fully involved in all discussion and interpretation. Questions are more valuable in leading patients to increase their understanding of their predicament than in increasing the therapist's knowledge:

'Can you see recurring patterns in your family?'

'Can you see similarities between the generations?'

'What effect has keeping this secret had on your family?'

'We can see that second children in each generation on both sides of your family have been divorced. Does this seem to have any influence on any of you?' 'Is there some fear that it will happen again in the next generation?'

These are some of the ways that the doctor can introduce the theme that, though observable patterns may occur, they may also be preventable.

In the family presented in Fig. 4.2, when the parents start quarrelling, Ian becomes sick — he develops asthma and thus diverts his parents from arguing. In addition, the picture shows a circular reaction within the family. From this perspective it may be possible for everyone to understand the rows between Ian and Jane as well.

Figure 4.3 gives another example, showing how the genogram can help to clarify family relationships and suggest therapy. Instead of treating the son, efforts might be made to work through problems in the marriage which may enable the parents to be more consistent and free Jill from an insecure 'clinging' relationship with her mother.

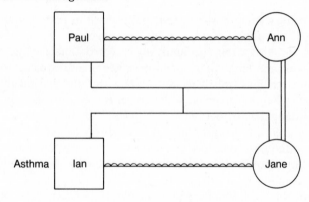

Fig. 4.2.

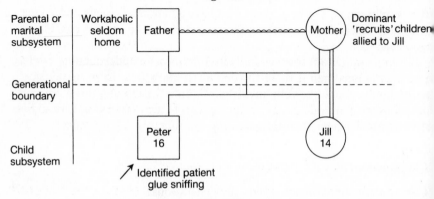

Fig. 4.3.

All the information gleaned in these ways can be reframed so as to make 'sense of the problem'. 'I see that your mother lost her first child and you have lost your first one too. How has that affected the way childbirth is seen in your family?' Or again, 'You see your family as a disaster because your father and brother are alcoholics. But in fact you come from a remarkable family—no divorces, no black sheep, no one unemployed!'

People do not change in the consulting room; seeds of ideas, problems, and situations, reframed in positive terms can help to make sense of current behaviour, and by pointing out patterns and actions that have been learned, and which can thus be unlearned, introduce the possibility of change. Thought can be stimulated about relationship, and permission given for changes to happen. These changes begin at home and continue in the days and weeks following a session.

A brief genogram can be constructed when a patient first registers with a practice, instead of a standard family history, or it can be used in the course of a routine consultation. The problems for which it has been most productive are listed in Table 4.1.

Table 4.1. *Problems for which genograms have been found particularly useful*

Depression and/or anxiety
Somatized problems (headaches, abdominal pain, and chest pains)
High attendance rates
Psychosomatic problems
Behavioural problems
Problems between family members
Step-families with problems
Obesity, alcohol, and drug abuse
Poor compliance

Evaluation

Genograms are used in many family practice centres both in Canada and the USA[4,5] and Rogers and Durkin[6] have described their evaluation of this process. Huygen[7] in The Netherlands has kept detailed records for over 30 years, and emphasizes the repetitive patterns of illness in the families which he has observed. Leiberman[8] has reported his experience using genograms in psychiatric practice, and has encouraged general practitioners to use similar techniques.

Family circles[9]

The family circle is another method of helping individuals understand their present predicament and of finding ways to change. By allowing individuals to draw a diagram of their family system, it rapidly explores their current life events and emotional status, and makes clearer the connection between emotions, life, and symptoms. The drawing can be completed in as little as two or three minutes. Once instructions are given, the presence of the therapist is not required during the drawing. The family circle drawings will often illustrate, in graphic form, patterns of closeness, distance, and power in a family, and the alliances and boundaries. They provide, at a glance, an overview of the family system as seen by the person who does the drawing. The drawings are a rich source of information concerning family dynamics and are useful for setting goals for changes in the family system.

Family circles may be collected from an individual, a family group (marital, sibling, parent, and child), or individually from all members of a family group in the presence of one another. The clinician draws a large circle on a piece of paper, blackboard, or flipchart (see Figs 4.4, 4.5, 4.6). The person(s) interviewed are instructed as follows:

'I am interested in you, your family and what is important to you. Let this circle stand for your family as it is now. Draw in some smaller circles to represent yourself and all people important to you and your family. Remember, people can be inside or outside the circle, touching or far apart. They can be large or small depending on their importance, and dead people can be included if they are still important to you. Initial each circle for identification. There are no right or wrong circles.'

Participants can also be invited to represent the important areas of their lives such as significant losses, work, vacations, and hobbies. Given this extra latitude, some participants will draw a picture of their entire life spaces including recreational activities, religion, and past events which are of current significance. Emphasis is always given to an appreciation of the individuality of these circles with a reminder that this is not a test.

Interpreting and understanding the family circle

The first step in the discussion of a family circle is for the person to describe and explain what has been produced. Inherent in this method is respect for the patient's interpretation of the circle, and thus the patient's control of the amount of self-disclosure and risk. Subsequent questioning may relate to intimacy and distance, power and decision making, closeness and communication patterns, and personal boundaries and space. The discussion may be directed towards any of these aspects of interpersonal relationship and the inquiry may be as brief or as long as is required. Completing the circle usually takes five minutes. The discussion may vary from three to 30 minutes.

Examples of questions which go into more depth are:

'How would you compare the circle you drew with the way you would like it to be?'

'How would you rearrange the circles or make these changes?'

'How would you accomplish this?'

'If one person in the circle (system) changes, what ripple effects will this have on others in the circle?'

'Who can you count on to help you in a crisis?'

This initial information provides a useful map for future discussions and continued relationship building.

In this way, the family circle method can be used for identifying and setting specific goals and increasing awareness of the dynamics of change in a system. It also aids in the development of a 'family' profile or database allowing the members to define their own concepts of family. The therapist does not interpret the drawing to the person or family. It is important to remember that the circles and their meanings belong to their originators and represent their subjective view of their own family system. The clinician's role is to ask questions in order to elicit the patient's viewpoint and also to help define areas of strength as well as of desired change. The dialogue can readily shift from assessment to goal setting.

In conjoint therapy, the family circle method is an ideal way to help patients understand each other's perspective. If each partner creates their circle separately and then the circles are discussed together, they will learn each other's view of many aspects of their relationship to each other.

This method is one of the least judgemental ways of approaching emotional and relationship problems, without focusing on individual pathology.

Certain typical family systems have special interest for health professionals, and are described below and represented in family circle form (Figs 4.4, 4.5, and 4.6).

The fused, enmeshed family   Fig. 4.4 is a family system in which members do not clearly separate their own feelings, anxieties, concerns, and identities. The members engage in a reverberating, soup-like emotional atmosphere which is shared by all. Boundaries between persons are very unclear. Sometimes, the therapist may unwittingly be caught up in the confusion.

These families often have members with psychosomatic disorders. On occasion a patient may draw another person's circle mostly overlapping or even precisely on top of his or her own.

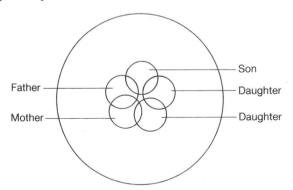

Fig. 4.4.   The enmeshed family.

The emotionally divorced family   (Fig. 4.5) In this family system the married couple has emotionally separated or 'divorced' while maintaining a common household. The husband and wife are distant and share few of their emotions. Living together may continue as a matter of convenience. Members of this system, including the children, are at risk of affective symptoms such as anxiety and depression.

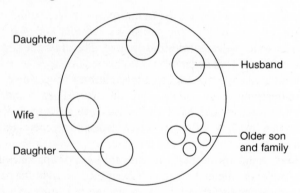

Fig. 4.5. The emotionally divorced family.

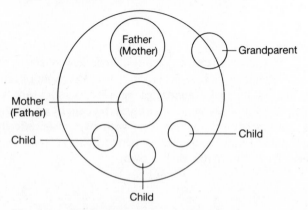

Fig. 4.6. The patriarchal or matriarchal family.

The patriarchal (or matriarchal) family (Fig. 4.6) Issues of power and hierarchy have great importance in this type of family. Sometimes there is one leader who wields power. However, real power may also reside with an apparently passive or compliant spouse. The assessment of the distribution of power in a family is not a simple matter. Sometimes a grandparent, or even a child, has great influence. The misuse of this concentrated power will sometimes play a role in symptom production. Physicians, as figures of high status and power to their patients, may unwittingly engage in a power struggle with the family leader, or may pre-empt the leader's role in case of sickness. At times the physician deliberately challenges the power system for therapeutic purposes.

As can be seen, the family circle illustrates certain family dynamics and systems at a glance. Other fundamental principles are not as easily represented in a static picture. Since families are changing, the individual has to be viewed as part of an interactional network system which is constantly evolving.

Conclusion

Very brief outlines of approaches to the family have been suggested. For those who want to try more formal therapy, an experienced co-therapist recruited from the primary care team, the local social work unit, or child guidance clinic will be both reassuring and helpful.

Occasionally couples can be helped in one or two short sessions, but often a longer time is necessary. An increasing number of practices have easy access to marriage guidance counsellors, clinical psychologists, community psychiatric nurses, and other counsellors who will help with particular problems, including family ones, or take patients over if requested.

Much work with families can be done without formal training, but it would be wise to try drawing up one's own genogram and circles with a colleague before using this method with patients.

References

1. Weakland, J. H., Fisch, R., Watzcawick, P., and Bodin, A. M. (1974). Brief therapy. Focused problem resolution. *Family Process* **13**, (2), 141–68.
2. Wallerstein, J. S. (1986). *Surviving the break up. How parents and children cope with divorce.* Grant McIntyre, New York.
3. Medalie, J. H. (1983). Family determinants of disease. *J. Fam. Pract.* **I**, (1), 9–13.
4. Doherty, W. J. and Baird, M. A. (1983). *Family therapy and family medicine.* Guildford Press, New York.
5. Mullins, H. C. and Christie-Seeley, J. (1984). Collecting and recording data—the genogram. In *Working with the family in primary care.* (ed.) Christie-Seely, J. Praeger, New York.
6. Rogers, J. and Durkin, M. (1986). The semi-structured genogram interview. *Fam. Systems Med.* **2**, (2), 176–85.
7. Huygen, F. S. A. (1978). *Family medicine. The medical history of families.* Dekker and van de Vegt, Nijmegen, The Netherlands.
8. Leiberman, S. (1980). *Transgenerational family therapy.* Croom Helm, London.
9. Thrower, S. M., Bruce, W. E., and Walton, R. F. (1982). The family circle method for integrating family systems concepts in family medicine. *J. Fam. Pract.* **15**, 451–7.

Further reading

Doherty, W. J. and Baird, M. A. (1983). *Family therapy and family medicine.* Guildford Press, New York.
Haley, J. (1973). *Uncommon therapy.* W. W. Norton, New York.
McGoldrick, M. and Gerson, R. (1985). *Genograms in family assessment.* W. W. Norton, London.
Minuchin, S. (1974). *Families and family therapy.* Harvard University Press, Cambridge, Mass.

Napier, A. Y. and Whitamer, C. (1978). *The family crucible*. Harper and Row, New York.
Skynner, R. and Cleese, S. (1983). *Families and how to survive them*. Methuen, London.

4.5   GROUP THERAPY

Few general practitioners will have had much experience of running groups within their practices, although some patients will have attended antenatal groups, weight watchers, or groups to help them give up smoking. Three different but interlocking types of group may be used in the general practice setting—mutual support, educative, and therapeutic. These are described in subsequent pages. The first two may be professionally led, the third will usually be so.

The advantages of groups are that:

● they are economical in time and resources because one or two leaders can help a larger number of people;

● they may be the best way of helping people to change attitudes and improve interpersonal skills;

● groups can generate resources from within their own ranks, both emotional and cognitive, and perhaps for some groups supportive as well;

● individuals come to the group as autonomous persons and work is done by them rather than to them.

One disadvantage is that the influence of the group may lead individuals to disclosures, or even behaviours, that they might subsequently regret. This may be a special problem if groups are held in small communities.

Mutual support groups

These groups use 'veterans', people who are themselves crippled, bereaved, homosexual, or members of some other stigmatized group, to provide help to others in the same situation. The advantages of this type of group are:

● peers have learned the hard way. Their experience is relevant because it is authentic.

● those who come for help may also find themselves giving help. This reduces the risk of them seeing themselves as 'sick' or 'helpless', and restores self-esteem.

- being outside the 'establishment' they can criticize and act as a pressure group to improve services;

- peers are less likely to patronize or be excessively sympathetic. They will see through attempts to manipulate or seek attention and will discourage unnecessary crippledom.

The disadvantages, which need to be continually borne in mind, are:

- veterans sometimes over-generalize or fail to recognize the differences between their own situation and the circumstances of others;

- they often lack the objectivity and special knowledge of the professionals and may decry the validity of that knowledge;

- some mutual help groups arise as a reaction to bad handling by professionals, and tend to become militantly anti-professional;

- mutual help groups are vulnerable to being taken over by their most vociferous or angry members, which may cause them to become paranoid and untherapeutic.

Many of the disadvantages can be prevented if professionals play a leading role within mutual help groups. The presence of a professional in a mutual help group, as in the groups run for bereaved parents by 'Cruse', may mitigate some of the difficulties but may lessen the effectiveness of the groups in some areas of activity.

Members of the primary care team (PCT) who offer themselves as group leaders to 'Mutual Support Groups' should avoid the temptation to attempt to provide solutions to the problems that emerge. The group will often turn to the professional as to an 'expert' who is expected to solve all their problems. In fact it is unlikely that our experience is any more 'expert' than theirs, and we may know less about the experience which the group shares than the participants themselves. Even if we have answers, it is better if these emerge from the other group members themselves who, in this way, enhance their own sense of competence.

The main function of the group leader(s) is to set reasonable limits — ensuring that the group does not go on too long, that everyone has a chance to be heard, and that no single person is permitted to dominate the group.

If the level of anxiety in the group rises too high, the leader can often lower it by one of the following techniques:

- making a humorous remark;

- acknowledging the feeling and thereby defusing it, e.g. 'We're all getting a bit wound-up about this issue aren't we?';

- promising to deal with the problem outside the group, e.g. 'I think this is too difficult (or complex) a problem to deal with here. Perhaps I could have a talk to Mrs Jones about it afterwards.';

- changing the topic, e.g. 'Well, I don't think we're going to get much further with this problem today. Are there any other issues that people would like to discuss?';

- giving verbal and non-verbal reassurance, e.g. if a member bursts into tears, getting up from one's seat and putting one's arms around him or her;

- suggesting that the group takes a break.

Occasionally the opposite seems to be happening. Groups chit-chat about trivial topics and nobody seems to want to talk about anything serious. This usually arises at an early stage of the group, when nobody has learnt to trust the others. The leaders can help by sharing some personal thoughts which reflect their own willingness to trust the group and respect the value of its member. Gentle coaxing will often encourage somebody to unburden themselves, and this will act as a catalyst to the rest. Silences need not be feared as they often create the gap which eventually prompts somebody to start talking.

There already exists a range of organizations (see Appendix II for a list of these) for patients with chronic physical or mental disabilities, for people in transition, and for those who live in particular disadvantaged circumstances. Many of these run support groups, and it is useful for members of the PCT to know about any which are available in their area and to encourage appropriate patients to join. Some conditions are common enough for general practitioners to consider encouraging a group based on the practice population. Diabetes, eczema, and asthma are possible examples. Antenatal groups already exist and are supported by the PCT. Young mothers' groups may usefully be set up for those who are isolated, lonely, or frightened about the task of rearing their babies, a group which the health visitor is likely to lead.[1]

The population is getting older, and older people continue to be looked after by relatives. The elderly need the support of the statutory services — meals-on-wheels, home helps, and nurses, but the carers themselves also need support. In some areas this need has been satisfied by the creation of groups for them, which provide mutual support, both emotional and physical, a forum for the exchange of ideas and help for the participants to realize that they are not the only ones with such a burden (e.g. Alzheimer's Association). Some of these groups will choose to exert pressure for better provision at a local or national level. GPs may be involved in the initiation of such groups, which hopefully will become autonomous, though often continuing to use resources from the primary care team, including social workers. Again, there may be pressure, and indeed a need, for the group leader to provide technical information, but again the temptation to de-skill, or compete with, members of the group must be resisted.

Educative groups

Some groups have been initiated to bring together those with health education interests, such as postnatal, smoking prevention, and looking after children. These groups are usually informative and are especially valuable in giving participants chances to discuss and exchange ideas.

Therapeutic groups

These may be divided into talking and experiential groups.

Talking groups

In most districts there already exist groups for the obese, for smokers, and for people abusing alcohol, some run commercially, some under the aegis of the primary care team. A few successful groups have been run for patients who are depressed or anxious, who have phobic problems or problems with social skills, and for patients with somatoform disorders[2,3] (see Chapter 6). The latter may be particularly worth considering for group therapy, in view of the low success rate of other methods of treatment.

Many volumes have been written on the practice of group psychotherapy, and this is a field for which special training is needed. Certainly, it is beyond the scope of this volume to do more than indicate what a patient should be told to expect from a group.

Therapy groups may be open or closed, for fixed numbers of meetings or for an indefinite period. These boundaries need to be explained in advance.

Patients are usually selected for a group on some clear basis, e.g. adults with sexual problems, and this, too, will need to be explained in advance, so that each knows why they and the other members are there. They need to know that there will be one (or sometimes two) group leaders who have special training for this work but that, even so, the group leader will probably say very little. The purpose of the group is to provide an opportunity for people to help each other and the leader's role is to facilitate this.

As in all forms of psychotherapy, patients will get out of it what they put in. They need to be prepared to put up with embarrassment, silences, personal remarks, and even criticism from others. It is better not to coax reluctant patients to take part, since they will seldom stick with the group and may spoil the chances of others to make a success of the opportunity which the group presents. Consequently, it is better to warn potential members of the group of the difficulties that groups can run into. Groups are not for 'fun'. They are powerful forms of therapy which, like other powerful treatments, should not be lightly undertaken. For the well-motivated patient, however, they can bring about profound benefits.

In general, 'talking' groups are most suitable for people who are able to express themselves verbally. For the inarticulate, experiential groups may be more effective.

Experiential groups

These groups are less concerned with treating disorders and more concerned with personal development which occurs as a result of the *experience* of being in the group. They include groups using a variety of methods, with names such as 'Contact' and 'T Groups', 'co-counselling', 'psychodrama', 'psychosynthesis', 'bioenergetics', 'drama', 'music', and 'art' therapy. In general, they are concerned with the 'growth' of the individual. By 'growth' is meant increasing individuals' sensitivity to the needs and potential of themselves and others, and increasing their awareness of their own emotions and their ability to express these appropriately. The groups aim also to increase participants' choice of behaviours and ways of relating to people, encouraging more honest ways of communication, and integrating the mind and body in an enhancement of autonomy. The experience of such groups may involve individuals in movement, dance, touch, massage, ritual, role play, catharsis, meditation, laughter, and tears. General practitioners are unlikely to initiate such groups in their practices, but should be aware of their existence, characteristics, and suitability for individual patients.

Difficulty with groups in general practice

Patients who know each other from outside the group may create problems within it, especially in therapeutic groups, when there is likely to be some disclosure of very personal information. Allied to this difficulty is the question of confidentiality which may not be easy for non-professionals to comply with. Groups often wish to meet in the evenings, and this may be awkward for professionals. All groups need some skills from their group leaders or facilitators, though this is more of a problem with therapeutic groups. There are advantages in two people leading interactive therapeutic groups, as if one gets embroiled the other can effect rescue and comment on the circumstances that lead to the difficulty. Two therapists, particularly if of the opposite sex, can model good relationships and provide group members with a choice of parent figure. In general practice it may be difficult for the therapists to find time to work together, and unless they are experienced they may be manipulated by the group. Ideally, one or more members of the extended PCT — GP, health visitor, social worker, community psychiatric nurse, psychologist, marriage guidance counsellor, or family therapist — may have been trained and be available for group work.

General issues regarding group therapy

The choice of individual or group therapy may depend on availability, and there are many patients who will do equally well with both. Given a choice, the following issues need to be considered:

- People who run away from social situations which they cannot handle will be unlikely to tolerate the criticisms and exposure of a therapy group (though they may benefit most). Others who have difficulties in the social sphere, but who are strongly motivated, may benefit greatly from the opportunity which groups provide to see themselves and the world through the eyes of others.

- Experiential groups can be a good way of helping people to unlock feelings that have been inhibited or repressed, and they often generate mutual support between members which is greatly appreciated by the lonely and the isolated.

- Passive, dependent people contribute little to a group and gain little in return.

- Psychotic symptoms will alarm the group and may be made worse by group therapy.

- Severely agitated and/or suicidal patients dominate groups and are better helped on an individual basis.

- Couples should only be included in groups in which all members attend as couples.

- Special groups may be needed for the treatment of alcoholism or drug abuse.

- People who know each other and live in the same community need to be aware of the special problems of confidentiality which govern the disclosure of personal information in groups.

- The dangers of 'acting out' and allowing the intense feelings (of affection or antagonism) that commonly spring up within a group to continue into the world outside the group are issues which limit their value in a local setting.

Practical considerations

We hope that this section will have helped members of the primary care team decide which patients might benefit from group therapy.

Some general practitioners will wish to create groups for their patients though, perhaps surprisingly, people who have tried to do so have found it difficult to collect suitable numbers from among the patients of even moderate-sized group practices.

Some will already feel able to lead such groups with or without the help of a co-therapist, especially the less interactive types of group. For others who are interested we suggest further reading and guidance from an experienced group leader.

Groups for doctors

Not surprisingly, doctors are prone to the same problems as their patients. Therapeutically, special groups for doctors with alcohol problems are available.

It may be difficult to separate the needs of doctors for learning, personal development, and support. Groups of the type originated by Balint help doctors to gain insight by discussing patients' case histories and analysing the emotions aroused in themselves. In this way they aim to achieve limited, but definite changes in the attitudes, assumptions, and methods of working of the doctors. Young doctors' groups may be educative and supportive. Experiential groups for doctors also aim to enhance their interpersonal skills in general, but particularly in the consulting room.

References

1. McKears, J. (1983). Group support for young mothers. *Health Visitor* 56, 16.
2. Hang, H. J. and Verberne, C. P. M. (1982). Experience with patient groups in a health centre. *General Practice International* 2, 75–9.
3. Trepka, C., Laing, I., and Smith, S. (1986). Group treatment of general practice anxiety problems. *J. R. Coll. Gen. Pract.* 36, 114–17.

Further reading

Weston Smith, J., Harrison, P. S., and Mottram, M. (1979). Group psychotherapy in general practice. *Update* 18, (7), 907–10.

4.6 CRISIS INTERVENTION AND TRANSITION COUNSELLING

Points of intervention

Because we can anticipate crises we can often help people to prepare themselves for the events that are to come. The times at which intervention may be possible are summarized in Fig. 4.7. Intervention at:

A. protects people by *educating* them about the nature of the changes that may occur in their lives and ways of coping competently with them.

B. is the point at which *anticipatory guidance* becomes possible. Individuals who are known to be approaching a crisis are informed and supported as described below.

C. is the moment of truth, the *critical event* over which doctors sometimes have a measure of control. Our behaviour at such times may mitigate some of the pain which occurs.

D. is the time when mental turmoil is likely to peak and the term *crisis intervention* is best reserved for this period. Although people are often aware of the need for help at this time, it cannot be assumed that all those who need help will ask for it. Some may be too fearful, too disorganized or too depressed to request help. Contrary to traditional medical practice, active steps may need to be taken to assess risk and offer help to those who need it (i.e. the doctor must become 'proactive' rather than 'reactive').

Because crises often affect more than one member of the family, and because the family is an important source of support, it is particularly important to make the family the unit of care whenever this is possible.

E. is the point at which most *therapeutic services* come into operation. By this time new patterns of thought and behaviour will have become established and, however unsatisfactory these may be, it will often be very difficult to

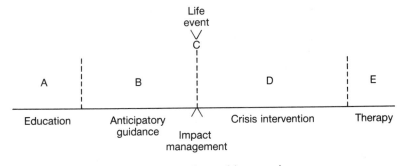

Fig. 4.7. The chart of intervention.

change them. Emotional expressions of distress are likely to be seen a
evidence of sickness by the patient and others, and a secondary train o
consequences (loss of employment, loss of confidence, loss of trust, etc.) ma
further complicate a bad situation. Because physical and psychologica
reserves are now depleted, psychophysiological and emotional symptom
develop. These may be aggravated by repression of feelings and othe
psychological defences. Time has passed and other life events have occurre
so that the connection between the initial life event and the present problem
may not be obvious.

For all these reasons, the traditional and rightly valued model of medica
services which waits for 'patients' to become 'sick' before they qualify fo
help, has its limitations. But there will always be some who will slip through
the net of prevention. We should try to minimize the risk by ensuring tha
help is available at all the points listed above.

A.   Education for change

Education that is conducted well in advance of the event, at a time whe
anxiety is low, is often more effective than anticipatory guidance that ha
been left until the last minute.

It is not unreasonable to regard most education as a way of preparing
people for the changes that are to come in their lives. Thus, par
of the function of schooling is to prepare children for the transition from
child to adult, and part of the function of training courses is to prepare
people for new jobs and responsibilities. Despite this, there are many majo
psychosocial transitions for which little or no education is provided. Most
married women will one day be widows, yet there are no 'schools for widows'.
Few people attend 'retirement classes' and even antenatal classes are ofter
poorly attended.

General practitioners and other members of the primary care team (PCT)
are sometimes in a position to prepare people for the changes, wanted and
unwanted, that are to come in their lives, but most of this teaching will remain
in the hands of others. However, our awareness of the importance of this
kind of preparation may enable us to educate the educators.

B.   Anticipatory guidance

This is most appropriately provided by the PCT when people are faced with
major changes in their lives as a result of illness or accident. Examples are
given in several parts of this volume, particularly those concerned with

reparation for surgery, when the need for guidance is very clear (p. 303), nd in breaking bad news.

Experimental studies with humans and animals show that the ability to ope with threatening events is increased if the events are predictable and ontrollable. Information-giving can increase this ability and patients have ad less pain and better outcomes in a variety of clinical procedures, e.g. ndoscopy and surgery, if given additional information in advance. Patients requently complain that they are given too little information or that they re given conflicting information; on the other hand, doctors are wary of iving information, particularly when in a position to give bad news about patient's condition. However, patients may also reject what they are not eady or able to bear.

People differ in their personal style of coping with stressful situations, some referring to seek out all possible information while others avoid information bout the threatening events. Those who seek information tend to have higher evels of anxiety and distress. Those who avoid it may cope better with short-erm stresses, especially if there is nothing that they can do to avert the angers; but in the long term they may show more signs of physical illness.[1] hese findings also have parallels in animal studies where animals subjected o chronic stress, with no available method of active coping, have shown igh levels of activity in the pituitary–adrenal cortex axis, resulting in athophysiological changes, disease, and death.

C. *Amelioration of the critical event*

his is best illustrated by the care which we give to families when a person dying (see Section 5.11). It is also needed whenever we are handling an cute medical emergency such as a coronary thrombosis. The essential omponents are gentleness, time, and emotional support. Expressions of istress should be expected and indeed facilitated. This means that a private lace should be chosen whenever possible.

D. *Crisis intervention*

rises come to our notice in a variety of ways. Most often a member of the amily will present with a symptom which is recognized as an indicator of istress. At other times one member of the family calls because of the ymptoms or behaviour of another. As soon as it is clear that more than ne person is involved in a situation which is causing acute distress, all relevant amily members need to be brought together with as many members of the PCT as require to be involved. The prime purpose of this meeting is to assess he situation and initiate a plan of management.

Family crises

Family assessment

This may seem a tall order when it is so much easier to see just 'the patient', but there are several dangers which arise if this course is taken.

(1)   Everyone's belief that 'the patient' is sick will be confirmed.

(2)   Family members who are in a position, and willing, to help will back away for fear of interfering with the doctor's treatment.

(3)   The needs for help of others in the family who are caught up in the crisis may be overlooked.

(4)   The needs of others may well undermine efforts to help 'the patient'.

If the level of distress is high and more than two family members are going to be present, it is a good idea for more than one member of the PCT to take part in the assessment. Not only are two heads better than one when trying to unravel the complexities of family dynamics, but a team of two can give more effective support to the family than one person alone. They can also support each other, an important thing to do when anxiety is running high and the family are demanding drastic solutions. This second person might be a health visitor, social worker, community psychiatric nurse, or clinical psychologist.

Sufficient time should always be set aside to allow the overall level of tension to subside and each member of the family to contribute to the assessment. We may, at first, find that we are expected to provide magical solutions to family problems. Demands for drugs or hospital admission may seem to provide easy answers to 'end of tether' behaviour. But these demands will often become less strident if the team can 'hold the line' until anxiety begins to diminish.

In a way we are acting like parents who, by remaining calm in the face of anger and fear, reassure the children that all will be well. When we do this the family may begin to consider other solutions to their problems. Members who have been reluctant to offer help for fear of being landed with more than they can handle, may make tentative suggestions for sharing support with others. Behaviour, which has been misinterpreted as 'mad' or 'bad', may be understood and accepted as a natural reaction to real or imagined difficulties. Trust may be re-established and self-esteem regained.

Management of family crises

The roles of the PCT are often quite straightforward. We act as impartial catalysts, encouraging discussion, but never taking sides. We help to clarify

he viewpoints expressed and the feelings underlying them by such remarks
as 'You seem to be feeling angry (or sad or frightened) about . . .' (whatever
the behaviour is that is giving rise to distress) and then referring the matter
to its supposed author, 'What do you think (or feel) about that?' A moderate
level of tension may stimulate discussion, but we may need to intervene if
this is becoming intolerable: 'Well, we clearly aren't going to reach agreement
on this, how about a cup of tea?', or 'We can come back to this later. I'd
like to ask about something quite different', or 'I'm beginning to realize how
hard things are for you at the moment; it's painful to have to feel this sort
of tension, isn't it?' These three approaches, taking a break, changing the
subject, and expressing sympathy can all be expected to lower the level of
anxiety for a while. By the time the family return to the issues that are
distressing them they may be able to cope rather better.

Doctors are more likely to find themselves reassuring people that they are
not sick than making psychiatric diagnoses. But even when a family member
is quite obviously sick, we should not collude with the family's wish to
dissociate themselves from the problem. Drugs and other treatments may
ameliorate symptoms, but that does not mean that family support is not
needed. We need to be scrupulously realistic and open about what psychiatric
treatments can be expected to achieve, to express our understanding of the
burden which may well remain for the family and to express our willingness
to support them.

Before we leave, we should have worked out with the family a plan which
is acceptable to them. This may well be of a provisional nature: 'This has
been a very helpful meeting. Why don't we leave things until tomorrow (or
next week) so that everyone can think over what has been said. Then we can
meet again to decide what's best.' Or we may be in a position to sum up
a plan that has emerged, e.g. 'We are agreed that there is no need for Bill
to go into hospital, but his older sister has agreed to take him home with
her for a week to give his mother a rest. We'll meet again in two weeks to
see how things are going.'

Team review

After the initial visit those members of the PCT who are involved should
normally meet, together with any other caregivers who are already involved,
or who need to be drawn in, to review the situation and to refine the plans.
It is sometimes useful to involve an outside professional at this meeting, even
if he or she is not going to be invited to see a patient or to take over.
Psychiatrists, senior social workers, psychologists, or community psychiatric
nurses can be of value if they are prepared to act in this way, and some
practices set up regular meetings with this in mind.

Subsequent plans may include further joint meetings between the team and
the family, or support from a particular team member to a particular family

member, e.g. 'Jim (the social worker in the team) will meet with Betty (whose husband is in prison) to give her a chance to talk through and share her grief at what has happened. Betty will take the children to visit their Dad next week. If any of you feel the need for another family session, let us know'.

Alternative approaches

Although, as a general rule, it is preferable to regard the whole family as the unit of care and to plan intervention accordingly, this is not always necessary, or possible. Some problems are not so serious that the family needs to be mobilized, and some people are isolated from their families and may refuse to allow them to be involved. Or they may permit their spouse to be involved but refuse to include the children. In such cases they will often prefer to be seen in the surgery rather than in their own home for fear of interruptions.

Again, the same general rules apply: we should encourage the person to 'talk through' their problem and provide the emotional support which will enable them to cope with the anxiety that this evokes.

Occasionally a family who have met to discuss a crisis become 'stuck'. We may sense that there are important secrets which need to be discussed but can not be shared in a family meeting. In such cases it may be appropriate to divide the family in two, and for one member of the team to go into another room with one or more members. Later it may be possible to bring the members together again and the team members may advise (through they can't insist) that the secrets be shared.

Jane's mother came to the surgery complaining that her teenage daughter was 'very sick'. When the doctor and social worker made a joint visit Jane was mute, withdrawn, and unresponsive. But when the social worker took the mother into another room, leaving the doctor alone with Jane, Jane began softly to speak of a relationship with a young man who had upset her by his ardour. Meanwhile, her mother was revealing to the social worker that she had intercepted and concealed ('for fear of making things worse') a proposal of marriage from the young man. Mother confessed how close she had become to her daughter since the death of her husband five years ago. At first she had felt suicidal and it was only her daughter who made life worth living. Since then she had recovered her self-confidence and purpose in life, but her daughter had remained insecure and seldom went out. After talking for about 20 minutes, the doctor suggested that Jane remain with her mother while the two team members discussed what to do. Both agreed that the root of the problem lay in the intense mutual clinging that had become established between mother and daughter. Each worried about the other, and their fears had become self-perpetuating. They proposed a series of further meetings at which individual and joint counselling would alternate.

In the event, only two more visits were needed. Once the mother realized that her daughter was not mentally ill, but was simply in conflict over her independence, she became less anxious about her. Following a frank talk together, Jane realized that her mother no longer needed her constant presence. A turning point occurred when the mother asked her daughter's permission to go out with a man. This recognition of her mother's sexual and emotional needs helped Jane to acknowledge her own needs and, although she subsequently rejected the proposal of marriage and broke off her relationship with the young man, it was not long before others took his place. She remains a quiet, introverted girl, but her relationship with her mother is now one of affectionate regard, rather than interdependence, and there are no signs of mental illness.

It is worth considering what might have happened if this case had been handled differently. A psychiatric referral, for instance, might well have given rise to a diagnosis of 'depressive mutism' and the prescription of antidepressant drugs; both actions which would have confirmed the mother's worst fears. If admitted to a psychiatric ward, Jane would probably have got better, but there would have been a real risk of recurrence when she returned home, and a pattern of reliance on medical care for a psychological problem would have become established. Of course psychiatrists are not unaware of this kind of possibility, and most will attempt to assess the family situation, but it is not always easy to appreciate what is going on at home when the patient is only seen at the hospital, and relatives are seldom given the support which they need in cases like this.

Despite other considerations, drugs are occasionally needed if we can find no other way of reducing distress to a safe level. A benzodiazepine may enable someone to 'stay with' a situation instead of avoiding it or running away. But we should make clear the purpose of the drug and insist that it is for temporary use only. Certainly, it should not be offered as a lasting solution to a problem. Likewise, people should be warned that the use of alcohol to master distressing feelings, or procure sleep, is likely to become a habit.

Suicide and violence

The risk of suicide and other hazardous behaviour should always be assessed in crisis situations. The simple way to do this is to ask 'Has it been so bad that you have wanted to kill yourself?' Some people are reluctant to ask such questions for fear of 'putting the idea into his (or her) head'. But this is illogical; someone who is very distressed is bound to have thought of suicide and by raising the issue we give them permission to talk about it. Given that opportunity, few of those who are at risk will conceal the fact. Further questions may be needed to elicit how serious is that risk and what method of suicide is contemplated. Those who are a serious suicidal risk will usually have worked out a plan. The same general rule applies to those who may be a danger to other people—it is always safest to ask.

The risk of suicide or violence to others can be reduced by:

● Removing the means, e.g. by removing from the house all drugs that might be used in overdose, and leaving only sufficient for therapeutic use. If dangerous quantities are left, they should be in the hands of a responsible relative or friend.

● Mobilizing the family in support, and warning them of the risk.

● Instituting a plan for emotional support and treatment of any psychiatric disturbance that is present (e.g. treating depressive illness).

● Admitting the patient to a psychiatric unit for treatment, preferably as a voluntary patient. This is seldom necessary, but we should not hesitate to make use of our powers under the Mental Health Act (see Appendix I) if this is the only safe way to ensure that suicidal or dangerous patients receive the treatment which they need.

These actions should be discussed with the patient and co-operation obtained whenever possible.

Parasuicide

Parasuicide refers to deliberate, non-fatal self-poisoning or self-injury—the former accounting for 90 per cent of events. Self-poisoning involves three components—a deliberate act, a quantity known to be excessive, and a realization that it may be harmful. Although the incidence of successful suicide has been falling gradually in this country since the early sixties, the incidence of parasuicide has increased. One study found a fourfold increase between 1962 and 1972 and a more gradual increase until the late seventies, when it seemed to level out. Suicide is more common amongst older males, compared to parasuicide which has a higher incidence amongst younger females. Many persons who attempt suicide repeat the attempt within the following year.

Various studies suggest that the incidence of parasuicide is positively related to:

● disturbed relationship with a key individual, frequently having had a recent quarrel;

● poor social conditions;

● high unemployment locally;

● large family size;

● early parental death;

● past criminal or anti-social record.

Associated factors include alcoholism, particularly in males, epilepsy, drug addiction, and subnormality.

Two-thirds of acts are impulsive and in another two-thirds patients give warning to someone in the month before the event. During this time the same proportion visit their GPs, and about a third are receiving treatment for physical disease from their general practitioner at the time of the attempt. In an Oxford study two-thirds of patients had been prescribed psychotropic drugs by their general practitioners during the three months before taking an overdose, and four out of five had used these very same drugs for their suicidal attempt.[1]

Assessment and management

Good assessment is the key to management. This helps to define those at risk of further attempts, those needing psychiatric treatment, and determines the strategy for further management. It may also allow patients to express their feelings and to clarify their problems. The following questions need to be answered:

What is the explanation for the attempt in terms of likely reasons and goals?

What was the degree of suicidal intent?

Is the patient at risk of suicide or is there an immediate risk of further overdose or self-injury?

What problems, either acute or chronic, confront the patient?

Did a particular event precipitate the attempt?

Is the patient psychiatrically ill and, if so, what is the diagnosis and how relevant is this to the attempt?

What kind of help would be appropriate and is the patient willing to accept such help?

The risk of repetition of the attempt itself may be assessed from the background factors, a detailed estimate of the seriousness of the intention and the degree of hopelessness. At greater risk are those where alcohol has been involved, those in poor health, those with disordered personalities, and those who have had previous in-patient or out-patient contact with psychiatric services or who have made previous attempts, particularly if these have not improved their social circumstances, and those who live alone and are older.

Further management will follow along the lines suggested earlier in this chapter. It is usually wise when assessing a patient, and often in therapy, to obtain permission from the patient to see key persons alone and then to try and include them in conjoint or family therapy.

Prevention

As about 60 per cent of patients attempting suicide see a general practitioner during the month before the attempt, there is considerable scope for prevention, assuming that the combination of background and trigger-factors are recognized. It is probable that counselling by the general practitioner or other member of the PCT will be effective in a number of instances. For reasons already stated, it is unwise to prescribe psychotrophic drugs to those who may be at risk.

Management of aggression and non-compliance

Psychiatrically disturbed patients are less often a danger to others than is commonly imagined. Even so, there are a few occasions when aggression may take place. Acute alcoholism is the commonest cause, particularly if associated with pathological jealousy (Section 8.5). Paranoid schizophrenics (Section 8.6) sometimes attack their supposed enemies, and manic patients (Section 8.4) may become excitable and aggressive. Confused patients (Section 7.2) sometimes misinterpret the behaviour of others as hostile, and may lose the inhibitions which normally prevent violence. Finally, there are a few truculent and aggressive psychopaths (see Section 8.1) who may become a danger to others. The treatment of these conditions will be described elsewhere, as is the legal position should compulsion be required (see Appendix I).

If agitated or aggressive patients need to be brought under control, it may be necessary to sedate them. Haloperidol, by intramuscular injection, at a dosage of 5-10 mg, repeated if need be ½-1 hour later, is an effective means of controlling most forms of agitation. It should be used at lower dosage and with caution if the patient has cardiovascular disease or parkinsonism, or has already been taking alcohol or other sedative or tranquillizing drugs. Patients should be advised to lie down after intramuscular injections of haloperidol because of the hypotensive effects of this drug at high dosage (see also p. 163).

Physical restraint should be kept to a minimum, but sufficient help needs to be available before any attempt is made to administer treatment. Because restraint often provokes retaliation, it should be discontinued as soon as its aim has been accomplished, even if the patient is still struggling. A violently struggling person can often be quietened by asking one's helpers to step back and by adopting a warm and friendly attitude. But it is wise to keep the helpers near at hand in case of further outbursts!

Co-operative family members can sometimes help to quieten a frightened or aggressive patient, but we should always explain to them exactly what we propose to do and why we are doing it, to obtain, if possible, their full co-operation.

The police are trained in the handling of violence and should be asked for help if needed. Their powers are, however, limited and they will seldom intervene in cases of domestic crises unless there is serious violence, steps have been taken under the Mental Health Acts, or they have a magistrate's warrant to remove the patient to a place of safety.

Management of psychosocial transitions

As we saw in the preceding chapter, many of the crises which come to the attention of a GP occur at times of psychosocial transition. In such cases it is necessary to ensure that people have the time and opportunity to express the distressing emotions that are a part of the normal reaction to these circumstances. In such situations it is difficult to avoid medicalizing the problem. 'Aren't you going to give me anything?' said one lady who had spent an hour pouring out her grief at the death of her husband. We need to make it clear that we do not regard such a person as sick, and that long-term medication would only create more problems for her. Time, a more precious commodity, is what we are giving, though this does not rule out the occasional short-term use of sedatives if distress is severe and persistent.

Because psychosocial transition takes time, it is advisable for someone from the PCT to meet those whose lives are most affected on a number of occasions. Having been given the opportunity to grieve, and being reassured of the normality of the physical accompaniments of strong emotion, the intensity of the sufferers' distress will begin to diminish and with it resistance to accepting the full reality of the change. At this point it becomes possible to point them towards the people (and situations) who will help them to discover the new direction which their life must now take. 'Veterans' who have come through a similar experience in the past and are now back on course have much to offer, and there are several special organizations which arrange meetings where people in transition can share feelings and learn how to cope (see Section 4.5 and Appendix II).

Because a world that has changed often feels dangerous and people in transition may feel insecure and alarmed, the general practitioner and other members of the PCT can help patients by expressing confidence in their strength and value, and by steering them gently but firmly towards new challenges.

Ending intervention

When the acute crisis has subsided, the team must decide whether or not to continue to provide support. In general, it is better to provide too little help than too much. People easily become dependent on well-meaning caregivers who may be reluctant to allow their charges to 'stand on their own feet'. There comes a time when a realistic plan and a date for ending therapy should be set, and this plan should then be adhered to, unless new circumstances arise which render it invalid. It is, of course, in the nature of general practice that contact can easily be made again if required — sometimes too easily.

Recurrent crises

Some multi-problem families go from crisis to crisis, and there may be little we can do to prevent this. Intractable mental illness, personality disorders, or life circumstances that are beyond remedy may leave people vulnerable to life events that most people would take in their stride.

We can perform a useful role by being available to such people in order to tide them through each crisis as it occurs. Sometimes we may reduce the frequency of such crises by this very means. Knowing that help is available may itself reduce anxiety and the need for help. At other times the seeds of the next crisis may be sown at the time of a current one — as in the case of a gambler who borrows money to pay his debts, or the alcoholic who binges in order to escape from a problem. Hence the need to help the person to find better ways of handling problems.

The tendency to repeat one's mistakes has been termed by Freud the 'Repetition Compulsion'. It takes many subtle and complex forms. These can sometimes be recognized in the context of family meetings, and they should always be looked for. One clue to the existence of a compulsion to repeat is a feeling given by the family that one is taking part in a play, the scenes of which have already been played many times. Rather than accepting that the players are trapped in their 'family script', we can help them to articulate the play and to work out alternative endings. Some therapists use psychodrama as a means of re-enacting critical family scenes and finding alternative ways of handling them.

An example of crisis intervention

Ann, aged 37, arrived in the surgery one day in great distress, threatening to take yet another overdose. With three previous overdoses in as many years, there was obviously a risk that she would act upon this threat. She reported that the present episode had resulted from a quarrel which had ended when her husband packed a bag and moved out of the house. Without him she was terrified and unable to cope with the needs of her two small children.

The doctor arranged for both partners to come to the neutral ground of the surgery later the same day to meet with him and a social worker in order to assess the situation. The story which emerged was not uncommon.

Ann had always been an insecure girl whose parents had had a stormy relationship. She grew up with a tendency to cling at times of stress. This had led to the break up of several previous relationships, following each of which she had become agitated, depressed, and suicidal. The overdoses had never been large enough to do her serious harm, but they had drawn attention to her plight and rallied support from the family.

Ann had married her second husband, George, a year previously. George was very fond of her, but perplexed by her moods. Their first baby had been born a month previously and George had hoped that this would 'calm her down'. But she seemed, if anything, more irritable and anxious since the birth of the baby, and kept phoning him at work and making unreasonable demands that he return home to deal with numerous trivial problems.

This story had emerged in the course of a joint meeting in which Ann had repeatedly blamed herself for everything that had happened. She confessed that he had only walked out because she had told him to go. She was half-convinced that her husband no longer found her attractive and had detected a note of annoyance in his voice when he tried to reassure her. Consequently, she had impulsively tried to 'test him out'. George, who had no idea how to handle the situation, had taken her at her word and left 'To give her time to cool down'. He could now see that this had been a mistake.

In the course of this meeting the atmosphere in the consulting room had gradually become calmer as each partner began to see the other's point of view. The doctor suggested that part of the problem arose from Ann's feelings of insecurity. Her own parent's marriage had not left her with much confidence in the security to be derived from attachments between husbands and wives, and the arrival of the baby was a major change in her life which made her feel all the more unsure of herself. Both of them would have to live with a measure of insecurity for some time to come, but there was no reason why things should not gradually improve.

At this point George came to his wife's support expressing his genuine love and admiration for her. He asked her how he should cope with her moods. Instead of answering this question the social worker asked him how they made him feel. He said, 'Helpless, if I do what she wants I feel I may just encourage her to be more unreasonable, but if I don't, she feels rejected and gets more upset'. The social worker remarked, 'It sounds as if both of you feel helpless when that happens', an observation with which both partners could agree.

Crisis intervention in this case made no great difference to the underlying problem, but it did enable the situation to be contained and left each partner with a better understanding of the situation and an appreciation of the other's points of view. Perhaps, in the future, they would be less likely to aggravate the situation by drastic 'solutions' and more tolerant of their own helplessness.

Reference

1. Hawton, K. and Blackstock, E. (1977). Deliberate self poisoning: implications for psychotropic drug prescribing in general practice *J. R. Coll. Gen. Pract.* **27**, 560–3.

Further reading

Hawton, K. and Catalan, J. (1987). *Attempted suicide.* Oxford University Press.

4.7   PRESCRIBING

The doctor as drug

For many doctors and patients, prescribing means giving the patient drugs to take. Whether the patient takes these drugs, or had expected to be given them, is another matter. Balint[1] coined the phrase 'The doctor as drug' and this concept applies not only to doctors but to the other members of the primary care team (PCT) who come into contact with patients. Every contact between humans has a consequence—for better or worse—and when considering the use of psychotropic drugs it is important to weigh their possible benefits against possible dangers and to bear in mind other alternatives. Will some form of 'talking treatment' be more helpful—and less harmful—to the patient than the prescription of drugs? Will it make the patient less medicalized, more in control of their own life? All doctors must have experienced prescribing a drug and having the patient come back a day or two later saying 'I didn't take the tablets because I felt much better as soon as I'd talked to you.'

In recent years there has been an increasing awareness of the risk of dependency on minor tranquillizers, and some of the problems relating to this will be discussed later in this section. Not only doctors, but informed, and misinformed, members of the public are now questioning the abandon with which drugs have been prescribed, and are turning to practitioners outside mainstream medicine, or are resisting taking the drugs which doctors offer. There are others whose blind faith that their doctor has a drug for every problem causes them to feel offended and rejected if their demands for medication are not met.

It is a basic assumption of this book that doctors can often help patients without prescribing drugs and that although drug prescribing has its place, it may also be an easy option and an effective way of ending a consultation, which only serves to postpone the time when the underlying problem must be faced. Is there evidence, then, that the kind of counselling/psychotherapy which may be available in the primary care setting is helpful to patients and reduces prescribing and consultation rates? The answer is 'Yes',[2,3] though, as with all psychological treatments, it is difficult to set up clinical trials with tightly defined criteria for admission and outcome.

In an interesting paper, Catalan *et al.* describe 91 patients with minor affective disorders who were seen in general practice.[4,5] They were randomly allocated to two groups, which were similar in all main variables, including GHQ scores (see Chapter 2), 80 per cent being classed as psychiatrically abnormal. One group was given anxiolytic drugs; the other was given support, advice, and reassurance of the kind GPs give as a routine part of their work, requiring no specialist skills. The GPs continued looking after these patients, whose psychiatric and social functioning were assessed after one and seven months. No difference was shown between the two groups; 30 per cent were still suffering some symptoms after seven months. Those patients who, on original assessment, had more severe problems, were equally represented in both groups. Of importance, too, was the finding that the group which did not receive anxiolytic drugs did not increase their consumption of alcohol, tobacco, or non-prescribed drugs, nor did they make increased use of the GP's time. It seems, then, that from the skills point of view, the basic trio of 'empathy, warmth, genuineness', present in the armamentarium of most GPs, is as effective as the prescribing of anxiolytics.

From the point of view of time, patients who feel that they have been inadequately treated have an uncomfortable habit of returning again and again, or calling the doctor out at inconvenient hours. A little extra time spent with such patients at the outset of management may save much time later on.

For patients who are more severely disturbed, the GP may call on colleagues with training in special techniques — psychiatrists,[6] counsellors (marriage guidance or other), social workers, clinical psychologists, or others, such as, for instance, psychotherapeutically trained nurses.[8,9] Over the past 10 years a considerable amount of work has been done on the evaluation of the role of such workers in general practice, and the reader is referred to the original reports for detailed summaries of findings — especially Waydenfeld and Waydenfeld,[8] Anderson and Hasler,[2] Earll and Kincey,[10] Ashurst,[11] Wyld,[14] and Robson *et al*.[7] Without exception, patients appreciated the counselling process. Most studies show a decrease in the use of psychotropic drugs and calls on the GPs time, but this difference is no longer significant a year after original entry into the trials. This may be because, in practice, many problems dealt with are of an acute and self-limiting nature; patients do get better on their own, and the effect of counselling is to make the patient get better more quickly and with the use of less medication. Also, patients who have been on psychotropics for longer than six months are more likely to get off them with counselling than without.[11]

When trying to wean patients off anxiolytic or hypnotic drugs, it is important to remember that the patient's acceptance of the need for intervention is a prerequisite for its success. All doctors have experience of patients who are adamant in maintaining their medication of these drugs — the moral is to try not to get the habit established.

Psychotropic drugs

General considerations

Most psychotropic drugs are easily absorbed from the gut, but because they are mostly metabolized by the liver, parenteral administration results in higher levels reaching the brain. Other concurrently administered drugs which induce liver enzymes tend to cause systemic blood levels of psychotropics to decrease. Drug metabolites are frequently themselves physiologically active and because of this, and the variable binding of active drugs to plasma proteins, measurements of the total plasma concentration of circulating drugs, as opposed to the measurement of the concentration of free, active compounds (which is not yet possible), give little help with clinical management.

Drug interaction is not a major problem with psychotropic drugs, with the important exception of monoamine-oxidase inhibitors (q.v.), though it is as well to remember that barbiturates induce liver enzymes and therefore their concurrent administration (e.g. for epilepsy) with chlorpromazine or tricyclic antidepressants reduces the other drug's blood level.

Some psychotropic drugs do not achieve their full effects for a matter of days, or in the case of tricyclic antidepressants, weeks, and on withdrawal there is a comparable time-lag before their clinical effects are lost.

Prescribing

It is advisable to use well-established drugs with which the doctor has become familiar. Two or three approved drugs in each category are usually enough, and adequate dosage is very important, bearing in mind that old people require lower doses. If a patient does not respond to a drug, there is little likelihood that another of the same group will be any better, though side-effects do vary and may justify such a change. It is usually better to prescribe single drugs rather than combinations and, if the latter, not the fixed ratios beloved of drug companies. It is better to use a sedating antidepressant such as amitriptyline if sedation is required in a depressed patient, rather than, for instance, combining imipramine and a tranquillizer. The side-effects of drugs need to be taken into account, and explained to the patient, especially the fact that effects such as dryness of the mouth, may occur with antidepressants long before the desired effect on mood. If this is not done, the patient may stop treatment prematurely. Once-daily dose regimes (always to be preferred, as they are easier to remember) are often possible with long-acting drugs such as antidepressants. Above all, the doctor needs to share with the patient the decision as to whether a drug should be used, and, if so, explain what the implications are regarding side-effects and length of treatment. Unless the patient's agreement is obtained, compliance is likely to be low.

Drugs used in general practice

Drugs used in general practice to deal with psychological problems fall into the following four categories:

1) anxiolytic;

2) hypnotic;

3) antidepressant;

4) antipsychotic.

These will be considered in turn. In addition, anti-parkinsonian drugs are occasionally used to counteract the side-effects of phenothiazines, but for the use of these drugs and detailed discussion of all drugs, the reader is referred to the *British National Formulary* or Martindale's *Extra pharmacopoea*.

Anxiolytics and hypnotics

These two groups are probably best considered together, as drugs that are anxiolytic in small doses cause sleep in large ones, and the drugs of choice for almost all purposes in general practice came from the benzodiazepine group.

Indications

Anxiety is a normal response to abnormal situations, as well as, at times, being an abnormal response to a normal one.

Benzodiazepines are effective in relieving anxiety, but the dangers of long-term problems makes it advisable to restrict their use as an anxyolitic to three clinical situations:

1) When the precipitating cause of anxiety is no longer present and the patient is trapped in a vicious circle of self-perpetuating anxiety leading to traumatic symptoms which then cause more anxiety. If other methods of anxiety management have failed (see Section 3.4), a short (less than six weeks) course of a benzodiazepine such as diazepam may break the vicious circle so that it is not re-established when the medication is discontinued.

2) When anxiety is preventing people from doing important things such as attending dental appointments, starting a job, or travelling for a holiday, a few doses of a benzodiazepine will often overcome this obstacle and restore confidence.

3) People who are agoraphobic are often afraid to leave home for fear that a panic attack will occur while they are out and they will be unable to do anything to relieve it. The provision of a small supply of e.g. diazepam 'for emergency use only' will give them added security, so much so that the drug may be carried but never taken.

In all of these cases the drug is one element in a total plan of anxiety management. It should never be given as a short-cut and we should be particularly cautious when prescribing for people with a tendency to become dependent on alcohol or other drugs.

The management of insomnia

When a patient presents with a sleep problem it is important first to take a full history. Disturbed sleep (with or without early waking), is often related to a depressive illness and this needs to be treated appropriately. The patient may be taking too much caffeine during the day in the form of tea or coffee. The patient's expectation of how much sleep is necessary may be unrealistic. A normally active person who has to stay at home with a broken leg may need less sleep than when active—and may need analgesics to help get what sleep is needed. The amount of sleep required decreases with age, and many old people don't realize this. Some people think they will become ill if they don't get their regular ten hours sleep. If the standard hot bath, hot drink and boring television programme or book doesn't work, or there is some transient crisis leading to restlessness, a sleeping tablet may be given, but again, a contract regarding the length of time and frequency of use should be made with the patient—preferably hypnotics should not be taken every night, even for a limited period of time.

Children almost never need hypnotics and sleep disturbances should be treated by other methods (see Section 5.3). The elderly should be treated with caution, as they often require smaller dosage and hypnotics may cause confusion and incontinence. Patients often come out of hospital having been given 'routine' night sedation. This should be discontinued as soon as possible—or better still, never started.

Drugs available

There is rarely any place for the use of barbiturates in the treatment of anxiety or insomnia. Short-acting benzodiazepines are the most popular choice, but as a hypnotic, chloral hydrate (and its related compound, dichloral phenazone) is of particular value in old people and is still occasionally used so is chlormethiazole, which probably has little to commend it except in the management of alcohol-withdrawal problems, when its anticonvulsant properties are useful.

Phenothiazines

These drugs will be considered in a later section. Their use in anxiety is restricted to patients in whom aggressive behaviour is unmasked by the use of benzodiazepines.

Tricyclic antidepressants

These will also be considered in the next section. Patients with depressive lness in whom anxiety is a major feature may benefit from the use of a sedating type of tricyclic antidepressant, such as amitriptyline.

Benzodiazepines

These drugs are anxiolytic in smaller doses and hypnotic in larger. They may be divided into short- and long-acting ones, and it is probably best for the clinician to use only one or two drugs in each category—effects are so similar that the oldest and cheapest are usually to be preferred.

Table 4.2. *Benzodiazepines*

Short-acting	Long-acting
Oxazepam	Diazepam
Lorazepam	Chlordiazepoxide
Temazepam	Nitrazepam
Triazolam	Clobazam

It is customary to use nitrazepam as a hypnotic but temazepam is less likely to cause residual effects the next day.

Side-effects of benzodiazepines are mainly due to their sedative properties, though they can reduce inhibition (like alcohol) and cause a release of aggression in people so inclined. Overdosage with these drugs is relatively safe as they do not cause respiratory depression, (unlike barbiturates) but their effects are additive with alcohol and patients need to be warned about this.

Recently, it has become apparent that benzodiazepines cause true physiological dependence.[7,12] A survey by Balter *et al.*[13] in 1984 showed that 5 per cent of adults in the UK had taken a benzodiazepine regularly for a year or more, so around 200 000 adults in this country may have been pharmacologically dependent on these drugs in that year. The delay in realizing that a true withdrawal syndrome occurs on stopping regular benzodiazepine treatment arose because the symptoms of withdrawal are similar to those for which the patient is often started on the drug—it can be difficult to distinguish anxiety due to withdrawal from a relapse of the underlying anxiety state. It is only the subsequent course of the symptoms which may distinguish their cause. Symptoms much more severe than those of simple anxiety may occur on withdrawal, the commonest being perceptual disturbances such as heightened sensitivity to all forms of sensory stimuli, depersonalization, nightmares, restlessness, and feelings of unreality. A few patients have even more severe symptoms, such as hypertension, hyperpyrexia, epileptic seizures, or psychotic behaviour. Heather Ashton,[12] in her 1984 paper, quotes a patient's own account of the harrowing process of benzodiazepine withdrawal and this is recommended reading. Overall, probably around 15 per cent of long-term users suffer clinically significant withdrawal symptoms on stopping treatment, although this figure rises to 50 per cent of those habituated to lorazepam (Ativan).

The question then arises — is long-term treatment with benzodiazepines harmful? Apart from general considerations of the inadvisability of unnecessary long-term medication of any kind, and the medicalization of patients, there is some, though no entirely convincing, evidence that benzodiazepines impair intelligence and psycho-motor functioning.

It is also common clinical experience that many patients on diazepines require increasing doses in order to maintain the same degree of symptom control. This tolerance to the drug may lead to escalation of dosage. If dosage is not increased, it is alleged that long-term treatment can lead to the occurrence of withdrawal symptoms despite the continuation of a constant level of medication.

Differences between drugs seem to relate only to the rate at which the blood level of the drug falls, which explains the length of action of the drug. Short-acting drugs such as temazepam and lorazepam are more likely to cause problems than long-acting ones such as diazepam. The moral seems to be not to start drugs unless there are good indications, and not to continue them for longer than necessary, an upper limit of six weeks having been suggested by the Committee on the Review of Medicines in 1980. Their recommendation probably still stands.

In patients who have been on treatment for a long time and who agree to cut down, withdrawal should be gradual but structured over, say, 2–4 months. Beta-blocker drugs, such as propranolol 20–40 mg tds may help to cover some of the physical effects of withdrawal, such as tremor. Behavioural methods may also help with withdrawal, for instance by the involvement of a clinical psychologist or relaxation therapist. A mutual self-help group ('Tranx', see Appendix II) can provide additional encouragement and support to those who choose to discontinue tranquillizers.

Antidepressants

The main groups of drugs used for the management of depressive illness are the tricyclic and related tetracyclic compounds. These are labelled according to the number of rings in their structure, to which different side chains are attached. Monoamine-oxidase inhibitors (MAOI) are less frequently used, and L-tryptophan will only be mentioned in this introductory paragraph. The evidence for its efficacy is far from clear. Lithium, used in manic depressive conditions, will also be considered.

The whole problem of whether to use antidepressant drugs, if so in what dose and for what length of time, is a difficult one. The label 'antidepressant' seems designed to make the doctor equate depression with antidepressants. The first problem is what constitutes 'depression' as opposed to 'sadness' or normal reaction to adverse events? This is considered in Section 8.4.

Research indicates that the best results with antidepressants are obtained when there are physical accompaniments to any mood disturbance, such as early waking, loss of weight or libido, diurnal variation in mood, and retardation of thought and movement. Antidepressants may also be of use in masked depressive states, such as backache, for which no other explanation or treatment has been found to be helpful (see Chapter 6). Nevertheless, the prescribing of antidepressants should be carefully considered in the light of possible alternative strategies — psychological, social, cognitive, or behavioural management. It should be borne in mind that if the decision to use antidepressants is not truly shared between doctor and patient, then prescription of these drugs may take away management control from the patient and give it to the doctor. A pattern of dependent behaviour may then be set for the future. The sensitivity of some patients to the side-effects of antidepressants means that the GP sometimes has to tread a thin line between prescribing too low a dose for effective therapy and a dosage which makes the patient feel peculiar. GPs on the whole tend to prescribe lower doses of antidepressants than hospital doctors and claim that these doses are effective. Recent research evidence supports this claim.[15] In most circumstances it is best to start with a dose at the lower end of the effective range, but to be prepared to increase this if needed. Side-effects which are experienced in the first few days usually wear off so that subsequent increases in medication are better tolerated. A once-nightly dosage regime for the sedating type of antidepressant has become popular lately, having the advantage of helping the patient to sleep and reducing interference with daily life.

Bearing in mind the delay in onset of action of most of these drugs, it is reasonable practice, when doubt exists as to whether a severely depressed patient should be put on drugs or not, to start. If, then, the patient gets better in a few days, the doctor knows that this has been due to factors other than the drug, which can then be stopped. In this way, time is not wasted in starting recovery as quickly as possible in those who are going to need medication. Patients responding to drugs quite often feel a sudden lifting of symptoms, around the 10th day of treatment, but sometimes much later. Treatment usually needs to go on for many weeks, sometimes months. The only sure way of finding out if the patient still needs drugs is to tail them off and see what happens. If the patient relapses, either alternative forms of treatment will have to be considered, or the antidepressants restarted. A very few need continuing treatment. Others, who relapse when antidepressants are withdrawn, may be helped by lithium (q.v.) even though they don't ever exhibit a manic phase.

Tricyclic and tetracyclic compounds

A large number of compounds are available, of similar activity but very variable cost. As always, doctors should familiarize themselves with only a few compounds. The main difference between the drugs is the degree of sedation they induce, their cardiotoxic effects, and their interaction with other drugs.

Of the older drugs, amitriptyline has a marked sedative effect, imipramine is relatively neutral, and protriptyline has a mildly stimulant effect. The first two of these drugs are probably sufficient for the large majority of needs. Both drugs are long-acting and may be used once daily, at night, building up from 25–150 mg depending on therapeutic and side-effects.

The newer antidepressants include mianserin, nomifesine, dothiepin, and doxepin. One of this group of drugs is enough to become familiar with — mianserin has milder anticholinergic effects than amitriptyline and is less cardiotoxic, so may be preferable for elderly people and those with glaucoma, though its effectiveness as an antidepressant is not as surely proven, it is much more expensive and it occasionally causes blood dyscrasias.

All antidepressants drugs have side-effects, which vary with the drug and the individual — hence the need to have more than one drug 'up one's sleeve' (see Table 4.3).

Table 4.3. *Side-effects of antidepressants*

Autonomic	—dry mouth
	—impaired accommodation
	—difficulty in micturition (particularly important in elderly men with prostatic hypertrophy)
	—increased sweating
Cardiovascular	—tachycardia
	—postural hypotension
	—arrhythmias
	—fluid retention and oedema
Neurological	—fine tremor
	—incoordination
	—epileptic seizures
Other	—skin rashes
	—jaundice
	—blood dyscrasias (rare)

Overdose with antidepressants can be extremely serious — another reason for being careful with their use, assessing the person's likelihood of a suicide attempt before starting, and maybe asking a relative to be responsible for the tablets during the early weeks of treatment. The toxic effects relate to the side-effects — the most serious are respiratory depression, cardiac toxicity, and convulsions. Most patients only require supportive care, but hospital monitoring is mandatory in all but the mildest overdoses.

Tricyclic drugs potentiate the pressor effects of adrenalin and related drugs — a potential hazard if local anaesthetics are used. Their rate of breakdown is increased by barbiturates but not by benzodiazepines, though there are very few occasions when both drugs should be used together. They do not interact with beta-blocking drugs, although they do interfere with the effects of bethanidine, guanethidine, and clonidine. Withdrawal of tricyclic drugs from patients on these hypotensives must be very slow in case blood pressure rises suddenly.

Monoamine-oxidase inhibitors

These drugs are not much used nowadays in general practice — partly because their antidepressant (as opposed to anxiolytic) effect has never been conclusively proven, and partly because of the risk of precipitating a severe hypertensive crisis if the patient eats cheese and certain other foodstuffs. They are never drugs of first choice and it is difficult to define indications for their use, except perhaps failure with other drugs. The reader is referred to the British National Formulary for discussion of side-effects including an extensive list of important drug interactions and a model 'Treatment card' which should always be given to patients on these drugs to warn them of possible problems.

Antipsychotic drugs

Alternatively called major tranquillizers or neuroleptic drugs, these are basically compounds used in the management of psychomotor excitement and schizophrenia — different conditions which do not necessarily coexist.

In general, these drugs may be used in the short term to quieten disturbed patients, whatever the cause, and they are useful in the long-term management of schizophrenia, where they alleviate, and help to prevent the recurrence of, florid psychotic symptoms such as hallucinations and delusions.

When using these drugs for acutely disturbed patients, chlorpromazine in a dose adequate to sedate (e.g. 50–100 mg intramuscularly) or haloperidol (see p. 150) will be effective whatever the cause of the condition. A fuller discussion of organic syndromes occurs later in this book (Chapter 7), but it should again be emphasized how important it is to differentiate between an organic and non-organic cause, in case a primary organic cause such as hypoglycaemia or a cerebral tumour is missed. A history from someone who knows the patient well is likely to be most helpful.

When the acute episode has come under control and a diagnosis made, treatment may be given by the oral route, using the drugs considered below.

Schizophrenic patients, who are unreliable tablet-takers, can often be managed best with depot preparations (e.g. flupenthixol decanoate, 20 mg by deep intramuscular injection every 1–4 weeks). This regime avoids the necessity for daily tablets and maintains a steady blood level. Patients have a tendency to forget to come in for injections, and practices need to establish some water-tight system for ensuring that defaulters are contacted. If necessary, the doctor or nurse may have to go round to the patient and give the injection. This is a situation in which the doctor must be authoritarian!

Side-effects

These are mainly extrapyramidal symptoms. The commonest is a parkinsonian effect, the most serious is tardive dyskinesia, a syndrome characterized by chewing, sucking, grimacing, and choreoathetoid movements. Generalized motor restlessness may also occur and is less serious. It is difficult to predict which patients will get side-effects—this seems to depend on the drug, the dose, the length of use, and the patient's own response. The parkinsonian symptoms may be helped by the concurrent administration of anticholinergic drugs, but these should not be used routinely as not all patients get these symptoms and anticholinergic drugs may make the development of tardive dyskinesia more likely. This latter condition is particularly serious as it may not respond to withdrawal of the antipsychotic drug.

Because of the serious nature of these effects, long-term treatment with antipsychotic drugs should only be embarked upon when symptoms are seriously impairing the quality of life, or patients are a serious risk to themselves or others. All patients taking the drugs should be closely monitored and reviewed at regular intervals in the hope that it will be possible to discontinue medication.

Antipsychotic drugs are liable to result in interference with temperature regulation and also to cause hypotension, so that elderly persons need careful appraisal before a drug is started, and smaller doses if it is prescribed.

Available drugs

Most of these drugs fall into the phenothiazine group but some belong to other groups. The choice of which drug to use depends on the degree of sedation required, and on the individual patient's response to the drug in terms of wanted and unwanted effects. For long-term management depot preparations, as already mentioned, are available.

Chlorpromazine is the most widely used of this group. It is markedly sedating, and so useful in agitated patients. In the elderly, the slightly weaker promazine may be a better choice.

Thioridazine is useful in the elderly as it seems less likely to induce parkinsonian effects.

Flupenthixol has a slightly mood elevating effect and may be used by the oral or depot injection route. It is perhaps the drug of choice for apathetic patients.

Fluphenazine is also available for oral or depot use, is more sedating, and is more likely to cause parkinsonian effects.

Haloperidol is useful for the rapid control of manic states.

The approximate equivalent dosage of these drugs is given in Table 4.4

Table 4.4. *Approximate equivalent dosages of antipsychotic drugs*

Chlorpromazine	100 mg
Thioridazine	100 mg
Flupenthixol	3 mg
Fluphenazine	2 mg
Haloperidol	2 mg

Lithium

Lithium is indicated in the treatment and long-term prophylaxis of recurrent mania (and occasionally depression). Lithium quietens the overactive patient, though in mania a more quickly acting sedative, such as haloperidol, is usually required at first. Because of the risk of irreversible toxic encephalopathy, antipsychotic drugs like haloperidol should not be given concurrently with lithium.

Lithium has the potential for toxic side-effects, and its dosage needs to be carefully monitored by regular measurement of plasma concentrations — rather like treatment with anticoagulants. The advised therapeutic range is 0.6–1.2 mmol of lithium/litre, though for maintenance, or in the elderly, the lower end of this range should be aimed for. Overdosage can cause many side-effects, including tremor, ataxia, dysarthria, and renal impairment. Sodium depletion, for instance through the concurrent use of thiazide diuretics, potentiates these side-effects. Lithium can also cause hypothyroidism, and this needs to be checked for regularly, e.g. every six months.

For all these reasons, the decision to use lithium needs to be carefully considered with regard to the likely benefits and risks in the individual patient. Most GPs will feel the need to involve a consultant psychiatrist in the decision.

Lithium is usually given as the carbonate, but the various preparations available (see the *British National Formulary*) have widely different bioavailability, which makes it advisable to stick to using one branded make.

References

1. Balint, M. (1964). *The doctor, his patient and the illness* (2nd edn). Pitman Medical, London.
2. Anderson, S. and Hasler, J. C. (1979). Counselling in general practice. *J. R. Coll. Gen. Pract.* **29**, 352–6.
3. Robson, M. H., France, R., and Bland, M. (1984). Clinical psychologists in primary care: controlled clinical and economic evaluation. *Br. Med. J.* **288**, 1805–8.
4. Catalan, J., Gath, D., Bond, A., and Martin, P. (1984). The effects of nonprescribing of anxyolitics in general practice II. *Br. J. Psychiat.* **144**, 602–10.

5. Catalan, J., Gath, D., Edmonds, G., and Eunis, J. (1984). The effects of non-prescribing of anxyolitics in general practice I. *Br. J. Psychiat.* **144**, 602–10.
6. Strathdee, G. and Williams, P. (1986). Patterns of collaboration. In *Mental health illness in the primary care setting* (ed. M. Shepherd, G. Wilkinson, and P. Williams). Tavistock, London.
7. Tyrar, P. J. (1984). Benzodiazepines on trial. *Br. Med. J.* **288**, 1101–2.
8. Waydenfeld, D. and Waydenfeld, S. (1980). Counselling in general practice. *J. R. Coll. Gen. Pract.* **30**, 671–7.
9. Marks, I. (1985). Controlled trial of psychiatric nurse therapists in primary care. *Br. Med. J.* **290**, 1181–4.
10. Earll, L. and Kincey, J. (1982). Clinical psychology in general practice: a controlled trial evaluation. *J. R. Coll. Gen. Pract.* **32**, 32–7.
11. Ashurst, P. M. (1982). Counselling in general practice. In *Psychiatry and general practice* (ed. A. W. Clare and M. Lader), Academic Press, London.
12. Ashton, H. (1984). Benzodiazepine withdrawal: an unfinished story. *Br. Med. J.* **288**, 1135–40.
13. Balter, M. B., Manheimer, D. I., Mellinger, G. D., and Uhlenhuth, E. H. (1984). *Curr. Med. Res. Opin.* **8**, (4), 5–20.
14. Wyld, K. L. (1981). Counselling in general practice: a review. *Br. J. Guid. Counsell.* **9**, 129–41.
15. Paykel, E. S. (1988). Personal communication.

4.8   COMMUNITY SERVICES

The primary care team (PCT) has a range of resources with which to meet psychological problems presented to it. The typical core team of doctor, nurse, and health visitor can tackle a large proportion of these, and it has been estimated that only one in 20 of such patients is referred outside this core group.

If the core PCT resources are not sufficient, referral can be made to social workers, marriage guidance counsellors, local authority educational psychologists, domiciliary occupational therapists, community psychiatric nurses, clinical psychologists, or a wide variety of lay therapists. The GP will still retain primary medical responsibility for the patient. Alternatively, responsibility for the patient may be transferred to a psychiatrist and the care of the patient to the psychiatric rather than the primary care team.

At one time this distinction between GP-centred care and psychiatrist-centred care implied a clear dichotomy between care in the patient's home and community, and care delivered from a central hospital or hospital-based clinic. Recent changes in the organization of psychiatric services have blurred this distinction, and for many years it has been Health Service policy to change the focus of psychiatric care from the hospital to the community.

The arguments for centring a range of psychological services on the PCT are strong. This is the starting point for most patients' care and, in addition, this arrangement makes continuity of care more likely. Also it ensures that the existing knowledge which the team has of the relevant familial and other environmental factors will be available, whether the GP or the psychiatrist is nominally in charge.

When the GP, or other member of the PCT, refers the patient directly to the therapist, waste of time can be eliminated. It is no longer necessary for patients to wait for out-patient appointments with e.g. a psychiatrist who may refer them on to another waiting list for assessment by, for example, a psychologist. Significant reductions in delay have been achieved in this way.[1] People can get help in a crisis or at the point when they are ready to accept help, rather than having to wait until the critical moment has passed. Also, considerable savings can be made in the time required for therapy, as the patient's problems are formulated by the referring member of the PCT and the therapist together, without going through an intermediate 'ordering' which may be incompatible with the final model of treatment.

Responding to this logic, psychotherapists,[2] community psychiatric nurses[3,4] and clinical psychologists[5,6] have been attached to PCTs. They accept referrals from the PCT, the GP retains overall medical responsibility, and the attached worker is clinically responsible for their own work and managerially accountable to their own profession. Social workers and psychologists are likely to adopt a rather different approach to psychological problems than psychiatrists, seeing them in the context of normal living rather than as an illness.

If this arrangement is to work, however, the members of the PCT need to have a good understanding of the uses, strengths, and weaknesses of the various statutory and non-statutory helpers available to them. These are likely to vary from district to district. Time and trouble taken to get to know how the local network of mental health services operate, and in cultivating a working relationship with the people found to be trustworthy within them, is time well spent.

Access

Some practices are experimenting with open access to all members of their team, and linked to this is the subject of open or personal doctors' lists. There are certain advantages and disadvantages.

The advantages are that:

● Some patients prefer to go straight to the therapist without seeing the GP, because of embarrassment at the nature of the problem or because of the GP's continuing relationship to them and their family.

● It saves the doctor's time.

- The therapist can see the patients before the problems have been 'structured' through talking to other members of the team.

- It gives autonomy to both therapist and patient.

- Patients can choose a doctor or other team member who is thought to have particular skills.

The disadvantages are that:

- Physical and mental illness may be left undiagnosed.

- Nobody sees themselves as responsible for the patient. Balint describes this as the 'collusion of anonymity'.[7] It applies not only between doctors and other members of the PCT, but also between one doctor and another. In particular, there is the danger that no doctor will grasp the nettle in the case of the difficult patient who may shop around doctors and the team.

- Patients may be divided into parcels, psychological problems for the psychologist, social problems for the social worker, and organic problems for the doctor. This undermines one of the greatest assets of the general practitioner, that the whole patient can be helped by one person.

- Doctors who have helped patients at length with psychological problems may feel hurt if patients choose a different doctor for their cough. Implicit in this disadvantage is the problem of confidentiality.

Teams will need to make up their own minds on this issue. Many feel that the advantages of personal lists and, perhaps, family lists outweigh the disadvantages, but that open access by patients to all members of the team needs to be available in order to safeguard freedom of choice.

Psychiatric care

Despite the policy of shifting psychiatric care to the community, there are few parts of Britain in which this can truly be said to be taking place. Psychiatric training is virtually confined to hospitals,[9] and the development of psychiatric units in District General Hospitals has only served, in some areas, to switch the focus from one kind of institution to another.

An outline of one possible form of organization was published in 1975 in a government publication *Better services for the mentally ill*. This recommended the division of each area into sectors ('Sectorization'), each of which was to be served by a separate community team including psychiatrists, community psychiatric nurses, and social workers. Although these teams were expected to take responsibility for most of the serious psychiatric problems that occur in their sectors, specialist teams would continue to have area-wide or region-wide responsibility for psychogeriatrics, child psychiatry, forensic psychiatry, and, in some areas, psychotherapy, alcoholism, and drug abuse.

Sectorization has now been introduced in many parts of Britain, and this has led to some improvements in the liaison between primary and secondary care teams. Sector psychiatrists will undertake all the domiciliary visits that are requested in their sector, and this enables them to get to know, and be known by, the GP and other members of the PCT. But there are many sectors in which psychiatrists seldom set foot outside their own hospitals, and the community psychiatric nurses remain answerable, and available, only to psychiatrists rather than to the PCTs.

Many publications have emphasized the importance of proper liaison between the primary care and psychiatric teams.[9,10] Although everybody pays lip-service to this ideal, it is seldom achieved within systems which rely on a referral model (p. 49). Liaison is usually limited to a letter which the GP sends to the hospital when referring a patient, and a report from the psychiatrist which comes in reply. The GP and the psychiatrist seldom, if ever, meet; they know little of the contribution which each team can make to the other, and they seldom collaborate in any real sense when caring for patients. Small wonder that they have got caught up in a game of 'pass the parcel'. Many GPs are dissatisfied with the help which they get from psychiatrists, and many psychiatrists take a poor view of the psychiatric care provided by GPs.

Psychiatrist liaison attachments

Rather than retreating into their hospitals, however, some psychiatrists are responding to this challenge by themselves making liaison attachments. By moving out of the hospital into the GP's surgery, they become easily accessible to all of the primary care team and attached workers who are concerned with the treatment of psychological problems (see Chapter 2 for further discussion and references). Often all that is needed to persuade psychiatrists to leave their hospital base is an invitation. In other cases a letter from the local medical committee to the District Manager and the Community Health Council may work wonders. An extension of this kind of regular consultation is the inclusion of trainee GPs and trainee psychiatrists. Thus, one of us (CMP) currently makes fortnightly visits with a trainee psychiatrist to a group practice with its own trainee GP. The GPs select a patient who is clerked by the trainee psychiatrist during the hour before the consultant arrives. This case history is then presented to the general practice partners and the consultant by the referring GP, the trainee psychiatrist reports his or her findings, and there is a general discussion on management. Final responsibility rests with the referring GP, since the consultant's role is simply to consult, but he does, of course, have access to the full range of psychiatric services if these are needed. Meetings of this kind not only result in improved care for the patient, but they also provide invaluable training for the trainees of both specialties.

Although consultations between psychiatrists and general practitioners are usually centred on the patient's problems and feelings, Michael Balint made an important contribution when he encouraged GPs to share with each other their own problems and feelings about their patients.[7] Whether this is done in special 'Balint Groups' set up for the purpose, or simply as part of the regular discussion process, for instance between partners, it is likely to lead to greater sensitivity to the ways in which patients influence their doctors and doctors their patients. It can also lead to increasing the GP's awareness of the psychological components in many presentations of illness by patients.

If referral is needed, care needs to be taken to refer the patient to the right person. This may be the psychiatrist responsible for the sector in which the patient lives, but there is often reason to choose a particular person for a particular problem. Over the years, GPs get to know consultants and can improve the chances of obtaining the treatment of their choice by referring the patient to a consultant who has a special interest in the approach they feel appropriate for the individual. Thus, some consultants favour psychotherapeutic approaches, others prefer 'organic treatments'; some make much use of behaviour therapies, others never use them; some admit many patients to hospital, others only a few.

These differences in practice reflect the personal preferences of the consultants and the fact that there are few certainties in psychiatry. By choosing a particular consultant, the risk that time will be wasted in cross-referrals is reduced. Sectorization should never restrict the freedom of GPs to choose the consultant they feel most suited to the needs of their individual patient.

Many units now have crisis intervention teams or emergency clinics which can provide urgent care. Domiciliary visits by sector consultants are worth considering in serious emergencies, and provide GPs with another opportunity to meet consultants and form a working relationship with them.

Clinical psychologists

The majority of clinical psychologists do some of their work directly with general practitioners, fulfilling recommendation 13 of the Trethowan Committee report on the role of psychologists in the Health Service: 'It is desirable that clinical psychologists should become more closely involved in the primary care setting with general practitioners.'

Apart from this official encouragement, there are reasons, to do with the way the profession works, for conducting at least some part of its activity outside hospital settings. New approaches to psychological treatment in the 1950s and 1960s put considerable emphasis on the patient's environment as a contributory factor to the development and maintenance of psychological problems. It seldom makes sense to try to treat the patient away from that environment and, indeed, the environment may be the target for change. Any approach which considers patients' problems to lie in their adaptation to the environment, rather than primarily within themselves, is at variance with the concept of the hospital as the preferred site for treatment, unless 'asylum' is required.

Delays occur if patients are first referred through a psychiatric clinic, and such consultations may lead patients to think about their problems in ways that subvert psychological treatment. For example, a passive illness model may work quite well when patients are treated pharmacologically, but does not prepare them for treatments which require them to take a more active part.

To some extent, the conflict of models used by clinical psychologists and psychiatrists may have led psychologists to seek more compatible working liaisons in order to offer better treatment, and to seek this with general practitioners who are more attuned to seeing patients as having problems rather than illnesses.

Methods of working

A number of surveys and reports have now been published describing and evaluating the work of clinical psychologists with general practitioners.[5,6] At the simplest level, GPs may refer patients directly to clinical psychologists without going through a hospital consultant. At the other extreme there are psychologists working in health centres as part of the primary health care team. A common variant is sessional work in the health centre combined with other work at hospital-based clinics. The psychologist may work directly with patients, or in an advisory capacity to the GP, the health centre nurse, the health visitor, or other member of the primary care team. All possible variations in style of working are currently in operation. Psychologists may, according to their expertise, specialize in work with a particular age group, such as children or the elderly. They may limit the patients they see to those with a 'psychological problem', or they may be prepared to contribute to the care of patients whose problems, although normally considered physical, may benefit from psychological treatment. Although the 'bread and butter' of their work is the management of patients with anxiety and phobic problems, and the cognitive treatment of depression (see Section 3.4), other ways of integration are possible. One recent success was for a psychologist, in conjunction with a health visitor, to run groups for the parents of children with sleeping problems. Not only was the group highly effective (results to be published) but, after the clinical psychologist's original input, the health visitor was able to continue running successful groups and was able to pass on her skills to other health visitors. In this way some of the psychologist's approaches and skills can be passed on to the other members of the team. Psychologists are frequently involved in teaching and in research in the practice.

With this variety of operations, it is important that the members of the team, including the psychologist, are aware of the different expectations which they have of each other, in order to establish the form of working which makes best use of their skills and best suits their needs. Case discussions, which all members of the team (including the psychologist) attend, are a valuable way of enhancing this understanding.

Community psychiatric nurses

Community psychiatric nurses (CPNs) were initially introduced to provide after care (tertiary prevention) for patients on discharge from hospital (checking on medication, and advising patients and families about other sources of help in the community), but many of them are now taking on much wider roles. Their training in psychiatric nursing makes them good listeners, most are able to make use of problem-oriented assessment and management plans, but they are also likely to be aware of the value of medication when this is needed and to recognize those patients for whom psychiatric consultation is likely to be of value. In other words, they can help with many of the problems met with in general practice and are of special value in working with the more intractable mentally ill patients.

Their training for community work will have extended their experience in the hospital setting but, like psychologists and psychiatrists, they vary in their special interests and skills. Many of them are now being trained in the skills of counselling and crisis intervention.[3] A few have special training in working with children and some CPNs accept direct referrals from GPs and other members of the PCT. A few visit general practices in order to consult about psychological problems, including the management of alcohol and drug addiction, a type of liaison which needs to be encouraged.

Social workers

Social workers are even more varied in the degree of psychological sophistication which they bring to their work. Because each district has its team of generic social workers, those attached to hospitals tend to confine their activities to the needs of patients attending the hospital. Social workers based in the community are more likely to make links with the primary care team, but they exhibit a variable knowledge of, and interest in, psychological problems and their management. However, their family orientation and knowledge of local services make them a valuable source of support.

Social workers are always involved in the proceedings necessary when taking a child into the care of the local authority, and they should always be notified when a child is thought to be at risk of physical or sexual abuse. Their interest in these areas makes them good people to help with many aspects of child care. With the advent of the 1985 Mental Health Act appointed social workers are made responsible for compulsory admission to psychiatric care, and programmes of training have been introduced to enable them to fulfil this role. They also have important roles to play in crisis intervention and many of them have an interest in the psychodynamics of families, which is particularly relevant in a PCT. Social workers with special training in psychotherapy can be especially useful if linked with general practice teams.[2] This is another area in which close liaison pays dividends within the PCT, e.g. through joint meetings for case discussion.

Logistics

There is, of course, an overlap between the roles and skills of psychiatrists, community psychiatric nurses, psychologists, and social workers. This means that, to some degree, they are interchangeable and GPs can adapt their plans according to the services available, and to the personalities, interests, and skills of the individuals. Inspired opportunism enables GPs to choose between the various resources which exist in their own locality. If a psychiatrist is not willing to visit the practice regularly, it may be possible to persuade a psychologist to do so. If all the services are overworked, perhaps each of them can be persuaded to visit once a month or every two months. The average consultant psychiatrist conducts four out-patient clinics per week, that is, one session for *c.* 15 000 population. A general practice team of six partners caters for up to the same number of patients. It is, therefore, reasonable and economic for psychiatrists to transfer part of their out-patient time (say one session per fortnight) to each of two group practices in the locality. Similarly, clinical psychologists can organize primary care attachments that maintain the balance of services.[1]

There may be conflict between the various professionals about the best allocation of resources. Psychiatrists are often perplexed and annoyed to see hard-won community resources slipping from their control. It is difficult enough to get psychiatric patients out of hospital at the best of times, they argue, but if the community psychiatric nurses are all treating agoraphobics in GP surgeries they can't be providing community support for discharged schizophrenics.

Yet it is surely GPs rather than psychiatrists who bear first-line responsibility for the care of people in the community, be they agoraphobic or schizophrenic, and it is they who should decide between competing priorities of care.

To exercise this function effectively they must have a close liaison with the specialist workers. If the local mental health professionals are not providing the service that is needed, GPs should not hesitate to make suggestions and to nag them until they respond. At the very least, the psychiatrists and psychologists will begin to realize that local GPs are interested in the psychiatric and psychological problems of their patients, and this may foster a better working relationship. GPs who take the trouble to visit their patients in hospital, and to seek out the doctors in charge, will become known and will learn something of the strength and weakness of the service. Hospital staff sometimes set up multi-disciplinary meetings or training sessions in their own districts, and these are useful not only for sharing knowledge, but enhancing appropriate skills on both sides of the 'divide'. Psychiatric staff seldom attend teaching events run by GPs, yet the value of multi-disciplinary team work is never greater than it is in the management of psychological problems, and this kind of training has special value.

Finally, just as the family should constitute a caring network to the mutual advantage of its members, so the community team should be a family system to its members. Each of these types of family exists to provide care, but they can only do this if they also look after each other. This means that each member of each team should become aware of the needs of the others with whom they work. By reaching out to each other we make possible the relationships from which effective patient care can spring, for in the final analysis relationships are what it is all about.

Referral process

Many reasons exist for the referral of patients by GPs to other professionals. The need for advice, the desire for the patient's care to be taken over by the hospital (especially for patients with serious behavioural problems or with risk of suicide), the failure to respond to the GPs treatment, the patient's own request for referral, and sometimes the need for relief of the GP.

The concept of the primary team being extended to include other professionals means that different forms of communication may need to be worked out — formal letters are no longer enough. The availability of GPs' records to peruse, and make entries into, enables relevant information to be available for all those professionally and confidentially involved in the patient's health care. Adequate summary cards containing family histories as well as past medical and psychiatric records, coupled with either family record cards or the filing of family records together, allows for a less formal method of referral, more akin to the internal referrals occurring between specialists in hospital or between members of the PCT.

Where no direct contact with the psychiatrist or other professional is possible, the GP contributes to the value of the assessment through the content of the referral letter. The recipient needs to know exactly why the referral was made, what the GP hopes from the referral, what kinds of difficulty the GP has been having with the patient and/or family, and any impression or information about them which might not otherwise be obtained. It is important to list all drugs that have been or are being prescribed, along with the response to them, and any side-effects that have occurred. Information about previous referrals for help with psychological problems may be useful.

GPs often know a family well and have visited the patient's home. In such cases they are in possession of information which will be of great assistance. Detailed repetition of the history is not necessary when the patient is referred to someone who will obtain the history from the patient, but the GP's general observations may be invaluable.

Finally, the other professionals will want to know whether the GP or other members of the primary care team wish to continue to be involved in the management of the problem, or whether they would prefer responsibility to be taken over. Such comments as 'I have got to know and like this person over the years and will be glad to continue to see her', or 'This patient has been a great nuisance to my partners and myself in recent months and we would be grateful if you will do your best to reduce or share this burden', are helpful.

A proper assessment takes time and will include very much more than the attribution of a diagnostic label. This may be the first time that a patient has taken a bird's eye view of their own life history and there are many who find this very helpful. In fact, Malan *et al*.[11] found that many patients referred to the adult department at the Tavistock Clinic were so much helped by the diagnostic assessment that they required no further treatment, a finding many GPs making their own assessments of patients would support.

Although most psychiatrists and psychologists make full assessments and take the trouble to communicate these to the GP by letter, time taken in discussion is time well spent, be it face to face or by telephone. Sadly, it is a reflection of the gap between hospital and community services that GPs seldom meet their hospital colleagues at case conferences at which their patients are discussed.

Non-statutory services

Although it is, or should be, the aim of the statutory services to provide a full range of treatments for psychological problems, there are deficiencies in many areas and there are some services, notably those concerned with counselling and prevention, which are rarely provided. There are also many patients who will not accept referral to the statutory services and who press for consideration of other alternatives. When all the varieties of 'fringe' activity are taken into consideration, the list is endless, but it is wise to limit referrals to a relatively small number of responsible services which we can get to know and trust.

Patient preference is an important factor and the PCT needs to familiarize itself with the services available to particular ethnic and religious groups in the locality. A depressed Indian housewife who speaks no English may not get much help from an English counsellor but may benefit greatly from being introduced to the local Indian mothers' group.

Private fee-paying services vary from those provided by private psychiatrist (who often lack the ancillary services available within the NHS), to relatively inexpensive non-medical psychotherapists or counsellors. Such practitioners should have received proper training and accreditation at a responsible institute and it is worth checking the credentials of any therapist who is not personally known. Anyone can be a self-styled 'psychotherapist' and there are some very dubious practitioners of this trade.

Voluntary services can often be relied on to provide sensitive and effective counselling. Volunteers often have time to get to know well the people whom they help. Bodies such as The Samaritans, Marriage Guidance Council (recently renamed 'Relate'), Victim Support Scheme, and Cruse (for the bereaved) take pains to select and train volunteers in particular types of counselling. Before long they become at least as 'expert' as the professionals at their particular type of activity. MIND (formerly the National Association for Mental Health) has branches in many areas. These provide various counselling and group activities for patients with psychological problems and their families. A range of self-help or mutual-help groups exist (e.g. Alcoholics Anonymous) at which people with particular problems can meet others who are in a similar predicament. The emotional support and practical guidance which people can obtain in such groups is very striking. Finally, there are a number of telephone 'hot-lines' and 'drop-in' services in most areas. These enable people to get immediate help with a variety of problems without the stigma of having to be designated as 'sick'.

Keeping an up-to-date list of available facilities in a surgery or health centre is time consuming but very useful. Some areas have local Councils of Voluntary Service to provide information and co-ordination of the various voluntary activities. In other areas, social workers and Citizen's Advice Bureaux are likely to be the best sources of information on what is locally available. Many practices are now setting out to computerize their own lists. A list (but only of national bodies) is provided in Appendix II.

A few general practitioners recruit and train their own voluntee counsellors. Others develop close working links with a particular agency who may even be willing to allocate a counsellor to work within the GP surgery. These links encourage much greater mutual trust than is usual, and enable

;Ps to widen the range of caring services which they offer. This kind of xtension of the primary care team is considered at a number of points in his book.

References

1. Johnston, M. (1978). The work of a clinical psychologist in primary care. *J. R. Coll. Gen. Pract.* **28**, 661–7.
2. Brook, A. and Temperley, J. (1976). The contribution of a psychotherapist to general practice. *J. R. Coll. Gen. Pract.* **26**, 86–94.
3. Marks, I. (1985). Controlled trial of psychiatric nurse therapists in primary care. *Br. Med. J.* **290**, 1181–4.
4. Paykel, E. S., Mangen, S. P., Griffith, J. H., and Burns, T. P. (1982). Community psychiatric nursing for neurotic patients: a controlled trial. *Br. J. Psychiat.* **140**, 573–81.
5. Earll, L. and Kincey, J. (1982). Clincial psychology in general practice. *J. R. Coll. Gen. Pract.* **32**, 32–7.
6. Robson, M. H., France, R., and Bland, M. (1984). Clinical psychologists in primary care. *Br. Med. J.* **288**, 1805–8.
7. Balint, M. (1964). *The doctor, his patient and the illness.* Tavistock, London.
8. Freeman, H. (1985). Training for community psychiatry. *Bull. R. Coll. Psychiat.* **9**, 29–32.
9. Tredgold, R. (1976). Collaboration between general practitioner and psychiatrist. *News and Notes of Br. J. Psychiat.* March, 8–9.
10. Brook, A. (1967). An experiment in general practioner/psychiatrist cooperation. *J. R. Coll. Gen. Pract.* **13**, 127–31.
11. Malan, D. H., Bacal, H. A., Heath, E. S., and Balfour, F. H. G. (1968). A study of psychodynamic changes in untreated neurotic patients—I. *Br. J. Psychiat.* **141**, 525–51.

5 The family life cycle and its turning points

5.1 INTRODUCTION

In so far as a person is secure, with a reasonable degree of self-confidence and trust in others, and a sense of being 'on course', that person's mental health will probably be good. This happy state is likely to arise when our current assumptive model of the world accords well with the real world in which we live and when our expectations of the future are positive, that is to say, we predict that those changes which come about will bring us closer to our goals in life rather than further away.

Conversely, anything which reduces security, undermines our confidence, destroys trust, or throws us 'off course' is a threat to mental health. Changes within us or in our environment may create major discrepancies between our life space and the internal models by which we recognize and relate to that world, and these are particularly hard to cope with if they are seen as making it more difficult for us to move towards our major goals in life.

Such psychosocial transitions are likely to arise at all the turning points in the life cycle and this accounts for the increased prevalence of psychological problems at these times. But times of change, as we have seen, are also opportunities for maturation and the person who successfully completes the transition from one stage to another will be better prepared for further changes than the person who has resisted change or been protected from the need to change.

The members of the primary care team are often consulted at times of change, either because they are involved in the process of change (e.g. at times of birth or death) or because they are asked for help with symptoms which arise out of the stress of change. Sometimes we can help people to anticipate a change and prepare themselves, at other times we only become involved after the change has taken place.

Many of the changes which occur as part of the life cycle are predictable, and people may spend a lot of time preparing for them. If the preparation is conducted in a realistic and effective way, the transition will be smooth. But there are many reasons why this may not be so and, at such times, problems are likely to arise.

In the chapter which follows we shall consider the particular difficulties which arise at each stage of the life cycle and in the transitions from stage to stage.

We have adapted as our model the life cycle which is still common, but by no means invariable, in our society. That is to say, the progression from:

- child at home;

- child at school;

- young person who has left home;

- young married person, making a home;

- couple with a home with children;

- couple whose children have left home;

- retired couple;

- elderly couple;

- widow or widower alone; and

- terminally ill.

There are, of course, many who do not follow this cycle, children without homes, parents without partners, couples without children, elderly who will never retire, etc. They, too, need consideration and, where space permits, we have tried to consider their special problems and possibilities.

Finally, in Section 5.12, we look at some of the unscheduled, and therefore unexpected, transitions which sometimes occur and which carry special risk *because* they do not allow for adequate preparation.

5.2   BIRTH

Although Otto Rank and other psychoanalysts have made much of the psychological stress (or 'primal trauma') which is supposedly inflicted on the baby during the birth experience, and some adult patients have been so thoroughly analysed that they claim to have recalled this event, the evidence for regarding birth as a major psychological trauma for the child is thin. Certainly there are a few children who suffer brain damage at the time of birth and they will be considered in Chapter 7, but the baby's brain is at an incomplete stage of development at this time and, although the fetus can respond to sensory stimuli, it lacks any orienting experience which might make sense of the changes in bodily sensation that occur. In the circumstances it seems unlikely that the baby will retain a coherent image of this event.

Not so the mother. Her baby has been an object of considerable concern for her throughout the previous nine months and the birth experience is one which will often have been anxiously, if eagerly, anticipated. For reasons which will be discussed in Section 5.7, pregnancy and the puerperium are times when emotional disturbances commonly arise in the mother, and these may well influence the way in which she cares for the child. There is also evidence for regarding the period which immediately follows the birth as a critical period for the development of the mother's attachment to the child. Mothers who are separated from their new-born babe at this time have been shown later to be less sensitive to the child's needs and messages.[1,2]

It follows that mothers should be given the opportunity to hold and to care for their new-born child as soon as it is possible for them to do so. They should also be given the emotional support which they will need before, during, and after delivery. Often the husband will be the best person to do this, but he too may need support, for the birth of a child, particularly a first child, is a major event for both parents.

References

1. Klaus, M. H. and Kennell, J. H. (1976). *Maternal infant bonding: the impact of early separation and loss on family development.* C. V. Mosby, St Louis.
2. O'Connor, S. W., Vietze, R. M., Hopkins, S. B., and Altemeier, W. A. (1977). Post-partum extended maternal–infant contact: subsequent mothering and child health. *Pediat. Res.* **11**, 380.

5.3   EARLY CHILD DEVELOPMENT

Small babies appear to be very fragile things and it is not surprising that mothers often require reassurance that their physical and emotional development is 'normal'. Table 5.1 gives a picture of the ages by which each of the common milestones are reached.

Allowing for a fair amount of individual variation, it is advisable to refer any child who is late in reaching any of these milestones to an expert, e.g. a paediatrician, unless the cause for the delay is clear and treatable.

More variable, and therefore more difficult to evaluate, are the normal milestones for emotional and social development. Because these are socially as well as psychologically and physically determined, behaviour that is 'normal' in one culture or one family may be deviant in another. Even so, there is a range of normality for such behaviour as clinging, aggressiveness, and shyness and the members of the primary care team (PCT) are often in a position to recognize problems which may have serious consequences if they are ignored.

Insecurity in parenting and some vicious circles

Young babies vary greatly in their crying, restlessness, and general sensitivity. Some start at the slightest sound and cry readily, others are placid and

Table 5.1. *Milestones of normal child development*

Age	Milestones

Birth	Sucks nipple or finger
	Follows moving light with eyes
	Grasps with fingers and toes
	Moro reflex: abruptly strike pillow —
	    baby extends arms, then brings them
	    together
	Rooting reflex: tickle side of mouth —
	    baby roots towards that side

1–8 weeks	Vocalizations increase Visually attentive
3–4 weeks	Eye-to-eye contact is established
c. 3 months	Smiles at face Holds head up when placed prone
c. 4 months	Enjoys being held upright Moro reflex ceases
c. 6 months	Smiles more at familiar than unfamiliar faces Eye-to-hand co-ordination
c. 7 months	maintains sitting posture
c. 9 months	Stands when held Crawls Repeats sounds Fearful of strangers
c. 1 year	Weight around three times that at birth 1–6 teeth Speaks a few words (e.g. Mama) Points to eyes (etc.) on command Throws ball
c. 13 months	Climbs upstairs (beware!)
c. 15 months	Starts to walk unaided Shows some comprehension of simple language
c. 18 months	Knows 3–50 words
c 2 years	Uses two-word expressions Runs, but falls on sudden turns
c. 2½ years	Bowel trained Jumps in air with both feet Builds tower of six cubes Seems to understand most of what is said
5 years	88 per cent have bladder control

sluggish. The mother–child unit is constantly changing. If the mother is anxious, this fidgets the child and may, in turn, agitate the mother. Vicious circles of anxiety and tension may result in feeding problems, failure to thrive, excessive crying, restless nights, fear of strangers, clinging behaviour, hyperactivity, whimpering, and irritability in the baby. As it grows older, bedwetting, constipation, aggressive behaviour, temper tantrums, delayed learning, night terrors, sleep walking, stammering, tics, mannerisms, and provocative and self-punitive behaviour may result.

In the mother, increasing tension may lead to irritability, impulsive physical and verbal abuse of the child, punitive behaviour, inability to touch or cuddle the child, or its opposite—excessive clinging, over-protection, and intrusive behaviour. Some mothers become so depressed that they withdraw from their children, show little affection, and give up proper care. Their behaviour can react on their spouse, just as his behaviour can affect them. Thus, the whole family unit may cease to be a source of mutual support and become a monstrous trap from which nobody can escape for fear of worse. A lot of damage is done by parents who take the view that 'You must stop that kind of behaviour (be it clinging, bedwetting, demanding the bedroom light on, or other signs of anxiety), before it takes hold or it will lead to more trouble'. The classification of all upsetting behaviour as 'bad' leads to punitive actions which only increase the child's insecurity. Mother and child get trapped in a mutually ambivalent relationship characterized by such confusing messages as 'I only slap you because I love you', or, 'If you keep on like that, I'll give you to the policeman (or kill myself)'.

This kind of rigid, punitive behaviour contrasts with its opposite, the mother who is quite unable to set limits. Some mothers are so scared of being accused of neglecting their child, or fearful of the child rejecting them, that they find themselves incapable of saying 'No'. Parents may need our permission to get angry, stick by their decisions, and punish their children when they step over reasonable limits.

While a mother was talking to her doctor, her 18-month-old baby pulled a tissue from a box on the table. Another tissue popped up to take its place. The baby, much delighted with this new game, grabbed another tissue and another. At this point the mother said, 'Don't do that dear.' She was ignored. Before long the floor was littered with tissues. The mother then took the box away from the baby who proceeded to cry lustily. The tissues were promptly returned and the game continued until the entire contents of the box lay on the floor and the child was crying for more.

Such behaviour turns the child into a little tyrant unable to control its own impulses because it has never had them controlled by others. 'No' does not mean 'No', it means 'Maybe if you make a fuss you will get what you want.' The child is being taught to use coercion as a means of getting its own way.

Inappropriate child management may be a reflection of differences between the parents. Often each parent was brought up in a different way and with quite different preconceptions of how to handle their child. This leads to inconsistent messages to the child and often conflicts between the parents, with the child caught in between.

In such cases it is important to see both parents together and encourage them to agree on management. Even if their agreed plan seems inappropriate to us, it will probably suit the child better than the previous confusion.

These self-perpetuating and self-aggravating problems are a common cause of symptoms that bring people to the attention of the PCT. Only by talking to *all* relevant family members can we expect to make a proper assessment of the problem. When we do this, many symptoms which had been perplexing begin to make sense to them and to us. Parents inevitably feel responsible for anything that happens to their children. Their guilt may make them touchy, reluctant to accept help, and inclined to exculpate themselves by blaming others for their difficulties.

'My baby is driving me mad, you must give him a sedative.'

'My husband doesn't understand, he won't do his share.'

'My wife is so preoccupied with this new baby that she doesn't seem to care for me and the older children.'

Complaints of this kind are likely indicators of a disturbed family unit, which may need our help.

Proper diagnosis includes a careful physical examination of the child, which usually enables the doctor to give positive reassurance and clear explanation to the parents. This itself is often sufficient to break vicious circles.

Other acts which may reverse the circular effect are:

- Seeing both parents and even the whole family together in order to make sure that all who need to be are involved (see also Section 4.4 on family therapy). Joint meetings ensure that responsibility for care remains where it belongs (in the family) and de-escalates patterns of interaction which are aggravating or perpetuating themselves. Fathers can sometimes be persuaded to take a more active part in child care, and mothers feel less guilty and anxious if responsibility is shared. At the same time, we should reassure the parents of their own competence and recognize their needs for support.

- Drawing in additional support from the extended family, perhaps by suggesting that the mother take a break or obtain help with the child.

- Putting the mother in touch with a mutual support group for mothers.

- Drawing in the support of a health visitor, social worker, home help, Family Service Unit, etc. as appropriate.

● Prescribing for the mother a few tablets of diazepam (2–5 mg) for emergency use only with appropriate warnings against over-reliance on these drugs.

● Providing a buffer for use if the parents should get to the end of their tether. This may be a simple reassurance that they should come back for further help 'before things get bad again', or a telephone number which they can phone if things build up.

Mrs A, an ex-ballet dancer with a forceful manner, an ineffectual husband, and a disorganized household, had just about coped with her first child, a daughter. A son was born three years later and was 'a problem' from the start. He wouldn't feed properly, wouldn't sleep through the night even after a year, and had recurrent upper respiratory infections. His mother became more and more distraught, and on one occasion consulted her GP with her daughter and son, both with colds, and she herself with thirteen symptoms! Her GP involved the health visitor, and over a few weeks pre-nursery school was arranged for the daughter, Mrs A was given help with ordering her son's eating and sleeping habits, and the confused husband was helped to achieve a useful role in the home. Frequent visits by the health visitor helped Mrs A to restore her self-confidence and ability to cope, and a year later she and the rest of the family were well and hadn't been near the doctor for several months.

Specific problems

Sleepless nights

Sleepless nights can be a 'nightmare' for the parents, the children, and the doctor. A vicious circle often arises in which the baby wakens, the parents attempt to deal with the problem in ways which are inappropriate, and the baby wakes more as they become more tired.

Causes

Breast-fed babies tend to wake more than bottle-fed, breast milk being more dilute than bottle milk, though it is more valuable in other ways. Being in a special care unit, birth trauma, developing an illness, or having to go into hospital, all disturb the learning of sleep patterns. This is difficult for the parents who may become anxious and convey their anxiety to the child. Irritability and anxiety are infectious. The child faced with an angry or anxious parent:

● loses its appetite;

● gets tummy ache;

● stays awake for the rest of the night.

Sleepless nights may also reflect disagreements within the marriage (e.g. about who is responsible for night feeds).

Parents commonly mishandle sleeping problems, rewarding the child's cries by cuddles and games, breaking routines and varying their approaches, so that the child loses any sense of security. In this way they perpetuate difficulties that might otherwise have resolved.

Management

A careful assessment of what happens will be the beginning of treatment, and a useful technique is to ask the parents to keep a diary. This will show them that we understand their anxiety and are prepared to help. Positive reassurance must be given about any fears for the health of the baby, and goals defined in terms of the parent's needs for rest (which are usually greater than those of the baby).

Children should not be expected to sleep all night, but can be expected to remain in their cots or beds throughout the night without disturbing their parents.

By creating a set of expectations and habits the child comes to know when bedtime occurs and gets conditioned to go to sleep given certain cues. For most families it is important to establish a ritual at bedtime, which should be relatively unvarying, particularly when the child is learning to sleep. It may involve a bath, being read to, etc. This routine should be adhered to (if the limit is one story there should be no exceptions). Some children will like an object as a cue to going to bed, perhaps a favourite toy or a musical box that is started just before they go to sleep every night. In many ways the cot is the cue to sleep. If there are sleeping problems, the cot should only be used for sleeping, and baby should fall asleep in the cot and not in its parents' arms. Sometimes the cot can be used in daytime more easily and then the conditioning transferred to the evening. If possible, the child should not fall asleep anywhere but in the cot.

Although some psychologists claim that crying is soon 'extinguished' if it is ignored, the loss of security which results in the child if it learns that nobody will respond to it's fears make this a dangerous 'treatment' and one with which few parents would comply. But this does not mean that parents must give up all attempts to control their child's fears. For instance, it is often possible gradually to change a child's expectations.

Shaping and gradual approaches

These are easier and less traumatic for both child and parents than extinction. As the title suggests, if the child is normally not asleep and in bed by 11.30 p.m., an agreement is made with the child (if old enough) that bedtime will start at 11.30, but will be brought forward by 20 minutes every second day, until an appropriate bedtime is reached. These approaches are slower than 'extinction', but easier. They must be kept to firmly and caringly. It is important that the child is reassured by the parent's presence and not by any play or interaction.

Children can be rewarded by parental approval and praise for positive thing. such as not coming into the parent's room, for staying in their own room, o for not crying at night. This is perhaps the most important element o management. It may be symbolically reinforced with stars, using a star chart or a series of small objects, such as transfers to complete a 'Batman' series It is important that the rewards are only given for positive behaviour and ther is *no punishment for negative behaviour*. The accompanying praise anc behaviour are important and eventually the tangible rewards can be reduced It is also important that rewards, once given, cannot be removed, howeve upsetting subsequent behaviour is. Nor must there be any bargaining or change

The response of children to drugs is very variable. Drugs have the addec disadvantage that a medical answer is provided for what is essentially ar educational problem. However, if some peace is essential, chloral hydrat (15–25 mg per kg) as an elixir, given 15–30 minutes before bed, is usuall the safest and best sedative. Alternatively, a sedative antihistamine such a trimeprazine tartrate (1.5 mg per kg, 1 hour before bed) may be preferred

Although these techniques all focus on the child, they have the secondary effect of reassuring the parents that something can be done, thereby reducing their own sense of helplessness. This will be reinforced if the doctor adopt a confident and reassuring attitude and encourages the parents to ventilat their own feelings and suggestions. Groups to help parents of children witl sleeping problems have been found helpful in the primary care setting anc are mentioned on p. 171.

Sleepwalking

This can be alarming to the parents but seldom does any harm to the child. Parents should be reassured that it is not a serious condition and advisec to lead the child gently back to bed, and to stay with him or her for a while They should avoid abruptly awakening the child, who may be distressed tc wake up in a strange place surrounded by frightened adults. Occasionally the child may need a sedative if the problem is recurrent.

Child-proof gates at the top of stairs are a wise precaution in an household, regardless of the presence of somnambulists!

Night terrors and nightmares

These need similar gentle handling. Some parents make the mistake o ignoring the child who cries at night. 'You mustn't give way to him', the say, 'He's only seeking attention. If we go up every time he cries, there' be no end to it.' Such attitudes can only increase the child's fears anc perpetuate the problem. On the other hand, the parents who go to the othe extreme by waking the child up and playing exciting games will end up witl a tired, grumpy child next day.

Children who wake, crying, during the night need someone to sit with them for a short while to reassure them that all is well. Most have forgotten their terrors by the next day. A low-voltage electric light that can be left on all night costs very little and will help the child who is afraid of the dark.

Some children wake in terror at the same time each night. This can be avoided by waking the child briefly about half an hour before the terror was due to occur.

Temper tantrums and breath-holding

The volume of voice produced by an angry toddler is out of all proportion to the toddler's size, and there are some children who can imitate the fictional Violet Elizabeth Bott and 'Scream and scream until I make myself sick.' More often, a series of angry sobs is followed by breath-holding which progresses to severe cyanosis. Alternatively, tantrums may lead to overbreathing, with carpopedal spasms resembling a convulsion.

Alarming and embarrassing as these phenomena may be, they are not an indication that the child is going mad or becoming epileptic. Mothers may need to be reassured on this score.

Tantrums often reflect and aggravate a disturbance of the mother–child relationship. They will diminish in frequency and severity if the overall level of security at home improves. Consequently, they are best treated by the means described above for providing support to both parents.

Stammers, tics, and mannerisms

These are a result of anxiety in the child, and often reflect marital conflicts in the parents. They are likely to get worse if they evoke anxious or punitive reactions in the parent. The injunction to 'stop screwing your face up like that!' draws attention to the problem and increases the anxiety that causes it.

John, aged seven, was brought to the GP by his mother with a stammer which had developed about six months previously and was getting worse. The school had suggested referral to a speech therapist. The GP was aware that there had been marital problems between the parents in the past, and, after the initial consultation, saw first the mother and then the parents together. It emerged that just before John's stammer had started mother had divulged to the father her unresolved problems over an incestuous relationship in her early teens. John was not seen again, but his stammer resolved during the parents' subsequent counselling.

Failure to thrive

Failure to thrive, if not due to organic causes, is usually a sign that the child is anxious and insecure. If the above forms of family support do not get results, it may be necessary to admit the child to a hospital or to send him or her to stay with a relative for a while. This will often lead to a rapid gain in the child's weight, and will give the mother a rest. Because this action can easily reinforce the mother's doubts about her own competence, it is important to emphasize her continued importance and to help her to recognize that some babies are more difficult than others. Having broken a pattern of anxious interaction and built up the baby's weight, it is important to ensure that extra support is given by father and other family members to the mother when the child returns.

Clinging

Clinging behaviour in the child often leads to rejecting behaviour in the mother, which perpetuates the clinging. She should be assured that she will not be 'spoiling' the child if she allows the clinging. In fact she can easily demonstrate that if, when clinging occurs, she takes the child onto her knee and holds it close, the child will soon begin to push her away.

The 'spoilt' child

Two very different kinds of family problem can give rise to accusations that a child is 'spoilt'. One is a form of concealed neglect. Parents who feel guilty for some reason try to appease their child by giving it toys, sweets, or other food. The child, who dimly recognizes that these articles are a substitute for love, may become greedy, demanding more and more food, toys, etc., yet somehow never be satisfied; 'goodies' are no substitute for love. Compulsive stealing in later life is thought sometimes to be a consequence of such relationships.

Another kind of 'spoiling' can take place if a child has come to be seen as especially fragile or important. 'Only' children who arrive when infertile parents had despaired of having a baby, those who are the first to be born after a miscarriage or still birth, or children who have survived a near-fatal illness in early childhood, may be singled out for special care. Parents who feel that they have failed to fulfil their own potentialities may invest high hopes in a child.

Such parents are often over-protective and over-intrusive, pressing their children into a mould that is unlikely to fit. On the one hand, these parents convey the idea that the children are fragile and in constant danger, and, on the other hand, that they are deserving of the love and protection of others as a reward for their superior qualities. To the children it may seem that only by constantly proving to themselves and others that they possess these qualities and deserve these idealized expectations can they hope to survive. Their search for praise is a desperate attempt to confirm an identity which, at heart, they may know they lack. This behaviour is likely to be interpreted by their peers as a bid for undeserved status, and to lead to rejection and denigration.

Anything that reassures them and their parents that they are neither as vulnerable as they feel nor do they have to be as perfect as they believe, will help to break the vicious circle of attention-seeking and rejection that tends to perpetuate the pattern.

Child abuse

Contrary to popular belief, most parents who assault and damage their children are not the heartless monsters they are made out to be. During much of their lives they are caring, concerned parents who show every sign of affection for their children. True there are a few who have taken a dislike to a child from birth, but more often their abuse of the child can be seen as 'end of tether' behaviour in people who have always had difficulty in controlling their impulses.

Most parents initially learn how to treat their children from their own parents' treatment of themselves. Bad parenting can be learned as well as good. In later life people may make a conscious effort to behave differently, to provide a better model of parenthood from the example of their own parents. But at times of stress they tend to regress. Most baby batterers were themselves battered as children and, though they loathe themselves for doing it, they seem doomed to repeat the same mistakes. If, in addition, they lack the support of an understanding partner or are faced with long-term situations which undermine their confidence and self-control, they find themselves behaving with excessive violence, shaking a baby or toddler, throwing the child against a wall, or shoving him or her downstairs.

Although child abuse is commoner amongst parents of low intelligence, it is by no means confined to this group, and GPs need to take seriously any injuries to a child which give rise to suspicion and to obtain a social report in all such cases.

Risk factors which alert to possible dangers and enable preventive action to be taken are:

- alcoholism in either parent, particularly if associated with violent behaviour;

- rejection or indifference towards a child at birth;

- a known family history of child abuse;

- marital violence;

- difficulty by health workers in obtaining access to a child;

- cowed behaviour on the part of a child when in the presence of parents;

- 'end of tether' behaviour in a parent, particularly if they are known to have a bad temper;

● positive answers to the question 'Have there been times when you have been afraid that you (or your spouse) might harm your child?' This is an important question which should always be asked when a parent is thought to be under stress.

General practitioners are often afraid to stigmatize parents by placing them on the Social Services Department's 'at risk' register, but this is a mistake. The register is confidential to a very limited range of people whose main aim is to protect the child by supporting and helping the parents. They are more likely to become stigmatized by their neighbours if they continue to maltreat their child than if they are given preventive counselling.

The primary care team are sometimes more acceptable to the parents as a source of help than are social workers or NSPCC inspectors. The main aim is to eliminate the circumstances in which a child is likely to be abused. This may be done by helping people to reduce the level of stress under which they are living, to resolve marital problems, to treat behaviour problems in the children or, if the danger cannot be reduced by other means, to find some way of separating the abuser from the abused. Parents whose child has been placed on the 'at risk' register will normally receive close support from a social worker. Between them, the social workers, GP, and other members of the PCT may well reduce the risk of further abuse by providing parents with someone to turn to when tensions begin to rise.

Sylvia, a young teacher whose parents often resorted to violence during their frequent quarrels, was herself happily married. Her expectations and aspirations for her 2½-year-old son were very high. When he went through a normal 'negative' phase, she interpreted this as reflecting her own failure and found herself with an almost uncontrollable urge to hit him. She realized how inappropriate this feeling was and came to her GP for aid. She was much helped by realizing where her irrational urge originated and was able to re-establish self-control.

Child abuse, like other causes of psychological damage to a child, is often more helpfully seen as the outcome of a family situation that has arisen than as the 'crime' of a particular person. When legal action is taken, it is more often to protect the child than to punish the parent. But in most cases this is neither necessary nor desirable. Child sexual abuse is considered in Section 5.4.

Feeding and bowel problems

These can be a great worry to parents. Eating and defecating can become the two great battlegrounds on which conflicts between child and parent are acted out. By refusing to eat and by refusing to defecate in the right place the child can express resistance and exert control over the parents. Many toddlers go through a stage of negativism in which their response to al instructions is 'No'. This helps them to discover their own strength and their own limitations. Parents whose self-confidence is threatened by what is perceived as tyrannical behaviour, may become equally tyrannical in response. Both they and the child must learn that frustration is a natural part of life and that it is possible, on the one hand, to give way without losing all control and, on the other, to establish limits without losing the love of the other person. Refusal to eat some or all foods are equally worrying to parents who often find themselves providing extraordinary dietary regimes in an attempt to find out what their child likes. Since some children show a distinct preference for coal, soil, slugs, or other unsuitable objects (pica), one may have to keep a close watch on them. A lot of food fads are situational; a child who refuses adamantly to drink milk at home guzzles it down when visiting grandmother. Many of these problems fade away if treated in a matter of fact way without threats or anxiety, so that mealtimes do not become a drama. If a child chooses not to eat a meal, that is their affair. Sadly, there are many parents who try to force sweets or other food on their child as a demonstration of love, and feel personally rejected if the child refuses. The seeds of obesity and anorexia in later life are often sown at meal times in childhood.

Many parents need to be told that it is harmful to feed children between meals and that sweets cause dental caries. The fact that their own mothers ignored this precept is no reason for them to do the same, but does make such elementary health education more difficult and may lead to problems between parents and grandparents.

One has only to hear the parental delight with which a stool in the potty is greeted to realize the truth of Freud's statement that 'Faeces are the child's first gift to its mother.' Hugh Jolley points out, however, that the mother then throws them down the drain. The child, who has no preconceptions on the matter, will soon begin to respond to the expectations and emotional attitudes of the parents. Children whose parents live in anxious dread that their children will disgrace them will probably live up to these negative expectations. They may even come to believe that they are the 'dirty boy' (or girl) that mother says they are.

Physical and psychological factors often interact. Thus the stools of a child who is wilfully constipated may become so hard that they produce a small anal tear. This makes defecation painful and increases the child's determination not to evacuate. Physical methods to produce a softer stool may be needed along with psychological support and reassurance to mother and child.

Other causes of constipation in babies which need to be considered and treated include febrile illness, underfeeding, anal fissure or stricture, Hirschsprung's disease, hyperthyroidism, and hypercalcaemia. In older children, lack of security, conflict with parents or siblings, and over-anxiety in parents are common causes. Less common is Hirschsprung's disease (although this is occasionally a result of 'voluntary' retention).

192 The family life cycle

Having excluded persisting organic causes of constipation, it may be necessary to initiate treatment with oral laxatives, such as Senna BP. Occasionally a suppository or enema is needed, but these are a last rather than a first resort and children should be weaned off all medication as soon as possible. A family meeting may reduce differences between parents and result in an agreed plan of management. If the parents can be led to become consistent towards the child and supportive of each other, the problem will soon resolve. Even so, it may take some time for the colon to recover its tone if a child has been constipated for a long time; new habits take time to establish.

Persistent soiling (encopresis) may result from constipation or arise in its own right. Like enuresis it may be caused by parents who show too little or too much concern for their child's bowel training. In the latter case, the child will often be found to have achieved bowel control at an early age, but to have lost it later. Inadequate toilet facilities, punitive or fastidious parenting, and, occasionally, sexual abuse may have to be considered. Older children may become very anxious about soiling, particularly if teased by parents and peers.

As with other bowel disorders, it is important to work with the parents and the child to achieve a more reasonable and stress-free attitude to the problems and to establish a new bowel habit.

Bedwetting

This is common prior to the age of five years and parents, whose other children may have been dry from the first year, often need reassurance on this point. If it continues after that time (primary enuresis), it may be the result of psychological or physical factors. Relapse occurring after control has been established is termed secondary enuresis.

Primary enuresis is commoner in boys and may result from absence of proper potty training (when a child fails to learn the virtues of continence) or excessively anxious or punitive potty training (when the baby often becomes almost dry at an early age but relapses later). Parents (especially fathers) often get angry with enuretic children. They need to be told that the child can't help wetting the bed, that he is not 'naughty' and that punishment will make him more anxious and more likely to wet the bed. If a simple regime of potting before bed and restriction of evening fluid intake, together with measures to reduce maternal anxiety, fails, and the child is over the age of five years, it is best to make use of one of the electrical devices which will sensitize the child to the need for bladder control by ringing a bell as soon as it starts to wet the bed. This form of conditioning makes the child more alert to the state of its bladder sphincter and cures most cases of enuresis in older children and adolescents. A tricyclic antidepressant such as imipramine is sometimes an effective treatment, but 60 per cent relapse within six weeks when stopped. Because imipramine can be fatal in overdose, parents need to be warned to take special care.

Secondary enuresis often has a physical cause, such as diabetes, urinary infection, neurological defect, nocturnal epilepsy, severe mental handicap, or can be due to emotional upset. A careful physical examination and urine test will exclude the organic causes.

In the end, the remarkable thing seems to be that most children do come through the first few years of life without lasting damage. This says much for the resilience of both parents and children and convinces us that parents do not have to be perfect, they only have to be 'good enough'.

5.4   LATER CHILDHOOD DEVELOPMENT

For many children, going to school is the first separation from parents and home. It is, therefore, likely to evoke anxiety on both sides.

Most parents regard their children's going to school as a blessing. Toddlers are a tie and parents, whose self-esteem derives more from their life outside than inside the home, may be tempted to place their children in nursery school at an early age so as to go back to work. At times their own needs may conflict with those of their children.

There are no fixed rules about such issues as the 'right age' to send a child to nursery school. Some children are so secure in their relationship by the age of two and a half that they will enjoy the adventure of a nursery school, others are less secure and may become very distressed and 'clingy' if sent so early. Parental feelings of anxiety, guilt, and anger further complicate the situation and may increase the child's anxiety; so that this form of care, which, if successful, becomes a good form of preparaton for full-time schooling, may only serve to undermine the child's trust in the world.

Success in handling the life change of going to school depends on skills and deficits already acquired. The experience is easier for the child who finds new situations exciting than it is for one who is made nervous by them. It is also easier for the mother who is confident that her child is aware of the dangers of traffic than for the over-protective one who is worried by any new situation.

Vicious circles of anxiety may easily be created; the anxious child may create anxiety in the mother who, in turn, evokes more anxiety in the child. Identification of such a vicious circle can be of great therapeutic value, because the spiral of anxiety can be interrupted, thereby helping to prevent such problems as school refusal.

Because the surgery is a strange place to the child, it is possible to make important observations of abnormal or unusual behaviour in this setting; the child may be cowed, clinging, distractible, uncontrolled, over-active, or passive. It is also worth noting who attends with the child.

Important general factors in understanding problems at this stage are:

Normal developmental variability

Some reported problems simply reflect an unrealistic expectation of what the child should be achieving, or of the range of normal development. For example, while the average age at which children are dry at night is three years, about one-fifth of six-year-olds will continue to wet their beds occasionally.

Parental anxiety

This can be important in two ways. First, it can be transmitted to the child; the mother who is anxious about her child entering new situations may teach her child to be anxious too. This can be useful in teaching the child to avoid danger, but the same learning process can lead to the child becoming inappropriately anxious. Secondly, anxious parents are more likely to consult about problems. Most parents deal with occasional bedwetting in a five-year-old by restricting evening fluids and waking the child to go to the toilet, but the more anxious parents seek a diagnosis, and make more of an issue of what may be within the range of normal behaviour.

Parental control

By school entry time, patterns of discipline will have been developed. The level of control achieved will determine how much support the family can give the school in maintaining constraints such as school attendance, arriving on time, or attending to teachers. The style of control adopted at home may also predict the type of control the child adopts with peers; where home discipline is maintained by an aggressive or coercive style, the child will tend to control other children by hitting, shouting, or threatening.

Skill learning

In school, all children are expected to learn skills, although not all are equally ready to acquire them. At home, learning is tailored to the child, and although schools attempt to achieve this, some children find it more difficult than others to sit still, to attend to the teacher, or to work alone. Bright children may be bored and others have specific learning difficulties. Emotional and behavioural problems may result.

Problems

General issues

Problems may be defined by how they present, or in terms of the assumed causes. Presentations as diverse as learning difficulties and fighting with peers may arise from the same cause, for example unhappiness due to parents' marital strife or lack of sleep due to poor housing.

The sources of the problem may lie in the child; they may arise from defects in the development of the central nervous system, resulting in developmental delay, cognitive deficits, or motor deficits such as inco-ordination (see Chapter 7), or they may arise from sensory deficits such as short sight and deafness. Alternatively, the child may have acquired fears, phobias, or styles of behaviour through earlier learning. Thus, the child who is afraid of dogs may find it as difficult to get to school as the child who is frightened of separating from a sick, depressed, rejecting, or vulnerable parent. Children can also learn to behave in aggressive, clinging, or sickly ways to achieve a degree of control over their parents.

The parents may have linked problems. They may experience difficulties in separating from the child, due to imaginary dangers to the child, or to sickness in the child. Their over-protectiveness may be part of a generalized anxiety state or a specific separation anxiety. They may mis-perceive the child as having problems when, in fact, it is their own inappropriate expectations that are at fault.

Parents may identify very strongly with the child. This can make it hard for them to dissociate enough to be objective about the child's performance, or to succeed in acquiring adequate control. They vary in the extent to which they are strict or lax, consistent or variable, in controlling the child. Consistency over time and between parents is most important. The style of control may depend on reward, punishment, or coercion, or a mixture of all three, and may be administered physically as gifts and punishments, or socially as affection, approval, disapproval, or rejection. Punishment may train the child in aggressive behaviour. Some use of social rewards would appear to be necessary if the child is to learn to respond to the normal controls exerted by society. Lax control may indicate parental neglect, and lead to the child responding by behaviour which attracts attention. Alternatively, a punitive parent may effectively be a child abuser (see p. 109).

Children may also have problems due to the world outside home. Teachers may not offer ideal learning conditions. They may be punitive or denigrating, or they may ignore the child in school. Peers may bully the child or be jealous and rejecting, especially of brighter children. The outside world may be so frightening that the child seeks to avoid it, or so attractive that home activities are skipped in order to be part of it.

The complex interrelationships between the presenting problems and the underlying causes can make it difficult to identify a starting point, and any analysis of a problem that does not include all relevant areas can appear glib.

In the sections which follow, emphasis will be placed on identifying the causes of problems and working out, with the child and parents, a logical approach to management which holds out promise of success. As in all other forms of therapy, however, it is often the interest and care which we give which gets results. Children who feel that their difficulties are being taken seriously, and parents whose own problems are understood, will tackle the difficulty in a positive frame of mind, which may itself be more 'therapeutic' than any clever therapies which we can devise. Conversely, an approach which is seen as too clinical, detached, or uncaring has little chance of success.

In discussing specific problems, only the commonest ones are considered, together with the management thought at present to be the most effective.

Specific problems

School refusal

This is one of the earliest problems to appear. It is useful to consider separately the child who resists going to school in the first few weeks and the one who resists at a later stage, having attended satisfactorily at first. Children who do not want to go to school initially may be frightened of leaving mother and/or frightened of the unknown school situation. Their distress is likely to elicit distress in parents, who may already be somewhat anxious about the child's attendance at school. Some apparent 'school refusal' may arise because the mother does not want to let go of the child. The most natural response, and in the short term the easiest, is to give in and allow the child to come home. After a number of days the limits of this approach become apparent.

School refusal at this stage can usually be overcome if the parents can adopt a confident, positive, and firm approach. If they appear to be worried about the child going to school, the child senses this concern and may reflect it. If he or she additionally senses that the parents may relent, then showing enough distress or being 'ill' may ensure that they all avoid the frightening experience of school.

Clare was a precious only child, whose mother had had a stillbirth two years after Clare was born. Mother felt her close relationship with Clare to be threatened if she went to school, and could not prevent herself crying when Clare prepared to leave in the morning. She realized that her behaviour was inappropriate, and when the GP suggested that she also went out in the morning to help with a local playgroup, the situation became easier.

Occasionally children may require direct help and the best approach is some form of 'desensitization', either by having the child stay in school for gradually increasing amounts of time, or by having mother remain in school with the child for gradually decreasing periods (see p. 67).

Children who have entered school successfully and later become school refusers present a more complex pattern and their behaviour may have different explanations. Most often children refuse because they do not wish to leave home for fear of leaving a mother who may be ill, unhappy, being beaten by father, or giving love and attention to a new sibling. Less frequently, they may not wish to arrive at school where they are being bullied by other children, frightened by the teacher, failing to keep up with others in lessons, or, in the case of a bright child, bored. There may even be a problem *en route* if they have to pass a barking dog or meet unpleasant adults or teasing children. It is important to understand the child's concerns, so that reassurance can be given where relevant or some appropriate changes made. Changes may be simple, such as finding an alternative route to avoid the local bully, or more complex, such as desensitizing the child to a fear of dogs. It may be helpful for parents to introduce changes at home. For instance, the boy who is concerned about a new sibling attracting mother's attention may be reassured if she spends some time with him when he returns from school. Similarly, there may be useful changes which can be made by the school.

Having established a reason for the school refusal and defused this problem as much as possible, the child should be gradually reintroduced to school. Even where no specific problem is identified, it may be possible to pursue this approach—by taking walks near the school at weekends, then during school time, and so on. Some physical symptoms may be the result of the child's anxiety and some an attempt to manipulate the situation. In either case parents may be confused by the child being 'too sick to go to school'. A firm line is desirable, giving minimal attention to symptoms and ensuring that the child attends school unless symptoms are incapacitating. The symptoms will disappear when actual experience of school reduces the fears that cause them, or when it becomes clear to the child that the symptoms do not enable the situation to be manipulated.

Mrs J had had an unhappy childhood. Her foster parents were remembered as being unkind and her school as hostile. She was determined that her daughter Jane would not suffer in the same way, so she over-protected her and her school attendance became erratic. A session with the family elicited and clarified this situation. Father was recruited to support mother and to take Jane to school himself for the first week or so; the problem resolved.

Truancy

Truancy presents a rather different kind of problem, the child avoiding school not because of fears, but because of a preference for being elsewhere. The truant's parents are less likely to know about it, as the child may spend the day away from home, often with peers. Truancy is often associated with delinquency and with poor school performance, but it is usually unclear which came first; whether school failure led to truancy and this free time became occupied with antisocial activities, or whether engagement in such activities led to truancy and subsequent failure to keep up at school.

Cases of truancy are most likely to be identified and dealt with by the school teachers, who may involve an educational psychologist in solving the problems. It is important that the efforts of the school and health care team are well co-ordinated, and a general arrangement between the two for the exchange of information is well worthwhile.

The father of a 14-year-old boy arrived at the general practitioner's surgery carrying a large brown paper bag containing many packets of cigarettes which his son had stolen from a local filling station. The GP suggested that he and the practice clinical psychologist talk to the boy. The boy readily confessed to other petty crime and to repeated truanting from school. Both boy and father agreed that the school should be contacted. The school had not marked the boy out as a truant, but their records revealed less than a 50 per cent attendance rate. From this point onwards both school and health care team worked together on a realistically assessed problem, which was far from a simple case of delinquency or truancy. It turned out that the boy was leading a lonely, frightened existence during the day and was consumed by disturbing thoughts. The family were seen together, both at the health centre and at home, and some simple work was done with the boy on his own, aimed at helping him to manage and reinterpret his disturbing thoughts. His school attendance improved.

Learning difficulties

These may reflect the child's intellectual difficulties or they may indicate poor adaptation to the class-room. If the child is unhappy in school, due to failure to get on with the teacher or other children, then school attainments may fall below the child's capability as indicated by intellectual assessment. Equally, the child who is unhappy at home may bring the problems to school and be unable to achieve full potential. Other children may be unable to concentrate due to lack of breakfast or lack of sleep, perhaps resulting from their responsibilities at home, or from watching late television. Some children may be lagging due to short-sight or deafness. Very occasionally, difficulties may reflect an organic disorder (see Chapter 7).

It is important that such difficulties be correctly identified and resolved, as problems are likely to be cumulative. It can often be useful to have a full assessment of the child's scholastic attainments and level of intellectual functioning. Where the child does have learning difficulties, supplementary teaching by the school or by parents can minimize the deficits. Clearly, this approach involves the school, together with either an educational or clinical psychologist.

Occasionally a parent's complaint regarding a child's learning difficulties reflects parental attitudes to scholastic achievement, rather than the child's performance. Such parents may need help in reconciling ambition with reality, or in finding a more satisfactory criterion against which to value their child.

Children's behaviour problems

These may occur at home or at school. The GP may be consulted by the parents after contact from the school concerning class-room behaviour.

If problems occur only in school, then they are likely to be resolved in collaboration with the school. Other problems may be present in both places, the child being out of control, disobedient, aggressive and overactive, or being withdrawn, shy and nervous. In each case, the child has learned to behave in this way to cope with the constraints of the particular environment, but the behaviour is not necessarily a satisfactory way of coping in the long term, whatever short-term gains may result.

The first group of problems (*acting-out*) are seen as behavioural excesses and are likely to respond well to consistent use of reward techniques for clearly specified behaviours. The school-aged child can be involved in setting the goals and agreeing the schedule of rewards — indeed they can be very creative in identifying their own valued rewards which they will work very hard to achieve. Wall charts and star systems can be helpful in making the targets and rewards explicit. It is important that targets be achievable and that rewards be appropriate and not over-generous.

Passive withdrawn behaviour may also respond to some form of reward but this must be very carefully tailored to the child. Where there is avoidance of specific situations — such as mixing with peers — it is important to find out why the child does this, in order to clarify misconceptions and, if appropriate, introduce some desensitizing approach. For example, the child might start by engaging in favourite activities with the least threatening of his peers before being asked to participate in group situations or in less enjoyable tasks.

Some behaviour problems only occur at home. This may be due to the parents' failure to agree with each other on a consistent form of discipline, with the result that the problem behaviours sometimes meet with approval and are rewarded, but at other times are punished. Some behaviours that the parents complain of may be the child's only sure way of getting parental attention, albeit of a chastising kind. For example, in a busy professional household, a daughter found that teasing her sisters and breaking things roused her parents from their inattention. Such situations point to the importance of social reinforcement — the attention, smiles, encouragements, and signs of approval we give each other and which lead to changes in behaviour. It can be useful to introduce programmes which identify target behaviours and use social and other rewards to alter these and help resolve problems.

One mother reported that her eight-year-old adopted daughter just did not like her and illustrated this by describing her failure to do what she was told, to tidy her bedroom and to get ready for school on time. It was not clear which behaviours the mother wished to change. In discussion with the daughter she described being sad that she could not do things to please her mother. Joint discussion led to a simple contract, in which clear tasks were identified on which both the girl and her mother agreed. Also a system of recording was evolved which ensured that the mother gave adequate signs of attention and approval, including involvement in joint cooking projects.

Physical symptoms

It is common for children to be brought to GPs with physical symptoms, such as recurrent abdominal pain or headache, which are a reflection of school or home problems, rather than signifying physical disease. The source of the problem may be the child's nervousness of peers, learning difficulties in school, mother's depression, or a whole host of other possibilities. Chapter 6 considers these psychogenic disorders in more detail.

The child is often presented by an anxious mother who is worried that there is a physical disease—'Could it be appendicitis?' Careful history-taking and monitoring of the symptoms—when and where they occur, who is present, and how they respond—helps to establish their psychological cause. For instance, abdominal pain may occur mainly on days on which games lessons are held. Possible gains which the child derives from the symptoms, e.g. missing games, help confirm the nature of the cause, and point to possible lines of management. First, the parents need to be reassured that there is no underlying disease, even though the child presents what are 'real' physical symptoms. This can be difficult to get across. The solution may then lie in trying to resolve the problem directly, for instance, by trying to overcome the child's problems with games. Alternatively, removing the rewarding consequences can be a very successful strategy; the child may be required to attend games even when the symptoms are present. Since avoidance of the situation contributes to the fear of the situation, getting the child back into it can help to overcome the fear.

Finally, some of these presenting problems will be best considered in the full family context. A few will benefit from more formal family therapy as described in Section 4.4.

Sexual abuse

The past few years have seen a large increase in the recognition of child sexual abuse, though it is not certain that this reflects an increase in incidence. Improved history-taking, using such methods as genograms, suggest a much higher incidence in the past than had been previously acknowledged. What might have been taken for fantasy is now thought often to have been reality. Although sexual abuse of male children occurs, it much more commonly involves females, happening between daughters and fathers, stepfathers, siblings, lodgers within the home, and a variety of outside contacts. It is most common with early teenage girls, and often several siblings have been involved, but it should also be remembered that it occurs in younger children. Prostitution and child-sex rings involve a certain number, who may be of either sex.

Sexual abuse is often associated with parental marital problems, alcohol, violence, and with opportunities, such as mothers going out to work leaving children unsupervised, or men, who are either out of work or working irregular hours, being in the house alone with the child. Not infrequently the mothers are aware of what is going on and may even collude, perhaps to avoid sexual advances towards themselves, or out of fear. Sexual abuse occurs in all social classes and, indeed, in all societies.

The long-term consequences of sexual abuse in children are loss of trust in adults, particularly males, sexual dysfunction, frigidity, and, later, promiscuity. In the short term the family may break up. Abuse by siblings is usually less damaging than abuse by a parent or other adult. Violence increases the severity of consequences. The victim may suffer a variety of feelings; feeling betrayed, dirty, soiled, unlovable, isolated, angry, guilty, lacking in self-esteem, and perhaps even sad at the loss of a lover. The rest of the family may be similarly affected.

Presentation

Direct presentation by either mothers or daughters is unusual, as they may both be too fearful of the consequences to tell anyone. The following symptoms should be regarded as alerting us to the possibility of sexual abuse; vaginal discharge, urinary tract infections, anal symptoms, anorexia, depression, and substance abuse. Any of these will be more relevant if accompanied by certain behaviours such as fearfulness, withdrawal, sullenness, avoidance of eye contact, and silence. Asking the child 'Has anyone ever done anything and told you not to tell anyone' will often disclose the situation.

Management

If the abuse is recent, immediate referral to a police surgeon is appropriate so that the necessary forensic tests can be carried out. Otherwise, at any examination, it is important to take note of the state of the hymen, any bruises, abrasions, or other signs of violence. Examination of the genitalia should be carried out towards the end of a general physical examination in order to allay the child's fear that we, too, are only interested in sex.

Because the consequences of abuse are so serious, the advice to the doctor must be that if suspicion is aroused, action of some kind must be taken, even though this will often precipitate anger, disbelief, or possibly the break-up of the family. In the case of young children the doctor should usually see the mother alone first. If she agrees, the family should be referred without interviewing the child, so as not to contaminate the evidence by putting ideas into the child's head. If the mother denies the possibility, an alternative is to ask to see the child alone or with a trusted adult. Older children are probably best seen alone. If there is more than a suspicion, discussion with the head of the local social work team is vital and it is usually better to leave it to the social workers to take over. The primary care team has a continuing role to play in supporting the family, particularly if the father is gaoled.

Sexual abuse is one of the few situations where the person who has sufficient suspicion, though no real evidence, may have to act in a way which risks alienating the family, who may well then be angry whether the suspicions were well founded or not.

A seven-year-old girl showed her diary to a school friend who reported to her own mother that the girl had twice been sexually abused by babysitters.

This mother informed the GP, who knew the family very well. The abused child's mother, a young widow, had a previous history of alcoholism and, on at least one occasion in the past, another child had been taken into the care of the local authority. Because of this, the GP thought it best to inform the local social worker.

The social worker visited the home but the mother angrily repudiated the child's claims and blamed the GP for acting on 'tittle-tattle'. The social worker, however, insisted on talking to the child, as a result of which the police were informed and two men subsequently pleaded guilty in court to charges of sexual abuse.

In the meantime, it became clear that the mother was still drinking heavily and she agreed to return to see the psychiatrist who had helped her in the past. Her child was placed on the 'at risk' register, which meant that she received regular visits from a young social worker whom she eventually came to trust. Between them the GP, the psychiatrist, and the social worker were able to convince the mother of their genuine care and concern for her and her child. She stopped drinking, returned to work, and is now thought to be a responsible mother to her child.

Further reading

Ciba Foundation (1984). *Child sexual abuse within the family*. Tavistock, London.
Herbert, M. (1981). *Behavioural treatment of problem children: a practical manual*. Academic Press, London.

5.5   THE TRANSITION FROM CHILD TO ADULT

By comparison with other species, human beings have a very long childhood. This enables them to stock their brains with a huge and elaborate model of the world and a set of assumptions about themselves and their fellows which will eventually allow them to survive and reproduce without the continuing protection of their parents.

The transition from childhood dependence to adult interdependence which takes place, or should take place, during adolescence, is associated with major bodily changes, all of which help to make this possible. There is a rapid growth in size and strength in both sexes (but to a greater extent in males than in females), males grow fearsome hair on their faces, and both sexes develop secondary sexual characteristics which are attractive to the opposite sex and which signal their biological readiness for reproduction. The orchestration of these bodily changes by the pituitary gland is associated with changes in other ductless glands, and with equally large psychological changes whose physiological origins are not always easy to distinguish from the effects of the social changes which are going on at the same time. For purposes of clarity, these psychological changes can be classified into those which increase autonomy and those which favour the formation of adult attachments and alliances.

Changes favouring autonomy

These include:

● reduction of reliance on parents for food, money, and other resources;

● seeking places in the various occupational and other hierarchies which enable a person to have control of resources of their own. This means competing with and, if necessary, fighting others, for status, territory, and control. The importance of aggressive behaviour in ensuring survival is more obvious among non-human mammals than in humans, but the same behavioural tendencies are present in our species and become very obvious during adolescence.

Changes favouring new relationships

These include:

● attenuation of attachment bonds to parents;

● emergence of powerful tendencies to seek and maintain new attachments.

These attachments commonly include sexual elements, but this should not blind us to the fact that they are also mediated by deeply felt needs for security and mutual alliance. These tendencies usually result in bonding to members of the opposite sex who can satisfy needs for both sex and security, but it is, of course, quite possible for people to seek sex from one relationship and security from another, and for either to be obtained from persons of the same sex.

The age of onset of these changes in maturation varies from one person to another, as does the intensity of the feelings which accompany them. Because all of these changes involve other people, the possibilities of conflict are numerous. Drives towards autonomy are often more powerful in boys than in girls, whereas drives towards new bonding are usually more powerful in girls. The waning of attachment to parents may or may not coincide with a corresponding waning on the side of the parents. To make matters yet more difficuilt, emergent aggressive tendencies are likely to complicate the conflicts which arise and make this a very stormy transition. Fortunately, the psychosocial transition of adolescence, like other transitions, will usually come to an end and there is then peace once more in the family, at least until the next transition!

Modern urban society presents particular problems for the adolescent. High population densities make it hard for boys to express their aggressive tendencies without running into conflict with society and the law. The costs and shortage of housing force many youngsters to remain at home against their inclinations and those of their parents, the need for further education keeps them at school, and although contraception enables them to have sex without the responsibilities to which this used to give rise, the complications in bonding which result are often painful. When accidental pregnancies do happen, the attachment and security which should support the inception of a new family are often lacking.

Adolescents are faced with the need to enter a world which their pre-existing models are unlikely to fit. In attempting to adjust to this new world, they have either to continue to use assumptions derived from the old model or to discover new ones. In so far as they cling to their old assumptions they are likely to be seen as 'childish' or 'immature'; in attempting to emancipate themselves from their parents they choose new models which are different from theirs, and are then seen as 'weird' or 'rebellious'.

For those who succeed in achieving a reasonable degree of autonomy, and in making reasonably secure new bonds, adolescence can be an exciting and delightful new period of life (in fact some will subsequently look back on it as the high-point). For others it can be a time of misery and failure; but for the majority it is a mixture of the two.

One thing is certain: the successes and failures which attend the transition from childhood to adult life are influenced by the preconceptions and expectations which arose from previous experiences, and they, in turn, colour the expectations and preconceptions which will influence the young adult in coping with future transitions. It follows that those who are particularly vulnerable, whose expectations are pessimistic or in other ways unrealistic, can often be identified before serious difficulties arise, and that any help which increases their chances of successful transition is likely to be of lasting benefit to them and their families.

Factors favouring successful transition include:

● secure attachments to parents which encourage reasonable autonomy;

● realistic and positive evaluations of the self which allow exploration with confidence;

● knowledge of the adult world and intelligence to use it to adapt in the face of new problems;

● physical strength and agility;

- sexual attractiveness and awareness;

- emergent drives/appetites which are neither excessively strong nor unduly weak;

- wise guidance from parents whose own needs don't conflict with those of the youngster;

- changes occurring at around the same age as in peers.

Conversely, difficulties are likely to emerge if:

- attachment to parents is insecure so that the youngster clings to them, or goes to the other extreme of rejecting them and all others in authority;

- self-esteem is low so that new or challenging situations are avoided or the young person gives up too easily;

- individuals are poorly prepared for the world which they are entering and the expectations placed upon them are inappropriate to their knowledge or intelligence;

- the youngster is physically weak or sees self (by comparison with peers) as impaired;

- the youngster is unattractive or perceives self as less attractive than peers;

- there are difficulties in controlling emergent aggressive or sexual impulses, there is lack of either of these by comparison with peers, or if the sexual impulses are seen as being disapproved of (e.g. directed towards the same sex);

- parents or parent substitutes block the youngster's development by clinging and rewarding childish or immature assumptions, or push the youngster out of the nest, or foster unrealistic expectations and assumptions which are doomed to disappointment;

- changes occur earlier or later than in most of their peers.

Problems

Many of the problems presenting at this time will reflect the uncertainties of the adolescent associated with establishing a personal identity independent of the family, and the need to try out different identities for fit. The parents may experience problems in relinquishing control at a satisfactory rate and so achieving a changing but appropriate level. Methods of discipline need to be adjusted to the individual offspring—what was suitable at an earlier age or for other siblings may not be right now or with this youngster.

At this time young people also make many significant educational an occupational choices, and aspirations which are too high or too low can b frustrating and lead to depression if not achieved. In this area, as in socia and sexual functioning, there will be a choice of role models; in the family at school, and in the peer group. Unsatisfactory role models can lead to poo educational performance, delinquency, drug abuse, promiscuity, and othe undesirable consequences.

In many of their choices adolescents will find themselves in conflic with authority figures in the shape of parents, teachers, police, o employers. This will be a problem both for the young people and for th authority figures.

The problems which are present are therefore difficult to disentangle an interpret.

Jim, an only child, was 16 when his father died and one year later, when his invali mother was on holiday, he held a wild drunken party in his house. The next da the health centre was contacted by no fewer than the neighbours, his aunt, the hom help, and his mother's social worker, all asking what they could do about Jim Fortunately, the GP had known him for many years and was able to go and see hir without formality. He found that he had still not come to terms with the death c his father and the subsequent change of his own position in the family, becomin the male his mother relied on both for household jobs and emotional support. Th pressures on his time hardly allowed him to go out and he felt increasingly isolate from his peers. The party had been a way of 'breaking out'. The doctor reassure him of the normality of these internal conflicts in adolescence and helped him griev for his father, and then seeing him with his mother, defused the crisis. Subsequently Jim was able to cope in a more socially acceptable way.

Behaviour problems

Behaviour problems at this age may be much the same as for younger childre but often with a flavour that reflects challenge to parental authority. Fo example, problems concerning staying out late or not coming home for meal are frequent, because the parents have been unable to let go and give thei offspring enough latitude to explore their own potential and wishes. Wis parents only make strict rules about things that really matter. As with politics the guiding rule must be the 'art of the possible'.

While the causes may derive from the adolescent's thoughts and confusions or from the social and family environment, the solutions are likely to be foun by altering the response of the family to the adolescent. Simple behavioura programmes, as used with younger children, can provide the uncertai teenager with clear, well-defined boundaries and also help the parents to asses the appropriateness of the controls they impose. At this stage, the join agreement of the adolescent and the parents to a behavioural contract ca also be valuable in developing more adult, negotiated relationships.

Mark, a 17-year-old, liked spending the evenings with his friends. The family usually ate at 8.30 and he asked if he could eat earlier. His mother resented cooking for him on his return from school but complied. However, his father insisted that even if Mark ate earlier, he had to help with the washing-up of the main family meal by returning at 9 o'clock. When he didn't, his father retaliated by stopping his pocket money, and Mark started stealing.

A few short sessions with the family allowed a satisfactory contract to be worked out. If he wanted to go out, Mark cooked his own meal on return from school, and washed up. He also promised that he would always be home by a previously agreed time. Peace was restored.

Some of the behaviour problems will have wider implications: juvenile delinquency (see p. 210) may bring the offender into contact with the law; sexual behaviour may lead to pregnancy, abortion, and sexually transmitted disease (see Section 5.6); and alcohol, glue sniffing, and drug abuse (see Section 8.5) may result in both physical and legal problems. Many behaviour problems will have associated mood problems.

Mood problems

Mood disturbances are also common at this age — indeed, moodiness is almost the hallmark of adolescence in popular writing. This can most readily be considered in the context of life events, stress, and psychosocial transitions.

While changing from child to adult, adolescents cannot be sure of their own resources and potential to meet new challenges, nor can they be sure what will be expected of them. At the same time, they meet many new and important challenges with apparently life-long consequences, such as passing critical exams, gaining paid employment, or meeting a future partner. Teenagers who fail to find a job on leaving school show a higher incidence of emotional distress on questionnaires such as the GHQ than their employed peers.[1]

The presentation to the GP may give some indication of the transitional nature of their status (see Section 3.3), as they may present by themselves, or with a parent, or the parent(s) may present the problem. Adolescents may report mood problems — feeling unhappy, nervous, irritable, labile — or they may report difficulty in functioning — lack of interest in what they are doing, inability to concentrate, not being 'themselves'. Alternatively, they may report physical symptoms such as lack of energy, headaches, sleeping poorly, or stomach upsets.

These complaints are quite normal responses to the typical problems faced by adolescents. The youngster and parents need to understand what these feelings are about, and the usual process of 'talking it through' will normally enable this to happen. It is important that these adolescents are not seen as 'sick', as this takes away from them the responsiblity for solving their problems, medicalizes them, and inhibits the normal processes of resolution.

Sometimes it will be helpful to involve a parent or the family, but at othe
times the opportunity to develop a private and confidential relationship wit
an adult outside and separate from the home may be very important. Th
GP may be ideal in this role, especially if it is made clear at the outset tha
total confidentiality is assured.

John, a clever 16-year-old about to take his 'O' levels, came to the doctor complainin
of tiredness and inability to work. He felt the need to go out in the evenings. Hi
parents disapproved — they felt he should be working. Both parents were kind bu
rigid and had high ambitions for him. It emerged in discussion that John was awar
of his parents' good intentions, but felt that he never received praise, only exhortation
to work hard for his own good. It also emerged that a few months before, whil
his parents had been on a visit to the USA, his grandmother had had a stroke, an
he had travelled 150 miles and stayed with her for a week, looked after her and nc
brought his parents home prematurely. This devotion had been taken for grante
by his parents.

Quite brief discussion with John and his family allowed the parents to acknowledg
his considerate behaviour and application to work, and transfer more of th
responsibility for organizing his life to John, who began to thrive.

Crises

Many of the crises which are particularly prevalent in adolescence are als
common in young adulthood. Some of these are associated with tests, whethe
they be exams, driving tests, or job interviews. It is hardly surprising tha
a number of adolescents in this vulnerable transitional stage, subjected a
they are to so many assessments of their abilities, develop acute anxiet
symptoms. These are associated with negative thoughts 'I'm bound to fail'
'If I fail I'll be flung out', 'It'll just prove I'm no good.' In addition to th
techniques of stress management (p. 75), GPs can help by discussin
previous performance in order to remind the young person of past success
or that previous failure did not lead to catastrophe. Careful planning of th
work during the period before the threatening test can bring structure to lif
and reduce the likelihood of panicky, ineffective preparation (see als
Section 4.6).

Other crises occur in the home as the adolescent challenges parenta
authority, for instance by threatening to leave home, to break up th
furniture, or to seriously menace the parents with violence. Yet other crise
are associated with the new relationships which are being developed: a possibl
engagement, a homosexual relationship, or an unwanted pregnancy.

In each case, crisis intervention is likely to be required and frequently som
continuing counselling, which the GP, or an attached member of the team
is in a good position to give. This avoids the stigmatization of hospital referral
and allows a continuing relationship with the PCT (primary care team) t
be built up. Future crises may then be defused at an earlier stage.

One exceedingly rare, but important, crisis which can occur at this age is the onset of a schizophrenic illness, sometimes triggered (though not caused) by experimentation with hallucinogenic drugs. While this should usually lead to a psychiatric referral, the GP will continue to play an important role for the family at the time of the crisis, and for the patient after discharge from specialized care. The symptoms of schizophrenia are discussed in Section 8.6. They are sometimes difficult to distinguish from those of the so-called 'identity crisis' which can occur at this age, due to confusion and uncertainty as to what kind of a person the young adult is becoming. The absence of lasting first-rank symptoms and the relatively rapid response to counselling will usually help differentiate. In other cases only time will tell.

Social skills/social phobia

New social skills are required of adolescents; it is unlikely that the approaches which succeeded at the Brownies or football club will be helpful at the disco. Apart from specific skills in verbal and non-verbal communication, the teenager may also have to decide whether the current situation is one in which behaviour from the repertoire of adult or child is most suitable. It is not surprising, then, that the peak age for social phobia is the early teens. It is characterized by nervousness of entering social situations, feeling that other people are watching and evaluating every action, and by expectation of failure. At the same time there is a strong wish to enter and enjoy the social situation, tempered by the inclination to avoid those that create too much discomfort.

It can be very helpful to emphasize that these ambivalent feelings are normal at this age. In the eyes of the nervous teenager, his or her peers appear to handle very complex interactions with no difficulty. If they can recognize that at least some of their peers feel the same sense of trepidation as they do, even though they may not show it outwardly, their own wariness can be seen in perspective. Also, they can see that the feelings are not incompatible with behaving effectively.

The second point to make is that avoidance does not help. As with all phobias, avoiding the frightening situation makes one feel better in the short term, but does nothing to overcome it. Gentle encouragement to participate may be all that is required, or it may be necessary to work on a graded approach, perhaps with the help of parents. If it is difficult to just turn up at the photographic club, it may be easier to telephone in advance and make a definite arrangement to meet the club secretary. If the thought of a whole evening at the disco is too terrible, it may be possible to go for an hour in the first instance.

While engaging in the threatening activity may overcome the basic difficulties, some people will require help with specific social skills. The most common issue is 'What will/should I say?', and teenage magazines frequently address this question. Since it is unlikely that the general practitioner knows the answer, it is probably best to offer the teenager the opportunity to rehearse possible approaches and allow him or her to decide what is the most appropriate. The main value of such discussions is in increasing self-esteem by showing the youngsters that they themselves can work out strategies which overcome their fear of the dreaded social situation.

Juvenile delinquency

The teens are also the peak ages for law-breaking. Property crimes reach a peak in the year prior to school-leaving age, crimes of violence are commonest at 17 and 18 (often associated with heavy alcohol drinking), and taking and driving vehicles are crimes of the late teens and early twenties. Fortunately, less than half of those found guilty of breaking the law as a juvenile go on to commit offences as adults. Boys are much more likely to be involved than girls in each of these types of offence. Delinquency is associated with social conditions, being far more prevalent in deprived inner-city areas, and also in families which do not maintain consistent affectionate pattern of discipline. The existence of a delinquent sub-culture makes it more likely that the next generation of youth will also engage in such activities. Each GP will be aware of the delinquency pattern in his or her own practice area.

The PCT may be consulted by parents who suspect or know that their youngster is involved in crimes. In such cases the help the PCT can give may be limited to emotional support for the parents. Parents can be encouraged to provide good structure and discipline at home and guide the youngster towards other, more rewarding activities and companions; these are likely to be highly sensitive areas. Sometimes the parents can do things with the youngster, to help develop more law-abiding approaches to society.

The GP who, despite the generation gap, is able to obtain the serious attention, if not the trust, of a young person may be as distressed by the situation as are the parents. It is often possible to indicate that while we cannot condone delinquent behaviour, we can hear and respect the cry of rage which it represents. By accepting the forbidden feelings which underlie delinquency, we may be able to help the young person to find more acceptable ways of expressing their aggression.

A similar stance can be helpful after the young person has been involved with the courts, though at that stage probation officers may also be involved. Liaison with the probation officer may be helpful—but only with the permission of the young offender and with the assurance of confidentiality.

Eating problems

By contrast, eating problems are more likely to occur in girls. Obesity anorexia nervosa, bulimia nervosa (binge eating and subsequent induced vomiting), and chaotic eating patterns typically start in the teens and can go on to have a very disruptive influence on life for years to come.

Obesity may become a problem, perhaps following on from eating disorders of childhood (see Section 5.3) or as a new problem in the teens. It can then continue as a lifelong difficulty. It may arise because appetite and bodily development do not keep pace, or as a result of emotional difficulties. For example, overeating can occur as part of the conflict with parents, or due to lack of confidence in relationships with peers. Eating may be a comfort which compensates for the other things that cannot be achieved, a gift of love to the self or a way of gaining the attention and concern of otherwise disinterested parents. Overeating and resultant obesity may appear to solve problems by providing the underconfident teenager with an excuse for avoiding, or a means of ensuring being avoided by, the opposite sex. Obesity may also bring its own problems, as this is the time in the whole lifespan when physical appearance matters most.

The approach to this problem is likely to involve both attempts to resolve emotional difficulties, and to control the eating pattern through dieting. However, care should be exercised lest the problem is exaggerated, reducing the adolescent's self-esteem and potentially laying the ground work for the development of anorexia nervosa or bulimia nervosa. It is worth remembering the existence, and transience, of 'puppy fat'.

Rather than encouraging 'crash' diets, following which patients rapidly return to their former pattern of eating, the aim should be to help the patient to acquire a new eating habit. Careful enquiry will usually elicit the time when overeating occurs—between meals or at a particular meal. It is important to break the habit, perhaps by giving the patient something else to do at these times. There is nothing worse than watching others eat!

Regular weighing in the surgery by a doctor or nurse not only enables us to monitor progress but to reward the patient for success. Often the only thing that stops the patient from eating is the fear of disappointing us! Group therapy can be obtained from various organization such as 'Weight Watchers'. Amphetamines and their derivatives should be avoided as appetite suppressants. A variety of low-calorie diets are available but they have problems with long-term use and it is best to have diets prepared individually by dieticians to suit the patient's own preference. Regular physical exercise is a good way of improving physique, but the increased appetite which results can make it harder to lose weight.

Anorexia nervosa is characterized by considerable weight loss. It involves the intention to lose weight, and a tendency to perceive oneself as fat, when, in fact, one is not. In other cases it can be regarded as a phobia of eating. There may be accompanying misuse of laxatives, and excessive exercising.

Menstruation is usually disrupted so that the girl either does not start to menstruate, or ceases to menstruate, usually when the weight has fallen to below 45 kg. It is likely that her parents will be involved in bringing her to the attention of the GP, as the girl will frequently perceive no problem and may, indeed, refuse to attend the surgery. The mother may report her daughter's weight loss, menstrual disturbance, distress, or general debility and tiredness. The girl herself may be more willing and concerned to consult a doctor about these symptoms than about weight loss.

Severe forms of anorexia nervosa need to be dealt with by a specialist unit, often as an in-patient. However, the PCT may wish to tackle less extreme forms by behavioural contracting, using a graded approach to eating, or by family or individual psychotherapy, or both. It is better to avoid plans which require the girl to report what she has eaten, as anorexics frequently deceive those around them. It is important, also, to monitor her weight to ensure that it does not become low enough to endanger her life.

Bulimia nervosa tends to present rather later and is also characterized by the wish to control weight. However, the bulimic girl is not necessarily much below her normal body weight, and controls her weight by vomiting regularly soon after meals. She is more likely to present with mood problems, usually of a depressive nature, often including elements of guilt and low self-esteem. Very often the doctor will be the first person she has told about habits that she is ashamed of and secretive about; ordinary counselling skills are therefore very important in assessing and helping with the problem.

In clinical practice, it is surprisingly effective simply to instruct the girl to stop vomiting. She should then be helped to develop a normal eating pattern, abandoning whatever devious eating style she has been using, be it eating alone, eating only carbohydrates, or eating only after 10 p.m. While getting control of her eating may be enough to re-establish her confidence and improve her mood, further work often remains to be done in some form of psychotherapeutic consultation, as these patients frequently have additional problems.

Mary, aged 25 and married with two children, presented to her GP with bulimia while her husband, John, was on a business trip to the USA. She had never told anyone about it before, and her husband was unaware of the problem. As a child she felt that her mother set great store by her eating what was put in front of her. At about 13 she asserted her independence by becoming mildly anorexic and later mixing with boys her mother didn't like. Father was a shadowy figure. When John had gone to the USA, mother had started to bring cooked dishes over to Mary, 'to help'. This brought back oppressive memories of her childhood which were so distressing that she sought aid. By involving John in the management of the problem, especially in helping her not to vomit, the situation came under control but brought out difficulties in her relationship with him, and men in general, which needed specialized psychotherapy.

Various theories have been put forward about the origins of these problems and, while the evidence is insufficient to confirm or refute them, it is helpful to see the eating disorder in the context of the family, as in Mary's case above—the girl's over-concern with food and eating is her attempt to control some part of her life in a family that exerts control over other areas. Another approach, especially to anorexia nervosa, is to see the weight control as an attempt to retain the child-like shape, and to resist entry to the adult role, of which menstruation and the ability to bear children is part.

It can also be useful to see these problems in the context of society's value systems for women. It seems that eating problems are far more common in societies which admire thinness in women and less common in countries, and at times, when a more robust figure is in vogue. Many of the attitudes which the anorexic and bulimic exemplify are also very common in teenage girls in general in Western countries today, and their problems may simply be an extreme form of the behaviour which these attitudes encourage.

In all eating disorders it is natural for doctors and parents to see the main problem as one of persuading the patient to eat. The patient, however, has quite different priorities. If we are to help to bring about any radical change, we must engage with the problems that matter to the patient. We may then find that the eating disorder disappears. Therapy of eating problems can be difficult, but is not always so, and there can be few therapies more rewarding than those which enable an ugly, anxious, and immature duckling to emerge as a mature swan.

Reference

1. Banks, M. H., Clegg, C. W., Jackson, P. R., Kemp, N. J., Stafford, E. M., and Wall, T. D. (1980). The use of the General Health Questionnaire as an indicator of mental health in occupational studies. *J. Occup. Psychol.* **53**, 187–94.

Further reading

Bruggen, P. and O'Brian, C. (1986). *Surviving adolescence. A handbook for adolescents and their parents.* Faber and Faber, London.

5.6 SEXUALITY AND SEX THERAPY

Sexual maturation

Sexual maturation accompanies physical development from babyhood onwards, gradually until adolescence, and then more rapidly. Defining

214   *The family life cycle*

maturity is difficult, but might run as follows: a sexually mature person is able to form a stable relationship with another person, usually of the opposite sex, which is both physically and emotionally satisfying and in which sexual intercourse forms an important, though not the only, mode of expressing love.

The early sexual and social development of boys and girls tends to follow a common pattern. By the end of the first year of life children of both sexes are usually closer to their mothers than their fathers. However, the stereotyping of gender roles starts from birth. By 3–4 years most children copy the parent of the same sex and become aware of the attributions which are made about them. Little girls mother dolls and younger children, and little boys play with objects such as footballs or trains; little boys are handsome and little girls are pretty. By this age most children are firmly identified with the sex role that has been assigned to them, and this is confirmed by the study of intersexes who have been incorrectly sexed at birth (due to malformations of the genitalia). If the mistake is not discovered until after the third year, it becomes virtually impossible to alter the child's sexual identity. This pattern tends to produce boys who are tough and girls who are tender. Some parents attempt to soften these stereotypes by giving little boys dolls and little girls swords, but the influence of the outside world, especially at school, tends to reinforce the traditional roles.

Masturbation is a normal expression of sexuality at all ages and in both sexes, though it may be coloured by guilt, often learnt in early childhood from adults. It is not uncommon for little girls to present to their general practitioners with sore labia, the result of masturbation, and the myths of acne and madness resulting from masturbation may underlie later consultations. It is also normal for little boys and girls to wish to see and explore the bodies of the opposite sex.

In early adolescence, when children are attempting to achieve independence from their parents and become part of the peer group, single-sex gangs are common, as are crushes on people of the same sex. The occurrence of such single-sex relationships is no predictor of the later establishment of homosexuality, being just one form of the normal search for identity at this age. Later, sexual relationships develop between the sexes, first on a tentative, almost experimental, basis, then more permanently as part of a wider relationship. At this stage a dichotomy may occur between the physical and emotional aspects of the relationship, especially amongst youngsters who have had a strict religious upbringing. The ideal girl is 'pure' and asexual, yet it is the physical which is the dominant desire. This leads to guilt and confusion. Gentle reassurance that both facets are important and 'good' in a relationship can be very helpful without in any way impinging on the young person's moral code. By the age of 18 the majority of both boys and girls have had some experience of sexual intercourse.[1]

Developmental difficulties

Difficulties created early in childhood often reappear in different guises during adolescence, but this may also be a time when new ways of feeling and thought become possible. Sexual development and personality interrelate. For example, introverted and shy persons, who condition more easily and are poor at self-assertion, are more likely to develop unusual expressions of their sexuality. In the same way, feelings of inferiority, perhaps engendered by parental attitudes or schoolteachers, may be reinforced by anxieties about physical development. Boys frequently worry about penile or general body size—either too big or too small. Girls may worry about hirsutism or the size of their breasts. Girls who develop breasts before their peers may be very embarrassed and wish to hide their developing sexuality, a trait which may persist into later life. Late development will tend to create feelings of inadequacy and inferiority. Much will depend on the parents' acceptance of these variations of normal development. Boys have similar difficulties. Of two 14-year-olds, one may have a tiny penis and a high voice and the other may be fully physically developed. The normal variation in age of onset of puberty needs to be stressed, as does the normality of boys developing transient 'breast buds' during adolescence.

From the earliest years, the behaviour and attitudes of parents will have a profound effect on sexual development. The development of trust and autonomy, and the ability to give and receive love, all of which begin in the first years of life, form the basis of a person's ability to experience a full relationship. An obvious later factor is the parents' attitudes to sexuality, which can vary from severe prudishness to flaunting exhibitionism. Even now, some parents seem unable to prepare their children for, or to be able to explain to them the changes of, puberty. In particular the parents' attitude to masturbation may determine feelings of enjoyment or guilt about sex. Sexual myths (see Table 5.2) may be acquired from parental models, from parental behaviour, and from the peer group.

Feelings of inadequacy, impotence, frigidity, and low libido may have their origins in the early teens. So, too, may eating disorders such as anorexia nervosa, which are thought often to result from attempts to avoid or repudiate adult sexual roles (see p. 210).

Incest by adults, particularly if it is repeated, and accompanied by coercion, can lead to frigidity, promiscuity, or prostitution. Sexual molestation by siblings may be less dangerous (see p. 200).

Homosexuality

Less obviously, the strength, weakness, or absence of a parent may affect both the strength of a person's sexual attachments and their orientation. A boy with a weak or absent father and a possessive mother may have difficulty

Table 5.2.   *Some common sexual myths* (from Hawton 1985[2])

1. A man always wants and is always ready to have sex
2. Sex must only ever occur at the instigation of the man
3. Any woman who initiates sex is immoral
4. Sex equals intercourse: anything else doesn't really count
5. When a man gets an erection it is bad for him not to use it to get an orgasm very soon
6. Sex should always be natural and spontaneous: thinking or talking about it spoils it
7. All physical contact must lead to intercourse
8. Men should not express their feelings
9. Any man ought to know how to give pleasure to any woman
10. Sex is really good only when partners have orgasms simultaneously
11. If people love each other they will know how to enjoy sex together
12. Partners in a sexual relationship instinctively know what the other partner thinks or wants
13. Masturbation is dirty or harmful
14. Masturbation within a sexual relationship is wrong
15. If a man loses his erection it means he doesn't find his partner attractive
16. It is wrong to have fantasies during intercourse
17. A man cannot say 'no' to sex/a woman cannot say 'no' to sex
18. There are certain absolute, universal rules about what is normal in sex.

in valuing his own masculinity and this may predispose him to seek homosexual relationships. Similarly, a girl who identifies strongly with her father may seek relationships with her own sex. Other factors which predispose to homosexual development are mistakes or ambiguity in child rearing, as indicated above. Young children are very sensitive to the expectations and other assumptions of parents and siblings. Once little boys have been labelled as 'girlish' or little girls seen as 'tomboys' it may be quite hard for them to shake off this identity. Most, however, will do this during their 'teens' when their secondary sexual characteristics develop. At this point social pressures to conform to the morphologically appropriate sex are considerable, but they can be 'turned off' the opposite sex by humiliation in a sexual encounter. Conversely they can be 'switched on' by members of the same sex if faced with particularly seductive experiences, or if heterosexual outlets are blocked.

Although the causes of homosexuality are not clear and some have postulated hereditory factors to explain a part of the variation, it does appear that, in many instances, in order for homosexual behaviour to persist and become the permanent preference, a person needs to have become disappointed or blocked in heterosexual relationships and have been successful and satisfied with the homosexual alternative. Despite this, there are some bisexual individuals who are attracted by both sexes, and many who have known 'as long as they can remember' that they are homosexual. In single-sex schools, prisons, and other circumstances in which heterosexual choice is blocked, many find themselves attracted by members of their own sex and, if opportunities present, may engage in homosexual behaviour. This can evoke considerable anguish in young people who mistakenly believe that such experiences mean that they are 'gay'. It is reassuring for them to learn that, in more normal environments, they may find heterosexual feelings arising when they meet members of the opposite sex.

It is not helpful to regard homosexuality as either a sin or a sickness. These attributions only add to the problems. Nor is any 'therapy' effective in changing the direction of peoples' sexual orientation. On the other hand, there is much that members of the primary care team (PCT) can do to help people to decide upon, and to come to terms with, their sexuality. We can explain that many overt heterosexuals have homosexual fantasies and dreams, and that about 5–10 per cent of both sexes have predominantly homosexual dispositions. Some choose to 'come out of the closet', declaring their sexual identity to the world and living with the consequences. Others prefer to keep their sex lives private, and there are many who marry members of the opposite sex and raise families, acknowledging to their spouse that they are attracted by their own sex. Although statistics on such matters are unreliable, there is no reason to doubt that such marriages can last and be reasonably successful. Encouraging the discussion of these issues in a matter-of-fact way, and without making value judgements, will do much to alleviate the burden of stigma and guilt which still shrouds the lives of homosexuals.

It seems that the threat of AIDS is changing the pattern of male homosexual behaviour, and it is certainly appropriate for the general practitioner to discuss the dangers with all known homosexuals and to recommend most strongly the adoption of safer sexual practices.

Whether homosexuals should, after careful counselling, be tested for HIV infection is a difficult question, bearing in mind that there is no cure available. It really hinges on the risk of others becoming infected if those tested were to be found positive and did not alter their sexual practices. Once they have been tested, they will need to declare this when applying for life insurance, and, even if they are negative, may find it difficult to get cover. If they are positive, they will need all the resources of counselling and physical management which can be provided to help them. While the PCT will, of necessity, be involved, it is advisable to refer such patients to a local clinic for sexually transmitted disease, and to put them in contact with the Terence Higgins Trust. This organization runs support groups for people who are HIV positive (body positive) and also provides befriending for patients who go on to develop AIDS (see Appendix II).

HIV-positive patients who continue to place others at risk are a menace. Since such behaviour is usually a reflection of aggrieved rage which has been stirred up by the awesome news, it is usually transient. They require intensive emotional support if they are to be dissuaded from this behaviour.

Anxiety about homosexuality is common in adolescents and often presents, thinly veiled, to the PCT. It may be exaggerated by prejudices against homosexuals in the peer culture and pressures to have relationships with the opposite sex. Amongst the issues to be discussed will be a reminder that we all have some bisexual potential. In general practice a straightforward counselling approach will usually be appropriate. Very occasionally, anxieties about sexual identity may be the first presentation of a psychotic illness.

Initiating discussion about the possibility of homosexuality can be difficult. Phrases such as 'In adolescence people have many thoughts and feelings about their sexuality and sometimes wonder in which direction their inclinations lie. Has this been the case with you, and if so would you care to tell me about it?' or 'Can you tell me about the relationship with your sexual partner?' may help.

Other forms of sexual dysfunction

The norms of sexual expression — vaginal intercourse, mutual masturbation, cunnilingus, fellatio, etc. will vary from culture to culture and from partner to partner, and any mismatch may need elucidating and counselling. Other uncommon pathways of sexual expression seldom present as problems to the PCT, perhaps because of the shame which is attached to them, but, when they do, they need a lot of help. Their management is also difficult.

People who cross-dress either in private or in public often have otherwise intact personalities, and this may be a normal, transient expression of adolescent confusion. Such people are often successful in the rest of their lives but, if married, may embarrass or confuse their spouses, so that marital counselling may be appropriate. Fetishes are in some ways similar, in that the rest of the patients' lives may be unaffected. Occasionally, however compulsion to steal underwear, or impose their fetishes on their partners may lead to involvement with the law or to marital distress. Fetishism may be traceable to specific sexually charged events in childhood. Treatment by behavioural psychotherapy may be helpful in limiting distress.

Flashers are usually inadequate, sad people who are unlikely to attempt rape or assault, unlike some rapists who do have very disturbed personalities. Some flashers have been helped by group therapy and some by behavioural psychotherapy. Any suggestion of violence towards victims, even if it does not lead to actual harm at the time, should be taken seriously. One violent act leads to another, and sexual sadism is very dangerous. The needs of the victims of rape and their consorts need to be remembered. Bestiality is often the result of loneliness, isolation, and alcohol.

Transvestites and transsexuals rarely present to general practitioners, perhaps because of the stigma, but if they do, they may request referral. Paedophilia usually presents through the Courts, but all sufferers and victims should be offered referral. Refusal to accept referral creates ethical problems, with a conflict between confidentiality and the risk to the children concerned.

Sexual dysfunction

Introduction

The term 'sexual dysfunction', though ambiguous, has here been reserved for problems relating to the sexual act itself.

There is a high prevalence of sexual dysfunction within marriages and couples[3] but its presentation to general practitioners is less common than might be expected, and its recognition depends on the skills and attitudes of the doctor. It may be presented openly, but more often it is part of a complex situation and so needs to be remembered as an underlying factor in relationship problems, depression, anxiety, or somatic symptoms.

Some patients will turn to the members of the PCT for help with sexual dysfunction because they are known, trusted, and make patients feel at ease. Others may feel embarrassment in disclosing sensitive problems to someone to whom they have previously entrusted only their physical health problems.

Categories

It is hard to give a definition of sexual dysfunction because what may be normal and satisfactory for one couple or individual may be a source of discord and unhappiness for others. Most problems present as dissatisfactions and may fall into any of the following categories:

- disorders of the desire phase—lack of interest in sexual behaviour;
- disorders of the excitement phase—mainly impotence in men and failure of relaxation and secretion in women;
- disorders of the orgasmic phase—premature ejaculation, retarded ejaculation, no orgasm in women;
- vaginismus and dyspareunia;
- ejaculatory pain
- sexual phobias

not considered further here, as specialist help is always needed.

Aetiology

Before considering psychological problems, it is well to remember that sexual function depends on satisfactory anatomical structures as well as normal physiological responses. Many illnesses and drugs cause sexual problems and are fully listed in Keith Hawton's excellent book.[2]

The more important drugs to remember are alcohol, which, while in moderation may reduce inhibitions and therefore increase performance, causes impotence when taken in excess. Of the hypotensives, bendrofluazide has been shown recently to cause impotence in up to 50 per cent of male patients, and tricyclic antidepressants can cause dry orgasms.

Of common illnesses affecting sexual function, diabetes often causes diagnostic problems. Impotence in such patients may be due either to the disease itself or to emotional problems. The occurrence of nocturnal erections makes diabetic neuropathy unlikely.

Psychological problems

Anxiety is the commonest cause of sexual dysfunction and sexual dysfunction causes anxiety, so the situation may become self-perpetuating. The associated causes of anxiety are:

(1)   intrapsychic—problems originating in the person's previous experience or personality;

(2)   situational—problems relating to where sex takes place;

(3)   interactional—problems relating to the relationship between those taking part;

(4)   performance—problems centred on perceived inadequacy in the performance of the sexual act.

Sexual problems may also be classified as primary or secondary, primary implying that the causes date back to childhood or adolescence, and secondary being the result of later experience. This division has implications for further history-taking and therapeutic strategies.

Intrapsychic

Whatever model of psychosocial development is used, anxiety often seems to date back to early childhood and to be deeply rooted. Freudians use the model of the Oedipal conflict, which assumes that children feel guilt at sexual feelings towards the parent of the opposite sex. This guilt is said to become repressed so that the person is unaware why it is that members of the opposite sex have become forbidden objects. The sexual ambience of the household is an important factor, and the sexually cold patient who describes the inability of her mother to talk about sex and menstruation is still not uncommon. Incest is increasingly being recognized as a reality and not only a fantasy, though either may be pathogenic (see p. 200). Other traumatic events, such as rape or painful first intercourse, are further causes of anxiety. Some people will be left with a feeling of disgust, not only about sexual intercourse, but about the genitalia of either or both sexes. Some may suffer guilt about past sexual activities, including masturbation.

A major source of anxiety can be the conflict between beliefs and attitudes (including those associated with religious and cultural groups), on the one hand, and sexual inclinations, on the other.

In addition to such causes, root problems of sexual dysfunction include fears of intimacy, rejection, or failure.

Secondary intrapsychic dysfunction often follows childbirth. Dyspareunia due to physical causes, such as a badly healed episiotomy scar, needs first to be excluded or remedied. Tiredness, depression, involvement with the baby, and lack of opportunity seem to be the commonest reasons given by patients for problems after childbirth, and are often allowed to drift on and become self-perpetuating.

A few couples find intercourse without the hope or risk of pregnancy unexciting. Fear of pregnancy may also have an inhibiting effect. As well as specific sexual difficulties, people's general self-confidence and belief in their own attractiveness are relevant.

Situational

Preservation of life takes priority over sexual reproduction. Any whiff of danger or fear is enough to deflate most men and, once intercourse has been unsuccessful, impotence may continue because of the fear of failure. Anxiety about privacy and interruption, or about discomfort, are influential: premature ejaculation may sometimes be a conditioned response from previous hurried intercourse caused by fear of interruption in difficult circumstances—for example, in the back of a car or in a parental home. Coitus interruptus or experience with a prostitute can have the same effect. For most people, the ambience and setting for sexual activity is best when it is not merely free from fear, stress, and symbols of stress, but is also romantic, relaxing, exciting, and unconstrained by time.

Interactional

Some men and women are capable of satisfactory sexual intercourse with strangers, but for most the success and joys of love-making depends on the couple's whole relationship. Some people are unable to have satisfactory sexual intercourse with a particular partner, but may be able to do so with different partners. Unresolved anger, irritation, suspicion, poor communication, and lack of love or trust may render sex impossible or unsatisfactory. Changing physical appearance due to age, trauma, or surgery for example mastectomy, may also be important.

Some couples are ignorant of the anatomy and physiology of sexual intercourse so that their mode of love-making is relatively crude, unsatisfying or painful. This is often combined with the inability to discuss openly the difficulties of sexual performance. Difficulties may also be a reflection of deeper conflicts in which experiences of early relationships, usually with parents, are echoed. Some people who view sex as a profane or 'dirty' activity can only enjoy it with a partner who is also degraded. Hence the people whose sex life stops abruptly on the day when they get married to someone they love and respect.

Performance

An isolated experience of failure, which is not uncommon, and which may have been precipitated by illness, alcohol, tiredness, or a new situation, may lead to a vicious circle of anxiety causing repeated failure. Less dramatically people may have anxieties about their performance and fantasies about the prowess and responsiveness of other people. Each partner may also be concerned about being seen as sexually inferior or not matching up to previous sexual partners. A man's fear of failure and of failing to please his partner can spiral to the point where intercourse becomes impossible.

These psychological causes of anxiety may be involved at any of the three phases of intercourse but, in general, disorders of the desire phase are more often associated with deeper problems. Given an appropriate stimulus, few people with normal physiology and anatomy, and free from drugs, lack desire. Where no desire manifests itself, it is often because it is suppressed at a very early stage. This suppression seems to protect against anxiety about sexual awakening, negative images, fears of letting go, or fears of rejection. The idea of a low sexual drive is probably less helpful than that of a suppressed one.

Disorders of the excitement phase are likely to be associated with fear of rejection as well as deeper problems. Disorders of the orgasmic phase are often related to ignorance, understimulation, spectatoring (the phenomenon of watching one's own performance), or concentration on control. Women may simulate arousal and enjoyment. Orgasm is essentially an autonomic function but, if observed, it can be inhibited. Distraction may allow release.

Management by the primary care team

Presentation

It is important that sexual dysfunction, however presented, be recognized as a problem in its own right, particularly as it may often be treated with elative ease. Such problems may be presented, overtly or covertly, to any member of the PCT, and the following notes are intended to help with the assessment of the dysfunction. Once this has been done, the person to whom the problem has been presented will need to decide whether to go on to attempt therapy. If the problems are thought too difficult, or rapport has not been well established, or one is uncomfortable in handling the particular problem presented, referral to someone else in the PCT (e.g. a counsellor) or to an outside agency may be wise. The decision whether or not to do this should be made before there is too much investment of time or energy on the professional's side, and before the patient has had to go through painful self-disclosures, which may then need to be repeated to someone else. Transfer to someone else, once a working relationship has been forged, may make the patient feel rejected.

Although people often present their sexual problems as personal ones, most of the common ones represent dysfunction within a couple and it is therefore usually more helpful to see couples together. Sexual problems also tend to be mixed with relationship problems and both parties may need help.

Occasionally improvement in the sexual dysfunction may encourage the general relationship to improve and vice versa. Often it is necessary to see individuals alone, at least once. A person may, for instance, have no regular partner, or may wish to disclose experiences and thoughts which they do not, at least initially, wish to share with their partners. What follows applies to couples in general, heterosexual and homosexual.

The motivation of both members needs to be ascertained. Both may be reluctant to give priority, time, and effort to the therapy, or one partner may be reluctant. If the reluctant partner can be engaged for one or two sessions, the experience may kindle enthusiasm, particularly when he or she discovers that the therapist is not in the business of apportioning blame. As in all therapies, the responsibility for change rests with the patient or patients, and the therapist is merely the facilitator.

The history

Before offering help with the sexual dysfunction, it may be wise to enquire about the relationship. As stated above, a relationship will sometimes improve if the dysfunction is relieved, but more often the dysfunction will persist until the relationship has improved. Continuing infidelity is probably a contraindication to therapy. Psychiatric illnesses may present as sexual dysfunction and, in particular, depression may present as a lack of libido. Pregnancy may be a particularly good, or particularly difficult, time to help couples. Questions should be asked to discover about relevant medical illnesses, past and present.

Having elicited that there are sexual difficulties, it is important to discover exactly what the sexual dysfunction is. This will enable appropriate management to be offered, and will reassure the patient that sexual matters can be discussed. It may be easier at this stage for either party to talk alone. It may be appropriate to enquire about wet dreams and morning erections, and sensations of arousal in women, all of which usually signify an intact physiology, though very occasionally nocturnal erections may still be present when there is a neurological reason for failure of the excitement phase.

While sexual therapy is concerned with the present, it may be important to take a sexual history as this may give clues to the origins of current beliefs, attitudes, and practices. This would include asking about masturbation, early sexual experiences, traumatic events, and the sexual history of the marriage. Because many people who have sexual dysfunctions are shy and embarrassed at talking about sexual matters, and because some doctors may not be at ease, this can be a difficult conversation. A framework of questions may help some, for instance 'Most people have sexual difficulties at some point, say after a baby is born, when they have worries, when they have rows; have you any such difficulties?', 'Most people have had some experience of masturbation, could you tell me about yours?'

Examination

Local physical examination may be important not only to exclude anatomical causes of dysfunction, especially in dyspareunia, but also because it helps to eliminate fears of abnormality which are often at the back of many patients' minds. The extent of any general physical examination will be determined by the history, but it is important to exclude neurological, endocrine, and vascular disorders.

Investigations

Again, these will be guided by the history, but in cases of impotence and loss of excitement it is sometimes helpful to estimate the serum testosterone, prolactin, and luteinizing hormone levels, as abnormal levels may signify a physical cause. If these are done at an early stage, the results may help silence any nagging doubts in both the doctor's and the patient's mind. However, it is equally important not to raise doubts about physical disorders when the solution is most likely to be found in the psychological area.

Treatment

After the history has been taken and examination carried out, a presentation of the therapist's formulation of the problem in terms which the patient or couple can understand will help to clarify the situation and may initiate a process of change.

This might comprise his or her understanding of:

● the nature of the problem (if only to make sure this has been agreed);

● the background factors relevant to the relationship;

- the factors which have precipitated the problem;
- the factors which have maintained the problem.

As stated before, disorders of desire are the most deep-rooted and the most difficult to treat, necessitating a mixture of behavioural, couple, and individual psychotherapy, while disorders of orgasm are the easiest and may often be helped by simple behavioural methods.

It is often surprisingly easy to help disorders of any phase by what may be termed superficial manoeuvres, without exploring the deeper aspects of the psyche. However, it should again be remembered that the treatment of sexual disorders, in general, frequently involves the delicate exploration of people's fears and anxieties.

Perhaps the greatest service a general practitioner or other therapist can do is to 'normalize' sexual experience. Many people have unrealistic expectations about such things as the normal frequency of sexual activity and the length of time it 'should' take, the importance of mutual orgasms, or the expectation of multiple orgasms in the woman. The patterns of sex are so infinitely variable that if the couple's pattern gives pleasure to both of them, they are unwise to measure it against any arbitrary standard.

The PLISSIT mnemonic is not only a convenient framework for thinking about helping sexual problems, but also suggests a logical order for treatment.

Permission
Limited Information
Specific Suggestions
Intensive Therapy

1. *Permission* Depending on the relationship with the patient, the GP may be in a good position to remove the restraints on sexual communication and behaviours which people have acquired over the years. The implication of this is that therapists need themselves to be free from restraints and hang-ups about sexual matters. As was said earlier, merely talking explicitly about sexual anatomy and experience helps to dispel myths, and can facilitate better communication between couples.

While it may be appropriate, if that is what the client or couple want, to give permission for digital stimulation of the clitoris and manual excitement of the penis, or for oral–genital contact to be made, it must be remembered that some activities will be distasteful for some people, and that pleasurable (and satisfactory) sex can be achieved without experiencing every possible form of stimulation. If requested, permission to masturbate may be given to the individual but other permissions are probably better negotiated with the couple. Permission can also be given to accept less than perfection. The couple should be encouraged not to turn sexual experiences which are not quite perfect into disasters, nor to minimize pleasures which do not include full intercourse and orgasm as valueless. These concepts of magnification and minimization may need to be brought into the open and discussed. Stereotyping needs to be broken through. Men need to be given permission to express such feelings as tenderness, compassion, weakness, and sensuality, regarded by some as unmasculine. The inability to do this can lead to very mechanical and distasteful experiences for women. Similarly, women may need to be given permission to initiate, take charge of, or orchestrate sex on some occasions. Some people may need permission and encouragement to use fantasy as an aid.

In this section we have repeatedly said that 'permission can be given to . . .' as if therapists have a divine dispensation. They may, indeed, have some authority and have parental powers projected onto them, but we have used this form of words as an abbreviation for 'with help the patient or couple can be enabled to give themselves permission to . . . .'

2. *Limited information*   It helps to have some diagrams or models to explain the anatomy and physiology of sexual intercourse; some people may be strangely ignorant. As well as limited information it may be helpful to discuss some of the popular myths (see Table 5.2). Although it is our thesis that sex is usually a natural and spontaneous event with wide variations, and that to medicalize it is a mistake, it is also true that sexual skills can be learned and improved. This is often difficult for some, especially men, to accept. Information may also need to be given about contraception, lubricants, the menopause and the feasibility of sex, or alternative methods of expressing sexual feelings in old age and in the disabled.

3. *Specific suggestions*   Before discussing specific sexual suggestions, it may be helpful to offer advice about the setting of sex within the hurly-burly of everyday life. Sex is usually more enjoyable when the couple are relaxed, and it is appropriate to offer suggestions about peace, warmth, a little alcohol, flowers, scent, cleanliness, lubricants, and perhaps music. Non-sexual massage, perhaps using attractive oils or lotions, is enjoyed by many on its own or as a relaxing prelude to sex. Some may need other sexual aids.

Sensate focus

Whatever the disorder, reducing the pressure to perform and creating a structure within which some sexual and sensual pleasures can be achieved is an advance. *Sensate focus* is a technique which is helpful in many dysfunctions. Initially, the partners are instructed not to attempt penetrative intercourse, but encouraged to spend an agreed amount of time together, pleasuring and caressing each other without genital stimulation. Some time needs to be spent discussing and experimenting with what actually does give each pleasure. Couples must speak to each other about what pleases them, and what doesn't.

At the next interview, if successful intercourse has not already occurred, as often happens in spite of the instruction, the caressing proceeds to genital stimulation subject to a veto on continuing to orgasm.

During the next stage the penis is inserted into the vagina with the woman in the superior position. She thrusts a few times, without the expectation of orgasm, and disengages before there is loss of erection or anxiety about performance. Male orgasm may then be achieved manually by either partner, according to preference. The woman may be given gentle digital stimulation which may or may not lead to orgasm. Attempts at full intercourse are still discouraged.

Subsequently, coitus is not attempted until the woman is well lubricated and is again best done with the woman in the superior position. In the final stage, orgasm is allowed with the man in the superior position. During sensate focus therapy, motivational and relationship problems may be highlighted and have to be dealt with.

Specific difficulties

Premature ejaculation Voluntary control over ejaculation is helped by increasing the patient's awareness and increasing his tolerance for the pleasurable sensation that occurs with the sexual excitement which comes before orgasm. It is usually unhelpful to suggest holding back, which may have failed so often before. Instead, the man can be encouraged to transfer his awareness to erotic sensation (see also p. 222).

The following method first described by Semans is frequently effective but relies on the couple being seen together.[4]

(1) The partner stimulates the man's penis, usually manually, until he is near orgasm. He tells her when this point has been reached and asks her to stop stimulation and to squeeze the shaft just proximal to the glans. A few seconds later, when he feels the intense sensations diminish, he asks her to start again. This is repeated until he is allowed to have his orgasm on the fourth stimulation.

(2) The stop/start stimulation of the penis manually by the partner is repeated, this time using a lubricant, e.g. KY jelly. This makes the experience more like vaginal intercourse.

(3) Stop/start stimulation is conducted intra-vaginally in the female-superior position. The man puts his hands on the partner's hips to guide her motions. She moves up and down until he feels he is near climax, when he tells her to stop. After a pause he asks her to start again and he climaxes on the fourth occasion. At first he should not thrust during this exercise. At a later stage, when intercourse is lasting longer, he proceeds to thrusting. When confidence has been reached in this

position, the side-to-side and male-superior position can be experimented with.

Orgasm problems   Orgasm is usually inhibited by the intensive observation of the act (spectatoring), associated with the fear of failure. Release may be obtained by distracting the attention from the performance and by achieving orgasm in different situations. Concentrating on the response and needs of the partner and not on one's own may be helpful. Some people can distract their attention by the use of fantasy and, for some, orgasm may be easier to achieve through masturbation. This provides a useful route for the solution of the problem.

Manual stimulation of the penis and the clitoris may be achieved with the aid of lubricants, fantasies, or vibrators. Once orgasm can be achieved alone by masturbation, it can be repeated in the company of the partner, unless there is strong resistance to masturbation. This shared experience can be repeated with increasing proximity and intimacy. Later, mutual manual masturbation can be tried, and finally intercourse. Sometimes, inability to achieve orgasm reflects deeper sexual conflicts which may require intensive treatment.

Excitement phase disorders   The inhibition of erection and excitement by performance anxiety is removed by reducing the anxiety and by avoiding making demands. The sensate focus technique is especially helpful.

Disorders of the desire phase   The simple measures outlined in the section on 'limited information' (p. 226), together with the sensate focus model, may be sufficient. Often, however, exploration of possible blocks, both intrapsychic and to do with the couple, may be necessary.

Although the above have been phrased to apply to heterosexual intercourse, the principles, and many of the specific techniques, are equally helpful in problems relating to homosexual activity.

Vaginismus   Here the therapist will need to advise the patient how to extinguish the spasm reflex conditioned by past fear or pain.

(1)   Limited information about vaginal anatomy is given, with the aid of drawings or models, and the patient is advised to study her own vagina with a mirror.

(2)   The patient is told to introduce her lubricated finger, or a small dilator, daily, when alone, peaceful, and relaxed.

(3)   Subsequently, two or three fingers or larger dilators are used.

(4)   The experience is repeated with the partner present and he is allowed

to insert one or two of his fingers without any attempt at sexual stimulation.

(5) The penis is inserted under control of the woman without thrusting.

(6) Full intercourse is achieved.

4. *Intensive therapy* Treatment of the less common or more difficult dysfunctions are not discussed here, as they are likely to need specialist treatment. The books suggested in the list of further reading are recommended.

References

1. Schofield, M. (1973). *Sexual behaviour of young adults*. Allen Lane, London.
2. Hawton, K. (1985). *Sex therapy: a practical guide*. Oxford University Press.
3. The Hite reports:
   Hite, S. (1976). *A nationwide study of female sexuality*. Dell, New York.
   Hite, S. (1981). *A nationwide study of male sexuality*. Dell, New York.
4. Semans, J. M. (1956). Premature ejaculation. A new approach. *Southern Med. J.* **49**, 353–7.

Further reading

Devlin, D. (1974). *The book of love*. New English Library, London. (Useful for giving to patients.)
Hawton, K. (1985). *Sex therapy: a practical guide*. Oxford University Press. (Particularly useful, brief, and clear.)
Kaplan, H. S. (1973). *The new sex therapy*. Penguin, Harmondsworth.
Storr, A. (1964). *Sexual deviation*. Penguin, Harmondsworth.

5.7 THE FAMILY HOME

The major transitions of young adult life, leaving school, starting in employment, leaving the parental home, and making lasting sexual relationships all move inexorably toward the founding of a new home. Home is, or should be, a safe place in which securely attached couples provide their young with the environment which will enable them to grow up physically and mentally healthy. Unfortunately, there are many obstacles along the way, and in this section we shall examine the nature of these and their implications for the prevention of mental ill health in parents and children.

The small nuclear family of two parents and one, two, or three children living together is a relatively recent phenomenon. Industrialization and the increased mobility which results from this effectively breaks up large family units. In the extended family, which still exists in many parts of the world, parents, grandparents, aunts, and uncles live together or in close proximity. This makes for greater flexibility in the face of temporary or permanent separations, enables roles to be shared more widely, encourages the old to remain useful, and gives the young support in their new responsibilities.

In industrial countries this is seldom the case. Parents may survive longer than they did, but they often live at a distance and, if they do move near, it is often because of their own needs for support. Links with siblings and other relatives are less close, and allegiances which can make 'the family' a real source of security and pride may not exist. This means that the nuclear family is more vulnerable than the extended.

Of course, there is another side to this argument. The industrial society is a much safer place than the Third World. Starvation and disease do not haunt the home and, except in a few inner-city areas, footpads do not haunt the streets. Social security and a good standard of health care have reduced many of the threats that made the family so essential in the past. Gradually, and almost imperceptibly, we have come to view the extended 'family' of the State as our principal source of security, and that massive network of interdependent social units has increased in complexity and organization to meet this assumption.

Because of this it is no longer possible or necessary for us to rely so much on the home, family, and neighbourhood friends at times of trouble. The church, which formerly provided strict control over the beliefs and rituals attending family milestones (births, deaths, and marriages), as well as supporting the sick, elderly, and widowed, has lost influence. The parish, as a living entity in the lives of its members, has dwindled in importance.

Sex roles

This change in the function of the home and family is associated with a similar change in the ways in which these functions are divided. Many women now see their status as deriving from their work, rather than their domestic roles. The word 'housewife' has for them taken on a pejorative meaning, and even 'mothering' is often seen as a hiatus in a 'career' rather than a prime function of women. Conflicts arise between parents on the extent to which parenting should be shared, and both may see child-care as a burden rather than a reward.

In most families prime responsibility for financial provision still rests with the man and this reinforces his traditional role as the 'bread-winner'. In the past his superiority in this role was enhanced by his superior physical strength, but in a society in which mechanical power has replaced muscle power this advantage is relatively slight. In fact, men often feel threatened by any superior brain power shown by women at home or at work. Whether or not men are, in fact, inferior to women in domestic and child-rearing roles, many tend to assume that they are, and those men who are forced (by sickness or unemployment) to adopt these roles usually feel emasculated and ashamed. Sports have taken on particular importance to men as one area of activity in which they can still excel.

As we saw in Chapter 1, there are biological differences between men and women which, despite the social pressures described above, push women towards child-rearing roles and men towards a more productive role to the whole family. This is reflected in the ways in which men and women express emotions. Women, in general, are more nurturant, express warmth and affection more openly, and are also more ready to express distress and to seek help than men. Hence, perhaps, their higher rates of consultation with GPs for help with depression and other 'emotional' symptoms. Men, on the other hand, tend to be more aggressive and assertive than women, reaching out and challenging external threats. They are more likely to repress, or avoid expression of, weakness or distress and find it more difficult to ask for help on their own account. At times of stress they often resort to self-prescription of alcohol in preference to seeking medical help. In their relationships with the opposite sex, men tend to be the more active and women the more passive partner.

There are, of course, many exceptions to these general statements, and individual upbringing, social, and family influences all play a part in explaining why some women are more 'masculine' than most men, and vice versa. Problems arise within and between individuals whenever the 'fit' between these many needs and the roles available conflict.

A woman who expects her spouse to play a greater part in child-care may be seen by her partner as a threat to his masculinity. Such women may compromise and know that their children are, to some degree, neglected, or they may sacrifice career success and feel that they are reduced in social status as a result. If they accept help, they are condemned as 'dependent'. If they insist on remaining autonomous, they are seen as 'butch'.

Men are peculiarly vulnerable to work stress and to isolation from support. The former arises from the very nature of the large organizations in which most work is now carried out (see Section 5.8), the latter from the compulsive self-reliance by which many men attempt to maintain their self-esteem.

Self-esteem, for either sex, arises from a confident assumption of personal worth, and this stems from a reasonably satisfactory fit between needs and roles. Even though not all needs can be instantly satisfied, we can tolerate this gap as long as we feel ourselves moving towards satisfaction. Many men today feel themselves helplessly caught up in an implacable machine over which they have little or no control. Because their control over their own world is limited, they find it particularly hard to give up what little control they have by asking for help. Self-control becomes a preordinate virtue, and any display of emotion a weakness and a source of shame. Physical disablement, because it reduces the individual's ability to control his world, is a particular threat to men. They may respond by ignoring the significance of the illness, refusing help, and minimizing symptoms. If their compulsive self-reliance fails to defend them and they are forced to acknowledge their incapacity, they may swing over to states of agitation, anger, or depression.

The transition from single to married roles

The psychological triggers for 'falling in love' are complex and poorly understood. Suffice it to say that the dwindling of attachment to parents which occurs during late adolescence is replaced by a powerful affiliative drive which tends to become focused on one person. This drive overrides the fear which maintains the boundaries between people and allows them to be penetrated. Some choose partners whose views reflect their own, others choose people who seem to complement them, and provide them with what they lack. Sexual intercourse is only one of the ways in which boundaries are dissolved, and those who 'fall in love' are often surprised at the experience of fusion and sharing of identity which results. The lover feels as if he or she knows the other person, as if they had one mind. This, of course, is an illusion. Lovers read into the other person an identity which is an amalgam of their own assumptions and hopes. Discrepancies tend to be ignored, hence love is indeed blind. Only as time passes will the discrepancies between romantic fantasy and reality become apparent. By this time a web of circumstances has usually reinforced the attachment.

Western society is so imbued with the assumption that love must precede marriage that we find the very idea that marriage should be arranged by parents obnoxious. Yet there are many parts of the world in which this is the norm, and Asian immigrants to the West continue to follow this tradition. Many Asians claim that parents are better qualified than young people to select partners who are suitable additions to their family, and that the attachments which then result are more likely to last for that very reason. The relative stability of marriages between Asians bears out this claim, but should not obscure the fact that the children of such marriages, living in this country, are confronted with conflicting assumptions which may be hard to reconcile.

Although the wedding ceremony is the legal and symbolic rite which establishes a couple as married, the psychosocial transition from single to married person starts before the wedding and continues for some time after it. This is reflected in the traditional period of engagement, in the honeymoon, and the later period of adjustment which follows.

Engagement is a time of preparation during which a couple begin to rehearse in their minds the implications of marriage. In so far as their plans are realistic, it is reasonable to suppose that the transition will proceed smoothly, but this is not always the case. Some people, as they come closer to the reality of marriage, experience rising anxiety and may shy away or develop tension symptoms (this has been termed 'engyesis' or 'engagement neurosis'). In such cases the GP is likely to be consulted and may have a role to play in helping the anxious party to talk through the root of their fears. We should not be in too much of a hurry to provide tranquillizers or facile reassurance, nor should we use our authority to push the person towards or away from marriage. By providing a non-judgemental space in which individuals are free to talk, we give them time to grieve for the real losses which may go along with marriages, and to have second thoughts about the wisdom of this step. Each partner may need to be seen, but it is advisable to see them separately at first.

Increasing numbers of people today adopt an alternative strategy, the 'trial marriage'. Instead of making a lifetime commitment, they enter into a period of cohabitation, without formal declaration of intent. On the face of it, this gives them the opportunity to discover how stable their relationship is before making promises. In fact there are other problems. Such relationships may be taken on without adequate reasons (one patient had moved in with his landlady so as to obtain the use of her toilet, truly a 'marriage of convenience!'), but, however lightly they may be entered into, it is in the nature of human relationships that they lead to attachments. Once an attachment has arisen it becomes increasingly difficult to sever, no matter how unsuitable, destructive, or painful it may be.

Whatever gains may accrue from marriage, it is likely that each partner will also lose something. During the honeymoon such losses can be disregarded and the couple can act out a fantasy of eternal bliss. Such problems as there are tend to stem from unrealistic expectations they may have of their own and their partner's sexual prowess (a good book on the subject of sex can be a great help, for example Devlin's *The book of love*[1]).

For many couples the realities of married life do not become apparent until they arrive home from the honeymoon. It then becomes more difficult to deny the stress produced by the need to learn a new pattern of life. Men, who may have relished the camaraderie of the pub and the football field, may find that these enthusiasms are not shared by their wives. Women with romantic notions of a home of their own may find themselves having to live as guests in the home of possessive mothers-in-law. Persisting attachments to parents give rise to jealousy and conflict.

Marital problems and their management

The security of the family may be undermined by the many stresses which arise in the early years of marriage. Each partner turns to the other in the hope of receiving support. Sometimes they get it, but at other times they may find that their partner's need for support equals or exceeds their own. Disillusioned, they turn back to the parents who supported them in the past. The marriage, they conclude, has failed. Alternatively, they may turn to another parent-figure, the GP, whose magic potions are expected to mitigate the symptoms of anxiety and despair. Marriage guidance counsellors are a valuable source of help in such cases, and some GPs have made arrangements for them to make regular visits to meet with the primary care team (PCT) and see clients in GP premises.

The question of referral to marriage guidance or other counsellors is one that has to be approached carefully so that the patient does not feel rejected by the doctor. If the doctor mentions early on in discussion of the problem that counselling is available, and that, if referral is made, the doctor will continue caring for the patient *with* the counsellor, the patient may feel more comfortable. In these situations it is also very important to stress that patients may define areas of strict confidentiality with each professional which the two will not share. But there are many couples who reject the help of a marriage guidance counsellor while continuing to seek the help of the PCT. They may imagine (incorrectly) that marriage guidance is only concerned with reconcilation, or that the professional or personal skills of the doctor are more appropriate to their case. The doctor's role in such cases must be to provide both partners with the time and opportunity to step aside from the pressing demands of the immediate situation and to take stock. It is advisable to see both of them together, unless it is clear that the relationship has broken down and that they will henceforth be leading separate lives. Individual consultations are divisive and it is not for any professional to press for a particular outcome, no matter how strongly we may feel on the matter.

Assumptions and myths

Each partner may have assumptions about the marriage and each other which stem from their experience of their parent's marriage. Children learn about the opposite sex by interaction with the parent of the opposite sex. They tend to over-generalize; thus a girl whose father abused her mother may treat all men with fear, a boy whose mother behaved like a slave will expect all women to be subordinate. Powerful myths may be involved and each partner may feel pressured towards an identity which does not fit. Peaceful individuals may be seen as aggressive, fearful as bold, children as adults, adults as children, lovers as monsters.

These projections are not consistent. A partner may be seen as a child at one moment and an adult the next. Particular situations which create anxiety may cause accusations of rejection and neglect which, at other times, are denied. This reflects the way in which images and assumptions from the past can be 'switched on' by later situations that evoke the same or similar feelings.

A man whose parents had been divorced claimed to trust his wife 'completely' but became pathologically jealous if his wife smiled at another man. Such action never failed to evoke extreme anger and reproaches which he later regretted. Seen in the surgery with his wife, he poured out a story of how, as a small child, he had been expected to act as 'look out' in case his father came in when his mother was with her lover. It was easy to see how feelings of anger and rage were being triggered by any situation which brought the betrayal to mind. By discussing this in the presence of his wife he found himself better able to control his feelings and those that did emerge were now understood. The wife, instead of feeling deeply hurt by his lack of trust, was able to tolerate the occasional spiteful words that continued to slip out.

Patterns of attachment

As we saw in Chapter 1, the nature and security of the attachments that are made in childhood sow the seeds of all later attachments. A person who has learned to cling remains a clinger, one who has become compulsively independent may grow up intolerant of closeness. These patterns persist into the marital relationship and influence the nature of the bond which arises. Sometimes the fit between partners may seem to work very well. A person who has always seen himself or herself as 'weak' may marry a partner who needs to be seen as 'strong'. Reciprocal interactions enable these myths to be confirmed and perpetuated. Two insecure people may cling together for fear of something worse. Each one's anxiety is perpetuated by being repeatedly confirmed by their partner; they withdraw into a 'hole in the ice' from which they gaze out, terrified, at a world which is seen as hostile. Partners who appear distant and intolerant of closeness are, at one level, hungry for love, and their attempts to get it sometimes lead to the so-called 'Yo-Yo' marriages in which they alternately come together only to break apart as one or other partner finds the increased closeness intolerable. Such marriages may be punctuated by outbursts of violence, and the outsider may be baffled by the persistence with which the injured party returns for more punishment. This sometimes leads us to label such relationships as sado-masochistic, as if the parties took pleasure in inflicting and receiving pain. But it is doubtful if this is the case. We should seek for an explanation of these recurrent scenarios in the childhood relationships which have set the pattern. Brought up in a world in which violence and threats of violence are 'normal', such partners may only feel 'at home' with people who are similarly inclined. A child whose only means of getting attention has been to provoke violence may later find him or herself irresistibly drawn into goading and provocative behaviour. The partner, who was teased and denigrated as a child, finds this behaviour quite familiar, an inevitable part of interaction which will henceforth become a normal part of the cat-and-dog marriage.

Such patterns are difficult to change, and the well-meaning professional who tries to act as peace-maker will often be disappointed. Even so, we are frequently asked to take sides or to deal with the aftermath of yet another outburst. If the pattern is clear-cut there may be little chance of changing it, but marital therapy (as described in Section 4.4) aimed at helping both partners to recognize the family script which they are enacting will sometimes help them to break out of these traps. We may also need to recognize that we, too, are written into the script. As parent figures we may be no more trusted than real parents and we, too, may find ourselves goaded and provoked. If we recognized the implications of this behaviour, we may be able to explain it to the patient.

The advent of the first pregnancy

The next major psychosocial transition is likely to be the arrival of the first child. During the pregnancy both partners have time to anticipate this event. However great the gain, there is also an element of loss. For the mother, the first of these may be the loss of physical attractiveness during pregnancy. This may seriously undermine her security, particularly if she is unsure of her partner's true feelings. Some pregnant women attempt to resolve this problem by denying its importance. They lose interest in sexuality and focus all their attention on their unborn baby. The husband may experience this as a rejection and develop feelings of antagonism towards his rival (the baby) which will continue to give rise to problems later.

Members of the PCT can help parents to acknowledge and talk through such difficulties, perhaps at antenatal classes. The husband may need to reassure the wife of his continuing care, and the wife to share her body and her baby with her husband.

Repudiation of sexuality during pregnancy sometimes reflects fear of damaging the baby. It is usually possible to reassure the mother on this point, and the whole question of sex during pregnancy is best brought up by the GP or health visitor during an early antenatal consultation, as patients are frequently reluctant to ask. Even so, it is common for primiparous mothers to feel extremely anxious about the safety of their unborn child and the increased responsibility may make them feel very insecure. Few are fully aware of the differences between a two-person and a three-person family. Henceforth, child-rearing will become a major preoccupation for at least one of the partners (usually the mother) and she will have to give up some established roles in order to accommodate the child. As already indicated she may have to choose between neglecting her career, her husband, or her baby. Of the three, her baby tends to take priority, but not without some conflicts, compromises, and often considerable guilt.

The realities of the situation frequently strike home a week or two after parturition. The excitement of the birth has worn off. From being the centre of attraction and congratulation the mother is now alone with her new demi-person. '*Maternity blues*' occur in 10 per cent of mothers and, in a minority (around 0.2 per cent), this may be so severe as to justify the term 'puerperal psychosis'.[2] Depressive reactions are most common after unplanned pregnancies, in those with a predisposition to depression, in those who have dependent relationships with their spouse, and in those who have previously had stillbirths and/or are disappointed with the new child (e.g. because it is 'the wrong sex' or, in some other way, imperfect). Sometimes the reaction is understandable in the light of an unsatisfactory life situation, at other times it seems quite inappropriate. The situation is made worse by the expectations of others that the mother cannot fail to be delighted with her new treasure. Even her spouse may be upset and annoyed by her reaction, which may undermine his own attempts to assure himself that 'everything in the garden is lovely'.[2]

In treating such mothers it is helpful to draw in the support of the family or others to relieve her of her immediate responsibilities and to give her time to think. If she is able to express her feelings, she should be encouraged to do so in an atmosphere of reassurance and trust. If depression is severe or there are psychotic or suicidal features, then antidepressant medication is likely to be needed and hospital admission may have to be considered.

Puerperal psychoses are thought usually to be causd by organic factors, and even if the psychotic symptoms are severe, the prognosis is good and most mothers will recover completely in the course of time. Situational factors are important; the absence of a caring spouse, a history of previous depressions, or prolonged illness or malformations in the child may complicate the situation. These are factors which should have caused the PCT to give extra attention to these mothers-to-be during the antenatal period and alerted them to the possibility of problems in the puerperium. As mentioned in Section 5.2 the attachment between mother and child is easily impaired by separations during early infancy, and depression can separate a mother from her child in a psychological sense. Mothers are sometimes frightened by the absence of maternal feelings towards their infant and they may even find themselves intensely hostile. (Infanticide can occur, though it is a rare occurrence.) In such cases the GP may be in a difficult position. Mother and child should not be separated more than is strictly necessary, yet there is a risk in encouraging too much proximity. In general, however, the risk is slight and can be eliminated if other members of the family are at hand and nobody tries to force the pace. Others should usually be encouraged to share in the care without taking the child away from the mother.

Sources of support for the mother

It is an important part of the role of health visitors to provide emotional support to new mothers, and they will usually take much of the burden of care from the GP. The GP needs to monitor the situation and to ensure that all that should be done is being done. One in five mothers who have suffered a psychosis in one puerperium will again become depressed if they have another child.[3] They may need extra support during and after all their pregnancies. Groups for young mothers can be a great source of support. They provide sympathy, encouragement, and understanding at a time when this is much needed. Members of the PCT can help to initiate such groups and to provide them with the professional advice which they will need from time to time. Once set up, they should be encouraged to become self-sustaining.

It is helpful if the PCT can provide a leaflet giving details of such organizations, as well as the crèches and other sources of support available to mothers.

Other members of the family

Of course, the mother is not the only person whose life may be changed by the birth of a baby. Husband, parents, and other children may all need to talk through the implications of this event if they are to revise their models of the world appropriately. The birth of a second child may change the role of the first-born from care-receiver to caregiver, and many an oldest daughter finds herself pressed into maternal roles while she is still a child. Some take this on willingly and may even come to rival their own mother as caregiver for the younger children. Others resent the loss of parental care for themselves and may become rivals to the new baby.

Fathers, too, may be surprised at the intensity of the jealous feelings which they experience towards a new baby who appears to have displaced them from their central position in the family. Far from supporting their wife in sharing in the care of the child, they may make demands which force the mother to choose between husband and child. Or they may go to the opposite extreme of 'spoiling' the child as a means of compensating for the affection they feel they are not getting themselves.

Children's needs and parents' needs

From the moment of its birth the new-born baby is the most important member of the family. In fact, it is not unreasonable to suggest that families exist mainly for the upbringing of children. Of course it may not feel that way to the parents. They may view their child as a plaything or an intruder. It is unlikely that this newcomer to their world will find his or her needs taking priority over theirs. Fortunately, as we have seen, babies are born with a powerful repertoire of tricks which ensure that, in most cases, their needs will be met.

From the adult's point of view the demands of the child and the difficulties which often arise may be seen as a severe restriction of liberty. Habits of life have to be changed. In most instances it is the mother who becomes 'chained' to the house, while the father goes out to work. The wife envies her husband his opportunities to 'escape', but the husband may not see it that way at all. He works all day for his wife and child, only to find them both irritable and unhappy when he returns. As reported in preceding sections, tensions in the parents evoke tensions in the children which in turn feed back to the parents. Vicious circles of this kind easily become self-perpetuating. They may give rise to symptoms in only one of the family members, but it is important to take a wider perspective. If doctors focus care on the presenting patient, they may underestimate the tensions which exist in other members of the family and fail to recognize the extent to which this distress causes other family members to undermine the patient. If, on the other hand, the family are seen together, preferably in the safe haven of their own home, it is easier to recognize the patterns which have grown up, to defuse the situation, and to help them, once again, to become mutually supportive.

Young couples, especially after their first baby, need some time together, to do the kind of things they were able to do before the baby came along. Arranging for a baby-sitter to allow the parents to go out to the cinema, a pub, or just a walk, may be very helpful in restoring a relationship.

There is no solution to the problem of competing needs. In the end, the best that most parents can achieve is a compromise. 'Give a little, take a little' is a reasonable-enough slogan for family life. Mothers don't have to be perfect mothers, just 'good enough'; likewise, the ideal wife, the ideal husband, the ideal worker, and even the 'ideal home' are figments to be admired not emulated. When faced with people who say they cannot cope, family doctors need to distinguish between the need for reassurance of the obsessional patient whose perfectionism makes them fearful of failure, and the need for positive guidance of the backward or inadequate person whose standards of child-care or home-care are dangerously low. Judgemental attitudes will do no good, but all will benefit from encouragement and, in the case of the inadequate parent, the guidance of an experienced health visitor will often provide them with a model of adequate performance which they can emulate. A family aide may be particularly helpful for people of low or borderline inteligence who may need to be taught to do things which most of us take for granted.

Moving home

Another psychosocial transition for the whole family is required each time they move from one environment to another. Although there are many who will take this in their stride, perhaps because they belong to a family which

has never stayed long enough to put down roots in any location, there ar
others for whom relocation is a major loss.

A change of home often means that friends are lost, leisure and all hom
activities have to be relearned, new social hierarchies must be entered an
a place established for each member of the family. For the children, nev
schools can be a major source of anxiety; for the parents, changes of hom
often accompany changes of job and links with the extended family ma
become more difficult to maintain.

Finding and registering with a new GP is just one of the many burdensom
tasks to be undertaken, and the fact that the new GP has no previou
knowledge of the family and, for a time, will not even have the benefit o
the case notes completed by others, places them all at a disadvantage
Awareness that this is a time of stress can make a big difference. The Gl
who recognizes that newly registered patients are often passing through ;
period of increased risk to physical or mental health and who takes the troubl
to meet them and to monitor their tolerance of the stress, may prevent mor
serious problems from arising and establish a basis for trust which will prov
valuable in later crises. For this reason, booking newly registered patient
for a longer appointment when first seen and constructing a 'database' i
the records is advantageous, and may save time in the long run as well. I
is even more helpful if a newly registered family can be seen together.

Marital breakdown

It is inevitable that GPs will sometimes find themselves dealing with the
casualties of separation and divorce. Both before and after separation there
is an increased risk to the physical and mental health of the partners and
their children. We may, at times, need to help them to consider the possible
consequences for their children, of a decision to separate or to stay together
but these issues are seldom clear-cut and there is no scientific data which
entitles us to assume that it is less harmful for children to be brought up
in an atmosphere of perpetual quarrelling, than for them to be brought up
in a 'broken home'.

Once the split has occurred, one or both partners may need individual help
in expressing the feelings of anger and grief which so often occur. As in al
forms of bereavement, they may need permission to grieve, but there may
also come a time when they need encouragement to stop grieving and get
on with the business of living a new life.

Children in divorce

Divorce, and the family situations which give rise to it, can have various
psychological effects on children. Children need their home to be secure i

they are to have the courage to explore and trust the outside world. Because parents are often preoccupied with their own problems at such times, those of the children may be ignored or misinterpreted until they bring themselves to our attention years later. Over one-third of children seen in child guidance clinics have parents who are separated or divorced. The PCT has an important preventive role to play in monitoring the risk and ensuring that proper care is given.

Problems

Many of these reflect grief and insecurity arising from the loss of secure parenting. Children often feel as if they have lost both parents, one having moved out and the other being so distressed that she (it is usually the mother who remains) may lean on the children rather than support them.

Children are often given little warning or explanation. Being at an egocentric stage of maturity they often blame themselves for what has happened. Alternatively, their grief may be expressed as unjust anger towards one or both parents. They may be caught between warring factions and expected to take sides. If they do this, they tend to 'monsterize' one parent and, since all children are, to some degree, identified with both their parents, they soon begin to hate and repudiate those aspects of the rejected parent which they see in themselves.

If they refuse to take sides, they may feel that they are losing the love of both sides. Either way, their sexual identity is likely to be impaired. They may cling inappropriately to non-parents or reject all members of the distrusted sex.

The development of autonomy in adolescence is easily impaired. Some adolescents become locked into an intense relationship with a parent which may be both protective and clinging. Others become compulsively self-reliant, while lacking the maturity for this. Overt sexual behaviour of a parent may give licence for sexual promiscuity in the adolescent, or it may set up an inverse reaction in which all sexuality is repudiated.

Management

Many of these problems can be prevented if the parents are aware of the risks and take appropriate action.[4,5] The members of the PCT do not have to wait for things to go wrong before they act. As soon as they become aware of the actual or incipient separation, they can try to set up a meeting with both parents in order to assure them of unbiased support and to help them to anticipate possible problems.

Parents need to be warned to expect disturbed behaviour in the children, but reassured that this is usually transient. If they understand that aggressive behaviour does not mean that they are not wanted, they will be less likely to withdraw their love when it is most needed. Likewise, if they can be persuaded to speak well of their partner in front of the children and to avoid any open or overt criticism, they will avoid splitting the child in two.

Children should not be used as messengers, or made party to secrets between parents. They need to receive the same explanation from both parents of the reasons for the separation, to be reassured that this is not their fault and that both parents will continue to love and to care for them. Frequent and easy visits to and from the separated parent are normally needed, and arrangements, once made, should not be broken.

Gifts are no substitute for love, and parents may need to be warned not to allow their pity for their children to prevent them from setting and keeping to reasonable limits, in this and other respects.

Many parents will benefit from an occasional talk with a member of the PCT, and they should be assured that we do not see this as inappropriate or a nuisance. Likewise, we should not hesitate to refer parents or children for child guidance, or to other sources of help, if our own attempts do not seem to be succeeding.

The one-parent family

Whether it is caused by the break-up of an existing marriage or by never marrying, the person who is faced with the need to raise one or more children without a partner is very vulnerable. Men rarely find themselves able to cope with this situation for more than a short while, and even those who do not remarry usually find a woman to act as a surrogate mother before very long. Women, however, are more likely to continue to struggle with the various demands that are placed upon them. Even if they are lucky enough to have adequate financial provision and the help of a caring mother, they are in for a hard time.

Often the one-parent family consists of an immature girl in her teens who has become pregnant 'by accident', and is unwilling to part with her baby. She receives little or no support from the child's father and her relationship with her own parents is highly ambivalent. Her pregnancy often represents an attempt to break away from parental ties, and both she and her mother resent the mutual dependence that is forced upon them by the demands of her child. Her mother, who had hoped that her own period of child-rearing was over, may find that the baby has been 'dumped' upon her so that her daughter can go out to work. Her father, who had expected that his daughter would soon be married and off his hands, may feel that she has wilfully spoiled her chances of matrimony by sinful behaviour and may react by withdrawing his support. The young mother is caught in a trap from which she sees no escape. Torn between the pressures of earning a living, caring for a baby, and depending on her parents, it is small wonder if she becomes anxious, irritable, and/or depressed. She may seek relief through drugs or alcohol and she will only too easily cling to others who offer her comfort, even if she knows them to be as insecure as herself. In doing so, she confirms her parents' worst fears and may lose their support. Occasionally a crisis at home will cause her to run away, in which case she easily becomes vulnerable to exploitation by unscrupulous employers, pimps, or drug-pushers.

For the sake of her child, as well as herself, unmarried teenage mothers and other lone parents need to have easy access to the emotional support and advice which will help them through this very difficult life situation. An assessment of the family networks available to them is a prerequisite, and it may be necessary to offer support to the supporters as well as the mother. Organizations such as Gingerbread, The Family Welfare Association, and the local social services have much to offer the GP whenever it is suspected that a one-parent family is at risk.

'The change'

Contrary to popular belief, the menopause is seldom a major hazard to mental health. Even so, it does remain a psychosocial transition which can increase the risk of psychiatric problems. Four factors contribute to this:

(1) The bodily symptoms which result from the menopause. Hot flushes are unpleasant and embarrassing and in some women they can be distressing. The decrease in vaginal secretions may make sexual intercourse painful unless a lubricant is used.

(2) There is considerable debate regarding the psychological effects of the hormonal changes which take place at this time. Some decrease in sexual appetite is common, but it is seldom possible to know how much hormones contribute to this and how much is due to other psychological factors. Depression is a rare symptom which is probably not directly influenced by sex hormones. 'Involutional depression' is probably a myth.

(3) For some women the menopause symbolizes the loss of feminine attractiveness, loss of sexual prowess, and the end of child-bearing. Those whose self-esteem depends upon these are likely to find the whole experience distressing.

(4) Popular myth about the 'change' may lead to expectations which are self-fulfilling.

The members of the PCT can help by dispelling myths and explaining the true facts of the situation; women do not necessarily cease to be attractive because their periods have stopped, nor do they necessarily themselves lose interest in sex. Any physical symptoms can be ameliorated by replacing the missing hormones.

For the treatment of the menopause with hormone-replacement therapy the reader is referred to Ann McPherson's book mentioned under 'further reading'. Whether or not reassurance and hormone replacements influence the situation, there may still be real causes for grief. Women who have hoped for a child may have to accept that this can never be, some of the effects of ageing may be irreversible, and, for many women, the menopause signals a mid-life crisis which must be faced if they are to move forwards to the next chapter of life in a positive frame of mind. The passing of youth can no longer be denied; what is left? Others may be involved in the search for an answer to this question; the husband, if there is one, may usefully be invited to take part in the discussions. It may be that he, too, is approaching the 'male menopause' and he may also need educating if he is to help his wife to cope with hers. Time, a chance to talk and to express feelings, together with the emotional support of a third party is likely to get them through this as through other changes of life.

References

1. Devlin, D. (1974). *The book of love*. New English Library, London.
2. Pitt, B. (1968). Psychiatric illness following childbirth. *Hosp. Med.* **2**, 815–18
3. Brockington, I. (1986). Puerperal mental illness. *Pract. Rev. Psychiat.* **8**, 3–5
4. Caplan, G. (1986). Psychological disorders in children of divorce. The general practitioner's role. *Br. Med. J.* **292**, 1431–6.
5. Caplan, G. (1986). Psychological disorders in children of divorce. Guidelines for the general practitioner. *Br. Med. J.* **292**, 1563–6.

Further reading

McPherson, A. (1988). *Women's problems in general practice* (2nd edn). Oxford University Press.

5.8   THE WORLD OF WORK

Work-related problems are of two main kinds: those that result from the psychosocial transitions which take place when a job is changed or lost, and those that reflect long-standing influences such as work stress or chronic unemployment. These should be differentiated from the depressed person's perception that work is a problem. The factory worker who complains about the monotony of his work, but who is also having marital problems, dislikes where he lives, or cannot get on with the neighbours, may be depressed rather than having a work problem. It is also possible that a work problem, or the cumulative effect of work and other problems, has precipitated a depression, which then further reduces a person's ability to cope with work.

Like other psychosocial transitions, those associated with work are life events requiring considerable adaptation both by the person employed and by those who live with, and are financially dependent on, the worker. Long-standing problems can arise from the nature of the work, relationships with colleagues and bosses, the journey to work, the status of the job, and the worker's ability to do the job. Acute problems may be precipitated by job loss or retirement.

Because of the imporance of work in people's lives, many GPs now enter dated details of patients' jobs in their summary record sheets.

Redundancy, retirement, and changing jobs

Except in the case of voluntary redundancy, losing one's job because either the worker or the work is no longer required is a very unpleasant loss. It usually threatens a person's standard of living, and it may introduce a major element of uncertainty if one cannot judge how long a period of unemployment will last. One may face the harrowing experience of looking for work. It often affects self-esteem, as one is no longer involved in valued work. Redundancy and retirement require a total change in the daily routine; indeed, they require the development of complete new routines. One's social contacts become more limited, with the loss of colleagues at work and even on the journey to work. One may be a nuisance at home, disrupting the routine by one's presence. Unemployment may even affect relationships with one's spouse, as normal patterns of working together are no longer viable.

Redundancy usually involves a period of anticipation. Beale and Nethercott studied the health of a group of men and women looked after by a Wiltshire general practice when they were threatened with redundancy and subsequently lost their jobs. They showed a 150 per cent increase in consultations and a 70 per cent increase in the number of episodes of illness. These changes began to occur two years before actual job losses started, when workers first learned that their employer was in financial difficulties.[1]

In another study, in the USA, the reactions of factory workers when the factory was about to close were monitored. In the two-month period prior to closure, there were signs of physical responses to the stress involved, in addition to the psychological distress. The men showed increases in blood pressure in the period before closure, and these were maintained for some time after they became redundant, especially in those who remained unemployed.[2]

Retirement has many similarities to redundancy in its effects on day-to-day functioning, and these are discussed in more detail in the next chapter.

Like redundancy and retirement, changing jobs is also stressful, as it requires considerable adjustment. Even a change for the better may place new and unknown demands on the individual, and life is generally less predictable; there is uncertainty about where one will be, who with, and at what times, and one may not be confident about small but important issues, such as the timing of tea breaks or the location of lavatories. New employees may be worried about their ability to do the job, to satisfy their bosses, and to get on with their workmates. The journey to work may be new and the change may have required a change of home and even a change of general practitioner. Indeed, many of the new patients joining a GP's list will have experienced such changes and this may result in higher-than-average consultation rates in recently registered patients, another reason for spending extra time with patients who come to register. While these new challenges are presented to the new employee, the stable, and perhaps supportive, base of their old employment has simultaneously been lost, and with that the protection this can offer against stress.

Failure to resolve the problems arising from redundancy or job changes can create difficulties which continue long after the critical period of change.

Enduring states

The nature of the work

It is widely accepted that certain jobs are more likely to lead to psychological problems, to symptoms, and to disease than others. Some occupations are described as stressful, and may even attract a higher salary on pay negotiations as a result, for instance, policework. There is ample evidence of differences in morbidity and mortality between jobs: doctors have high rates of suicide, policemen have high rates of coronary heart disease, and publicans have high rates of alcoholism. Differences have even been shown between monks carrying out different functions; those who had more responsibilities had a higher rate of coronary heart disease than those with fewer.[3]

This type of evidence is difficult to interpret, as people with different health characteristics may choose different jobs. The results may, therefore, be due to unhealthy people choosing the jobs we describe as stressful, rather than the nature of the work resulting in ill health.

This is equally true of shiftwork, which is associated with poorer physical and mental health, and especially with symptoms of insomnia, fatigue, and digestive problems.[4] The nature of the work clearly contributes to these symptoms, as they are all capable of disrupting the circadian rhythm, but such symptoms may also be more common in people who choose to do shiftwork. It is easy to bring to mind examples of men who work night-shift to avoid marital discord or to overcome a financial crisis.

In a similar vein, it is a common observation that low job satisfaction is associated with emotional disturbance, with anxiety, and with depression. Is it simply that emotionally vulnerable people choose unpleasant jobs? Or that nobody will employ them in pleasant jobs and they are left to choose amongst the worse jobs? Some studies suggest that, in addition, the job can be responsible for the disturbance. It has been shown that student nurses show increases in psychological symptoms when they work on wards that are independently assessed to be stressful ones. In another study, improvements in the organization of the work led to reductions in the symptoms of the workers. As a result of such research, Broadbent[5] argues convincingly that job characteristics can cause symptoms.

There is reasonable agreement about the critical factors, although studies to date deal mainly with male workers: jobs that are stressful and are associated with mental and physical ill health are those that require the worker to work hard but with little control over the work that is being done. These two factors each contribute separately to the strain experienced. Executives may be in very demanding jobs, working long hours, but the detrimental effects on their health may be moderated by the amount of choice they have about what work to do. There are parallels between the effects of work effort and control, and other types of stress. As noted in Section 1.2, it has been suggested that stressors that are threatening elicit different physiological responses from those that involve actual loss. In the work field, workers in highly demanding jobs show high catecholamine levels; where the worker has little control over the work, for instance when working on a fast production line, cortisol levels are high. These endocrine changes are similar to those found in animals in experiments on stress, and may offer at least a partial explanation of the increased symptomatology of stressed workers.

In addition to these physical effects, job stresses may lead to psychological distress, most commonly observed as increases in anxiety and depression, and reduced job satisfaction. It would appear that the pressure or pace of the work leads to anxiety symptoms, but not necessarily to depression or to low job satisfaction. Depression is more common where there is a lack of social interaction or social support in the job, mirroring other findings that people can cope with considerable stress without showing ill-effects if they have adequate social support. Job satisfaction depends on the worker's motivation as well as job characteristics; if the work is undertaken simply for money, satisfaction is not affected by the pace of the job, and anxiety symptoms are less likely to develop, even in a demanding job.

Damaging effects of job stresses are much more likely when signs of strain spill over into other areas of the worker's life. If he or she continues to feel anxious or dissatisfied during leisure time, the cumulative toll on health is greater than if he or she can switch off on leaving work.

Thus, the worst effects are seen when the worker is subject to enduring work stress, with continuing serious excess demands which he or she is in no position to control or compensate for, where there is little social support in the job, and where the detrimental effects of the work situation permeate the worker's private life.

Unemployment

Psychological problems are more common in people who are unemployed and seeking work than in those who are employed. Unemployment is also associated with higher rates of physical ill health and even mortality. However, these results are difficult to interpret when trying to understand patients' presentations: are they ill because they are unemployed or vice versa? One study, which throws light on this issue, observed unemployed school-leavers; they showed similar signs of distress to the unemployed who had previously held jobs. Another cohort of school-leavers was studied prior to leaving school, i.e. before entering the job market, and the same group was reassessed some time later when some had jobs and some were unemployed. The results showed the expected differences between the employed and the unemployed—the unemployed were higher on measures of psychological distress. The earlier assessment, at school, showed no difference between the two groups. It would appear that the psychological problems had arisen as a result of unemployment rather than caused it.[6]

As noted above, the effects of unemployment are greater if the person continues to have difficulty in finding a job than if the period of unemployment is brief. Initially, people search for work hopefully and energetically, but with continued failure may develop a form of learned helplessness, becoming dispirited and unable to persist in their efforts. The extent to which the individual comes to terms with unemployment and the ability to maintain or regain self-esteem will determine the long-term impact.

The effects of voluntary redundancy are usually less traumatic than are those which arise when redundancy has been forced upon the worker. In this case, anticipatory planning will allow a new assumptive world to be created and the transition may constitute a relief of stress rather than its imposition. Even so, Brown and Harris's work[7] suggests that lack of work *per se* may increase the likelihood of psychological problems; they found that women with no employment outside the home were more vulnerable to depression than those who had jobs.

The above discussion on unemployment and on the nature of work hints at the features of work that are critical for satisfactory psychological functioning. Work is clearly necessary to earn money and therefore limit financial threats. It also provides a source of social support. Self-esteem can be increased or decreased as a result of work and a person's place in the status hierarchy is largely determined by their occupation. People whose expectations exceed their achievements may be perpetually dissatisfied. The expectations of parents, spouses, and others can have a similar effect, so that some people come to see themselves as failures. In addition, work fills the day, providing a routine and reducing the number of decisions and uncertainties about how to behave. For one person, the main damaging aspect of unemployment may be financial; for another, lack of social contacts; for another, loss of self-esteem; and for another, under-employment, lack of purpose, and boredom. Unemployment may appear to be a homogeneous state, but is in fact many states, depending on its impact on the individual.

Presentation of work-related problems

Symptoms of work-related problems can be mental or physical. Patients may describe problems as work problems — feeling unable to do the job, being under pressure from the boss, or being threatened with redundancy. Alternatively, they may present with symptoms which are worse at work. If in doubt, it can be useful to ask the patient to keep a diary of the problem; the patient who feels better on Saturdays and Sundays may well have a work-related problem. However, severe work problems, are likely to have their impact on home and leisure time too.

Other patients may present the normal pattern of anxiety symptoms, including subjective feelings of tension, pains, especially headaches, and difficulty in getting to sleep; or they may present a more depressive pattern — lack of interest or pleasure in normal activities, irritability, inability to concentrate, and early morning waking.

All sorts of symptoms may be aggravated by work problems. It is well established that high rates of absenteeism are associated with low job satisfaction. If work is unattractive, symptoms which one may normally ignore can be perceived rather differently. A wide variety of presentations seen in general practice can be of this nature.

The endocrine changes occurring under conditions of work stress may also add to vulnerability. Increased cortisol secretion can disrupt immune functioning and leave the stressed worker more susceptible to infection.

Clearly, it is not helpful to see every problem that presents as due to work. On the other hand, work may be the cause of many otherwise inexplicable problems — after all, the full-time worker spends about one-third of waking time at work, emphasizing again the need for GP notes to record work details.

Management of work-related problems

Occasionally the opportunity arises to anticipate acute transitions, in the context of other consultations with workers or their families. As with other transitions, preparing for emotional consequences, as well as mentally rehearsing appropriate methods of coping with anticipated difficulties, may soften the impact of the event. Thus, a routine blood pressure check may offer the opportunity to enquire about job satisfaction and prospects, and how any anticipated changes are viewed.

More commonly, the event will have occurred, and the individual will present with symptoms. Apart from immediate symptom relief where appropriate, the two main avenues are cognitive and behavioural. If the primary problem is low self-esteem or despair about, for instance, ever getting a job, then cognitive restructuring may be useful, (see Section 3.4).

An Indian man had been sent to England at his father's expense in the expectation that he would obtain a university degree. Ten years later he had no degree and was working as an assistant librarian. He presented to his GP with chronic depressive symptoms and very low self-esteem. The GP refused to see him as a failure and helped him to recognize that his achievements as a husband to his wife and father to his children were quite as good as most peoples' and better than many. He came to realize that his own father's ambitions for him were a reflection of his father's need for vicarious esteem and that this was father's problem, not his.

If the focus is financial or social, then it may be more helpful to use a problem-solving strategy, encouraging the patient to identify behavioural alternatives and the pros and cons of each. As part of this strategy it is useful to invoke the patient's existing social network, as it may have been forgotten or seen as rejecting at the time of crisis; for example one of the alternatives might be 'to discuss the financial problems with my wife', or 'to discuss my loneliness and where I could meet friends, with my mother'.

With chronic work problems, the main task is likely to be the identification of the source of difficulties. This may be in the work itself—it's nature and quantity, too much or too little; in work relationships—with fellow workers, bosses, or subordinates; in the environment—poor seating, artificial lighting, distance from home; in the adequacy of payment; or in the status and opportunity associated with the job. Once the problem is identified, solutions can be considered and the best approach may be to learn greater assertiveness skills, to learn to relax in committee meetings, to interpret a colleague's behaviour differently, to request more pay or a better desk, or even to leave the job. This problem-solving approach seeks a solution compatible with the patient's existing resources while seeking to develop them, for example by relaxation or assertiveness training.

References

1. Beale, N. and Northcott, S. (1986). Job-loss and morbidity in a group of employees nearing retirement age. *J. R. Coll. Gen. Pract.* **36**, 265–6.

2. Kasl, S. V. (1984). Chronic life stress and health. In *Health care and human behaviour* (ed. A. Steptoe and A. Mathews). Academic Press, London.
3. Henry, J. P. and Stephens, P. M. (1977). *Stress, health and social environment: a sociobiological approach to medicine.* Springer-Verlag, New York.
4. Weinman, J. (1987). *An outline of psychology as applied to medicine.* Wright, London.
5. Broadbent, D. G. (1985). The clinical impact of job design. *Br. J. Clin. Psychol.* **24**, 33–44.
6. Banks, M. H. and Jackson, P. R. (1982). Unemployment and risk of minor psychiatric disorder in young people: cross sectional and longitudinal evidence. *Psychol. Med.* **12**, 789–98.
7. Brown, G. W. and Harris, T. (1978). *The social origins of depression.* Tavistock, London.

5.9 THE TRANSITION FROM WORK TO RETIREMENT

Although the ending of paid employment is one of the major turning points of life, research into its effects on physical and mental health do not show it to be uniformly damaging in its effects. Certainly, there are some studies which show an overall detriment in health after retirement, but others show no such change and a few suggest that retirement may even be good for our health.[1] To make sense of these findings we need to look more closely at the phenomenon of retirement. Retirement means different things to different people. For some it represents relief from the stress of a boring unpleasant job, for others the 'scrap heap', for some it is the beginning of a well-earned holiday, for others evidence of decay and one foot in the grave. Some retire voluntarily, some are compelled, some retire on grounds of age, others because of ill health, and some because they have no hope of getting another job. These factors all need to be considered if we are to explain the discrepancies between different studies.

Allowing for some fairly thorny methodological problems, it seems that the following factors are likely to predispose to poor psychological and/or physical health after retirement:[2]

- poor health before retirement;

- negative attitude towards retirement;

- unrealistic expectations;

- low income;

- absence of a spouse;

- low status;

- involuntary as opposed to voluntary retirement.

These are the types of factors which we would expect to influence the outcome of any psychosocial transition. They are important both because they enable us to identify people at risk and because they suggest ways of reducing the risk. Two of them, negative attitudes and unrealistic expectations, are potentially modifiable and constitute an argument for anticipatory guidance to people who are approaching retirement.

Mr L, 60 years of age, with a dull job in a car factory, was offered redundancy payment if he took early retirement within the next four weeks. At first he was glad and accepted this offer and enjoyed the initial period of freedom, but he soon became bored and aimless. He tried fruitlessly to obtain another job. During this time his attendance rate at the health centre, which had been below average in the past, rose to 12 per year. He developed aches in his joints and chest pains on exertion. All investigations were negative.

Mr J, in a similar job, did not take redundancy, but prepared for his retirement by attending evening classes in furniture restoration (in which he had long been interested). When he did retire four years later he pursued this interest, made some money, and remained in good health and vigour.

The effects of retirement are not confined to the retiree. The spouse may also be affected by the change in the partner's life; a wife who has long-established routines and territorial rights may find them seriously disrupted by a husband who insists on claiming his own space. As one put it, 'I took him for better or worse but not for lunch.'

General practitioners are often involved, either with the health problems that bring about, or are brought on by, retirement. This provides us with opportunities to aid the process of accommodation by encouraging those affected to talk through the implications of the change and to share their feelings about it. It also enables us to advise people about the areas in which problems may arise at this time of life, such as diet, exercise, and drug and alcohol consumption. Perhaps because retirement is often seen as a time when normal constraints are loosened, it is also a time when bad habits easily become established. If, on the other hand, the person is encouraged to see it as a time when attention to health can greatly improve the quality of life, we may be able to prevent later problems from arising.

For most people retirement marks the end of middle and the beginning of old age, but this does not mean that this period of life is not capable of being a rich and satisfying time. In fact, there are many aspects of 'young old age' which can make this a more contented time than any other. Freed from the need to compete for promotion, relieved of responsibilities towards dependent children, and settled into habits of life which may be less exciting, but are also less upsetting than those that precede them, the 'young old' often experience a growing sense of security and contentment. Lifelong anxiety symptoms often improve at this time, and even those problems that must be endured seem less agonizing than they did when there was no hope of change. For those with an active mind there is a wide choice of leisure activites which can be pursued and which help stimulate and maintain interest. Even physical manifestations, such as raised blood pressure, may remit and it is often possible to reduce or discontinue antihypertensive drugs after retirement.

It is these prospects that make the transition from work to retirement a challenge to the approached in a positive rather than a negative way. Retirement classes are one method of preparation which the primary care team can help provide, but any activity which encourages people to prepare themselves for the next chapter of their life deserves consideration before retirement comes about. A gradual reduction in working hours is something possible and older employees can be encouraged to relinquish some responsibilities to younger people. Unfulfilled ambitions may need to be grieved for, but having accepted the inevitable, people who retire can begin to relate to the new world which they are now entering and which may even create new challenges.

For those whose work has been stressful, the first year of retirement is often a holiday. 'I just wanted to put my feet up and take a rest, but there comes a time when the holiday has to end. I realized I was beginning to stagnate, when my wife told me it was about time I thought of getting a little job!' Feelings of discontent may emerge and some people become depressed at this time.

This delayed reaction to retirement may account for the increased mortality that has been reported in the third and fourth years after retirement,[1,3] and there are some grounds for providing routine checks on health at this time. Again, the opportunity to talk through any problems that arise may be sufficient to get a person through any disillusionment that arises.

As in so many transitions, our faith in our patients' intrinsic worth and their capacity to come through may act as the spur which will enable them to do just that.

References

1. Martin, J. and Doran, A. (1966). Evidence concerning the relationship between health and retirement. *Sociol. Rev.* **14**, 329.
2. Heidbroder, E. M. (1972). Factors in retirement adjustment: white collar/blue collar experience. *Ind. Geront.* **12**, 69.
3. Haynes, S. G., McMichael, A. J., and Tyroler, H. A. (1977). The relationship of normal, involuntary retirement to early mortality among US rubber workers. *Soc. Sci. Med.* **11**, 105-14.

5.10   OLD AGE—A TIME OF CHANGE

Although old age is a time when people are more vulnerable to depression, suicide, and a wider range of illnesses than they are at other times in their lives, it should not itself be regarded as an illness. Too often, patients are told that any symptoms which they develop are simply due to '*anno Domini*', doctors shrug their shoulders, there is 'nothing to be done', and patients are made to feel that they are wrong to complain. Likewise, depression and other distress is seen as incurable, and old people are not thought suitable for psychotherapies. This pessimistic view of old age is infectious. Under its influence the old themselves give up looking after themselves, treatable conditions are neglected, and many people settle for a twilight existence that may be quite out of keeping with their potentialities. There is probably more unnecessary crippledom and sick-role behaviour in this age group than in any other. Yet much of this is preventable.

Contrary to popular belief, most old people do not decline steadily and inevitably into a state of senile dementia, nor are they incapable of learning new things and looking after themselves. Their thinking may slow down a little, their memory may not be what it was, and their physical mobility may be reduced, but these restrictions do not imply that they are incapacitated and should not bar them from contributing usefully to the community in which they live, provided the community is prepared to acknowledge their needs. In most communities it is the primary care team (PCT) who are most aware of the needs of the elderly and best able either to meet these needs or communicate them to other competent agencies. Some needs reflect permanent changes and will continue, but many are transient. Arthritis may prevent an old lady from doing her own shopping, but the grief to which the realization of this fact gives rise will pass if she is given the physical help and emotional support which she needs. All members of the PCT have important roles to play, but it can be useful for one person to take a special interest. In some teams, health visitors have developed special competence and may even work exclusively with the elderly in the practice.

Health screening

There is much to be said for the idea adopted by many PCTs of screening all patients who reach the age of 65. Often very little physical disease is uncovered but such screening presents an excellent opportunity to assess any problems.

The multiple problems of old age and the liking of old people for familiar faces are two of the strong reasons why general practice is relevant in an increasingly specialized world.

Psychosocial transitions

Old age is a time of change. A period when psychosocial transitions, most of them unwanted, are frequent, and when the capacity to cope with such changes is flagging. Friends and family members die off, new friends are difficult to make, roles are lost, the range of territory which can be commanded shrinks and with it the reserves of money, authority, and strength by which mastery of life space is achieved.

The process of ageing seldom proceeds steadily. Old age comes in fits and starts. A fall, or a small vascular incident, will upset a precarious balance of adjustment. Some external event over which the elderly have no control, such as the marriage of a daughter or migration of a son, may suddenly bring about a major change; thus the death of an ageing spouse sometimes eases the burden on the survivor rather than aggravating it, while another event which seems trivial to the outsider can have profound consequences. An old woman who has prided herself on her ability to cope without help may lose her nerve if her handbag is snatched in the street. She may become too frightened to leave the house and suffer a profound loss of confidence in the world and in her own ability to cope with it. Similar consequences can result from a fall on a moving bus, a fainting attack in a crowded supermarket, or an unusually painful ingrowing toenail.

One event can trigger another which may set in train a ripple effect, with devastating consequences.

A minor infection caused a widower to take to his bed for a week. When he got up, he was so stiff and weak that he fell downstairs. The fall aggravated his arthritis and undermined his sense of security. He became depressed and irritable, taking it out on his daughter who lost her temper with him and walked out. The old man responded by taking a serious overdose.

Multiple problems often interact in this age group. Deafness, osteo-arthritis, visual impairment, and general frailty may undermine confidence and reduce an individual's ability to cope with emergent events. As one elderly amputee put it, 'If anyone talks to me about Douglas Bader again, I'll kick his teeth in.'

Yet the very prevalence of minor disabilities in this age group often seems to make them more bearable, and many old people are able to lead worthwhile and contented lives despite severe restrictions on their motor and sensory capacities. How can this be and what can be done to foster contentment in the elderly? With so many problems it seems unlikely that there are simple solutions. Even so, the general rules which have been found to aid other psychosocial transitions continue to have relevance in old age.

Anticipation and preparation

Changes which have been anticipated and appropriately prepared for are less traumatic than those which arrive unbidden or for which inappropriate expectations are held. This enables many old people to plan their lives on an assumption of diminished expectations. 'When my arthritis gets too bad, I shall move into a small flat near to my daughter', is a typical plan which will work, provided the daughter does not then move to another place and the plan includes recognition of the fact that the piano will not fit into a smaller flat. Old people should be encouraged to make and review plans well in advance of probable changes, rather than adopt an 'ostrich-like' attitude.

Disengagement

One commonly reported feature of old age is 'disengagement', a term coined by Cumming and Henry to describe the way in which old people progressively lose interest in the wider world and focus their attention on their immediate environment and themselves.[1] Like young children they are often accused of becoming self-centred, and it is certainly true that to others the elderly often seem preoccupied with their own problems and ailments.

There is much controversy among researchers and clinicians regarding the question of whether 'disengagement' is a normal aspect of ageing or a pathological reaction which should be treated or warded off. Those who see it as normal point out that 'disengagement' is a reasonable consequence of the physiological consequences of ageing. As people get older and thought processes slow down, they find that the world moves too fast for them, new information is difficult to assimilate, and it is appropriate to shrink the sphere of control to manageable proportions. Old people have less stake in the long-term future of the world and less need for long-term plans. Seen in this light their 'disengagement' is a realistic way of altering their focus and coping with less and less.

Opponents of this view point out that old people who are faced with stimulation and challenge can be induced to remain 'engaged'. The staff at some old people's homes are very proud of the number of 'O' and 'A' levels acquired by their residents, and the old person who has recently learned to speak Spanish may be rightly admired.

Interestingly enough 'disengagement' is not confined to the elderly. It is a common reaction to bereavement[2] and seems to be one of the ways in which people, faced with a need to grieve and to reorganize their internal models of the world, often lose interest in non-essential and peripheral matters for a while. Only when they regain their confidence in their ability to cope with their immediate needs do they begin to reach out again, to re-engage.

Viewed in this light, 'disengagement' can be seen as a normal consequence of the losses attending old age, but also as potentially reversible given time and encouragement. The brain, like other organs, benefits by being used, and environments or circumstances which discourage initiative and encourage passive conformity probably hasten 'disengagement'.

The important question would seem to be, what is it reasonable to expect of the elderly? Old people may be put in a situation (by retirement, their family, etc.) where little is expected or possible. They may respond by disengagement. They get little opportunity to exercise their mental abilities and may come to think more slowly, and be less able to cope with problems as a result. Yet old people, like the rest of us, thrive when they are stimulated, cared about and admired. In one study, old people were presented with either a budgerigar or a begonia. Those who received the budgerigar were subsequently found to be more contented and their mental health generally better than those who received only the begonia.[3]

Evidence from old people's homes shows that residents who are involved in decision-making are less depressed, and that programmes that favour engagement result in improved intellectual functioning.[4] The more we expect of people the more they will respond, but our expectations must be realistic. At times of change old people need emotional support and time to grieve for what is lost before they will be ready to cope with new challenges. Unreasonable expectations can be tyrannical and undermine morale.

Old age and the family

Doctors are commonly invited to restrict the activities of the elderly, 'Tell him he's too old to go on cooking for himself, I'm terrified he's going to set light to the place' is a common injunction. Conversely, they may be asked to act as a spur, 'He just sits and mopes doctor, tell him he's got to get out more.' Both injunctions may be reasonable or unreasonable according to circumstances. Before responding, members of the PCT need to find out more, not only about the elderly person but also about the rest of the family. The psychosocial transitions of old age may change the lives of an entire family, and their reactions may need to be taken into account. 'Tell him to stop smoking', may translate as, 'I can't stand his grief since my mother died'; 'I'm terrified he's going to set light to the place', may mean, 'I've been wishing him dead for months and have to over-protect him for fear that my wish might come true.' In such cases, rather than condemning the family as unreasonable, we need to understand why. The son who can't stand his father's grief may be unable to cope with his own grief. The daughter who is wishing her father dead may need permission to express the frustration and rage to which his behaviour is giving rise.

We sometimes hesitate to enquire into the family's needs for fear that we shall be opening the door to fresh problems, and it is certainly true that the provision of support to a family requires time and effort. Yet the consequences of failing to provide support can be even more expensive and time-consuming. The family are often the primary carers of the elderly and we are likely to find ourselves saddled with the main responsibility for care if we fail to give them the help which will enable them to continue in this role. Pressures to prescribe drugs or provide institutional care are often a sign that the family are coming to the end of their tether, and it is better to intervene before this happens than to wait until reserves of energy, hope, and affection have become exhausted. Families are often accused of cruelty and neglect of elderly relatives. In our view the opposite is more often the case. People will sacrifice their own plans and go to great lengths to care for severely disabled or mentally impaired old folks rather than sending them 'into a home'. On those occasions when neglect occurs, it is often because the family have been pushed beyond reason by the unjust expectations of an elderly person or their medical attendants. Sometimes each relative holds back from offering help for fear of being left with the entire burden of care, yet they are very willing to share the burden provided others play their part. A family meeting is often necessary to enable each person to have their say and to work out a joint plan.

Group support for people who are caring for an elderly relative at home is provided in many areas through local social workers or voluntary organizations such as Age Concern (see Appendix II). They enable carers to share their problems with each other and ensure that they become aware of the full range of supportive facilities that are available to them. An excellent booklet for careers, *Taking a break*, was published by King's Fund Publications in 1988.

Social networks and loneliness

If the family is the first line of support for the elderly, the community of old people is the next. Older people have a lot to offer to each other and there are many 'young old' who find satisfaction and esteem from supporting the 'old old'. Both by visiting the homes of the less mobile, and by bringing the more mobile together at luncheon clubs and other social gatherings, volunteers of all ages can help to maintain interests and activities. The employment of volunteer organizers for the elderly is an economical and effective way of maintaining mental health in this age group.

Many research project have revealed that loneliness is the besetting problem of old age. Left on their own at home for most of the time many old people sink into a chronic state of loneliness, irritability, and depression. In theory it should not be difficult to remedy this problem; if people are lonely, bring them together. In practice it is not always as easy as that. Old people who have been home-centred for many years are often reluctant to go out. 'I don't like old people', they say, thereby belittling their own identity and revealing their reluctance to face up to the implications of their life situation. Clearly, they need help in grieving for the youth which they have lost if they are to enjoy the age that is given to them. 'I don't think of myself as old', they say, or 'You're as old as you feel.' By restricting the definition of old age to the sick and the demented they attempt to postpone the things they most fear. Such remarks are often treated as if it were a virtue to deny reality. Young people, who themselves may dread old age, are encouraged to believe that it can be indefinitely postponed by an act of will. Old people then feel the need to prove their youth by competing with the young in ways which are sometimes pathetic and which will eventually lead to failure and distress.

By contrast, those who are able to face up to the realities of old age will grow old 'gracefully' and with dignity. They can be helped to do this if younger people treat them with the respect which their seniority deserves, but sadly this is often not the case. The rapidity of social change in our society has made redundant much of the accumulated knowledge of the old. People are devalued because they are old, much as an old car is assumed to be inferior to a new one. This assumption, which is only held in rapidly changing societies, means that even useful knowledge is devalued and, because old people themselves share the assumption, it leads to much self-denigration.

Organizations such as Age Concern do much to change this negative image by reminding old people of the real value of their experiences. If people can be helped to accept the limitations of old age, they can also be helped to enjoy the blessings. To do this they must be encouraged to take advantage of modern technology. Radio and television have already proved themselves to be a boon to the old and immobile; computers, microwave ovens, electric hoists, electric wheel chairs, and many other aids to living and means of communication hold out promise of a more rewarding life. It is not true that 'You can't teach an old dog new tricks'. It just takes a little longer. Old people may need a lot of coaxing and encouragement if they are to be persuaded to make use of these new things.

A caring PCT is most important in the life of an elderly person. Good health can no longer be taken for granted and personal security often depends on knowing that you have health professionals you can trust. Once trust has been established we may find ourselves consulted about issues concerning which medical training seems quite irrelevant. 'Should I sell my house and move into a flat near my son?' 'I feel so lonely since my wife died', 'Please tell the children to stop making so much noise outside my window.' Some physical complaints seem trivial until we recognize that they are simply an excuse to get our help with some more important problem. Discovering the problem behind the problem is not usually difficult once we start to look. Finding solutions may be harder. 'What can't be cured must be endured' applies to problems as well as symptoms, but even the recognition that a problem is insoluble may help, and an expression of understanding and sympathy reduce the feeling that nobody cares. As one arthritic old lady put it, 'I can put up with the pain most of the time, but once in a while it gets me down and then I go to the doctor. I know there's nothing he can do for me but it helps to have a good grumble'.

Grieving and grumbling are necessary ways of working through the discontents and psychosocial transitions of old age. They sometimes go on for a long time and the team may find their patience tested. Mutual support within the practice will spread the load and help us to 'hang in'. When we do this the end result is often gratifying.

This brief outline can do no more than highlight some of the issues which arise in the care of the elderly. Others will be covered in our discussion of the special problems associated with bereavement (Section 5.11), disablement (Section 5.12), dying (Section 5.11), depression (Section 8.4), and dementia (Section 7.2). Each of these topics has particular relevance to this age group and provides the PCT with chances to mitigate some of the saddest chapters of life. Yet, despite these sadnesses, old age can be a time of peace and contentment, and in one survey of an English suburban community, those aged over 65 were found to be more satisfied with life than any other age group.[5]

References

1. Cumming, E. and Henry, W. E. (1961). *Growing old*. Basic Books, New York.
2. Parkes, C. M. and Weiss, R. S. (1983). *Recovering from bereavement*. Basic Books, New York.
3. Mugford, R. A. and Comisky, M. (1975). Some recent work on the psychotherapeutic value of cage birds with old people. In *Pet animals and society* (ed. R. S. Anderson). Baillière, London.
4. Rodin, J. (1986). Aging and health: effects of the sense of control. *Science* **233**, 1211–16.
5. Parkes, C. M. (1971). *Chorleywood conglomerate: report of a local survey*. Chorleywood Community Arts Centre, Herts.

5.11   THE TRANSITION FROM LIFE TO DEATH

There is, perhaps, no greater test of the quality of primary care and no greater opportunity to help people through a psychosocial transition than that which faces us when a patient is dying. At the very time when curative medicine has nothing to offer and many of our colleagues regard the case as 'hopeless', we have no alternative but to commit ourselves to stay close and to reach out, not only to the patient, but to all those family members whose lives will be disrupted by a death in the family. For dying is a social event and the trauma of bereavement is probably the greatest mental stress that the family will meet. Anything which we can do to mitigate this trauma, both before and after it takes place, will reduce the risk of further sickness and distress.

At such times we probably feel very inadequate, our own knowledge and training seem irrelevant, the very fact that the patient is dying is evidence of our failure. Our helplessness may be a pale reflection of the patient's own feelings and this, strange to say, can act as a link between us. Rather than deceiving them by pretending that we have everything under control (a lie which will eventually be found out), we may do better to acknowledge the limits to our powers and to help patient and family to live with the uncertainty that results. We can make the uncontrollable more acceptable by acknowledging its existence and in doing so increase our own and the patient's sense of being in control.

Terminal care

Although 'terminal care' is usually taken to mean the care of the patient with advanced cancer, cancer is not the commonest cause of death and care should not be limited to the cancer patient. Many kinds of death cast their shadow before. Patients and their families often find it just as difficult to cope with chronic heart disease or with cerebro-vascular accidents, as with the more predictable course of an incurable cancer. One study has showed that the spouses of patients who died of cancer came through their bereavement with fewer problems in physical and mental health than people whose spouses had died from other causes.[1] It seems, then, that the anticipation of bereavement, painful though it is, does something to prepare a person for that event. If this is so, then it seems likely that the care which is given to a patient and family before bereavement will have a significant effect on that family's later adjustment.

Breaking bad news

As doctors, we do not like hurting people and we find it hard to do this when we are in possession of information that will cause pain if it is communicated to patients and their families. It is tempting to tell as little as our duty demands. We wrap things up in such a way that they will easily be misunderstood. As one patient said, 'Well, thank you doctor, I'm glad I'm not dying of anything serious!' Yet these are the very times when we may have the opportunity to prepare people for the disappointments and losses that are to come.

But there is more to breaking bad news than simply telling the truth in language which people will understand. If people are told too much at a time when they are unprepared to take in the full significance of what they are being told, they will either become excessively distressed or, more often, defend themselves by forgetting, misunderstanding, or not hearing what they are told. In order to communicate effectively, we must try to induce in the other person a receptive frame of mind, and we must tell them as much as they are ready to be told, but not more.

A receptive frame of mind comes from trust in the informant and their personal emotional support, so that the recipient feels safe enough to face the unsafe truth. It is not difficult to find out what the other person is ready to know by asking them what they know already and then inviting questions. This puts the other person in control of the interaction and enables them to monitor their own input of information. We should beware of forcing information on people who make it clear that they do not wish to be told any more.

This means that it takes time to break bad news and we may need to go back several times to check out what has been understood and to help people to extend their understanding. By doing this we enable them to work through and grieve over each aspect of the losses they are suffering and, in doing so, to come to terms with them. Illnesses such as cancer tend to follow a stepwise course and each turning point in the illness is another cause for grief and another opportunity to face facts.

Given our continuing support throughout the illness, a relationship of trust can be built up which maximizes the chances that both patient and family members will be 'in tune' with the real situation and with each other. This makes it unnecessary for families to suffer the added stress of concealment, as when a couple, who may never have had secrets from each other in the past, find themselves unable to talk about the most important problem in their lives.

Mr and Mrs P were looked after by different family doctors. Mrs P had told her doctor that Mr P had incurable cancer of the lung, but that he did not know, and therefore she could not discuss things with him. Some time later Mr P's doctor retired and Mrs P's doctor took over care for both. On his first visit to Mr P, his new doctor asked if he knew what was going on. He said 'Oh yes, I heard the hospital doctor talking about me as having cancer of the lung months ago, but I didn't like to worry my wife.' When Mrs P was asked to come into the room and was told of this, the couple fell into each other's arms and cried with relief at the barrier having been broken.

Communication about dying

Communication is complicated by the varied meanings which accrue to words such as 'cancer' and 'death'. To many people 'cancer' means 'death in agony' and 'death' is the epitome of suffering. The fact that, in decent circumstances of care, pain should always be relieved does not prevent people from being terrified. This is reflected in the way many will confess 'It's not being dead but dying that frightens me.' In a society in which few people ever witness the death of another person, our image of death comes from its dramatic representation in the mass media. This is often coloured by the horror stories which get passed from mouth to mouth about cousin Joe who 'suffered terribly' and auntie Maud who was 'hideously mutilated'. Peaceful deaths are not news and tend to be forgotten.

Consequently it is important, when talking about illness and death, to find out what the other person means by the words that they use. 'Have you ever known of anyone with this condition? What do you imagine it's like?' are good questions which usually enable us to give some good news along with the bad. 'Well you don't have *that* kind of cancer', or 'I can promise you that death is nothing like that.'

Dying

Most people who die of a debilitating disease slip quietly into unconsciousness before they die. For them death is not the dramatic event it is made out to be. As consciousness ebbs quietly away and people drift back and forth in a twilight world between waking and sleeping, neither they nor we know when their last conscious moment has come.

Given adequate control of pain and other physical symptoms (see Saunders[2] for an account of the physical treatments in use at St Christopher's Hospice for the palliation of symptoms of advanced cancer) illnesses such as cancer result in a gradual erosion of all of the appetites—for food, information, sex, even life itself; it then becomes easier for the patient to accept the prospect of his or her own death. Tiredness and apathy are common symptoms in late-stage cancer, but they do not necessarily cause great suffering.

The family at the bedside often imagine that the patient is suffering more than is actually the case. They seem to project their own suffering into the patient and find it hard to believe that it may be easier to die than to survive. As long as the patient is alive they tend to deny their own needs, and will often put up with great stress in order to be seen to go on caring. This is, after all, their last chance to get things right, they need to be able to look back on this period and to say, 'I did everything possible'. For this reason it is wrong for us to over-protect the family. We may thing that there is nothing that they can do for an unconscious patient, but they may suffer great remorse if they have allowed themselves to be persuaded to go to bed when, unexpectedly, the patient dies in the night.

Home, hospital, or hospice?

Most healthy people, asked where they would prefer to die, will say 'At home'. But dying patients often have a different opinion.

Home can be the best or the worst place to die. If unpleasant symptoms are controlled, if the doctors and nurses are readily available and trusted by the family, and if the patient and family caregivers are not unduly anxious, then it is best to provide terminal care at home. But there are a lot of 'ifs'. One of the commonest reasons for seeking admission to a hospital or hospice is reflected fear, the fear which the patient reads in the eyes of the people around him. Pain causes fear and fear pain, in fact all symptoms are worse if levels of anxiety are high.

This means that emotional support of patient and family must be a high priority for the primary care team. Frequent supportive visits, meticulous attention to symptom control, and a reliable back-up service that is available 24 hours a day are essential. And if our efforts do not prevent the escalation of anxiety, then prompt admission to a good, caring ward, either 'to give the family a break' or for terminal care, should not be regarded as a defeat.

Hospices are rightly proud of the quality of care which they provide, but they will never need or be able to serve more than a fraction of the people who die. Alternatives need careful appraisal, but there is no reason why good quality care cannot be provided in community or general hospitals if home proves unsuitable.

In many areas specialist home care nurses are available to advise primary care teams who are caring for patients with advanced cancer (sometimes under the aegis of the local hospital or hospice). Even if the intention is to seek admission, they can serve a useful function by preparing patient and family members for this, and they are a valuable source of skilled help in an area of service which is developing rapidly.

The Hospice Advisory Service* is also a useful source of up-to-date information about any aspect of terminal care. It keeps lists of addresses and telephone numbers of special facilities for late-stage cancer care in all parts of the United Kingdom.

The dying child

For caregivers as well as families, the death of a child is a harrowing experience. Parents tend to become very over-protective at such times and, while desperately needing our help, they may find it hard to trust us to communicate with their child, and may be wary of our treatments.

When a child is sick, healthy siblings are often neglected and this can cause serious problems if the sickness continues for more than a short space of time. Sometimes the family splits, with father taking on the care of the healthy

*The Hospice Advisory Service, St Christopher's Hospice, Lawrie Park Road, London SE26. Tel. (01) 778-9252.

children so that mother can devote all her attention to the sick one. When eventually the sick child dies the mother may have lost her place in the family.

All of this implies that support to parents is essential, and time spent in talking to them and helping to prepare them for the probable outcome is time well spent. Mothers often try to deny the seriousness of the situation, clinging to unrealistic hopes and dragging the child from one doctor to another. Rather than being offended by this we may need to assure them of our continued care and availability if, as we fear, their efforts are fruitless. At times we shall be the object of unreasonable blame—'If only the diagnosis had been made sooner . . .' There may be little we can do to counteract such outbursts, except to indicate our concern and willingness to 'hang in' if wanted.

Children are often more matter-of-fact than their parents. By the age of 2–3 years most children know that sick people sometimes die, and those with chronic disease may even have met others with similar conditions who have died. But they are unlikely to be told much about their condition by adults. This can be very confusing for them, and may leave them frightened and unable to communicate their fear. Without denying the parents' right to decide what the children are told, it is often possible to encourage the children to talk about their preconceptions, and to feed these back to the parents, so that they are aware what the child is thinking. Death games are part of the child's way of coming to terms with the realities of death, and parents need to understand that these constitute opportunities when support can be given.

Because of the stress on the parents of nursing a dying child at home, periods of ward care may enable them to take a rest from time to time. This is provided by some paediatric wards and by Helen House, in Oxford.

The special problems of miscarriage, stillbirths, and neonatal deaths will be considered in Section 5.12.

Bereavement

The death of a loved person may have been anticipated but there are few people who can say that they are fully prepared for bereavement. Yet most will come through the stress of this event without suffering lasting damage to their physical and/or mental health. It is important for members of primary care teams (PCTs) to understand the differences between healthy and unhealthy grieving if they are to assess the risks of bereavement and identify those bereaved people who may need special help.

Components of grief

Three conflicting psychological urges interact throughout the process of grieving and determine how grief will be expressed. Each of them is present at all times but it is likely that, at any particular moment, one will predominate.

The urge to search

It seems that whenever one person is separated for more than a short period of time from another to whom they are attached they experience an impulse to search for some form of contact with the lost person. This urge, which is present in many animal species, explains the powerful impulse to cry aloud, to lose interest in other activities, and to devote one's attention to a restless rehearsal of events leading up to the loss as if, even now, some way could be found to prevent it from happening. In pursuit of this quest people feel drawn towards places and objects associated with the lost person; they misidentify sights and sounds as indicating the presence of the lost person, and they carry a clear mental image of that person in their minds.

The urge to avoid

The intelligent human adult knows that it is no use wandering the streets searching for a person who is dead; that would be irrational and antisocial. We have been taught not to cry and any unrestrained expression of distress is likely to be interpreted as a 'breakdown'. Consequently we do all in our power to restrain our grief, avoid reminders of what has happened, and shut ourselves away from those people and situations that threaten our precarious control.

The urge to review and relearn our place in the world

A major bereavement produces many changes in the assumptive world. Quite suddenly a married woman has become a widow; new responsibilities and roles are required and a thousand assumptions about the world have to be changed. The event which has brought this about may be over in a moment, but it takes a considerable time before the bereaved discover what they have lost, let alone learn how to cope with the new demands of their life situation. The psychosocial transition which follows bereavement is the more difficult because it is unwanted, and often unanticipated (we don't 'look forward' to the things we don't 'look forward' to!).

The process of grieving

The intensity of these components of grief varies greatly from one person to another and, over time, within the same person. Thus it is most difficult to restrain the urge to search during the first few weeks of bereavement, and it is hard to relearn the world until the most intense preoccupation with searching is over. Although distress is most intense during the first few weeks of bereavement, there are some people whose need to avoid grieving is so strong that they shut off their feelings altogether. Some experience a period of '*numbness*' or 'blunting' when they may feel very little. This is most likely to arise following sudden and unexpected bereavements, but is not uncommon after any major loss. 'Numbness' does not normally last for more than a few hours or a few days and is then succeeded by the so-called pangs of grief.

Pangs of grief are episodes of acute pining accompanied by anxiety and its physiological accompaniments. They are brought on by any reminder of the loss, and usually reach a peak 5–14 days after the death. Between these pangs there are long periods of apathy, bewilderment, and general *disorganization and despair*. Feelings of irritability, shame, and loss of self-esteem are very common, people lose all of their appetites, sleep is disturbed, and limbs feel heavy. There is a tendency to sigh, sweat excessively, and to complain of indigestion, headaches, and other symptoms reflecting chronic anxiety and tension.

As time passes, the intensity and frequency of the pangs of grief grow less, but it is usually many months before people who have suffered a major bereavement begin to look forward and find a purpose in life. The first anniversary brings back the pangs of grief in full intensity, and people find themselves going over in their minds the events of a year previously. Once the first anniversary is over there is often an improvement; the next year cannot be quite so bad and the sufferer may begin to look to the future rather than constantly bemoaning the past. During this year there are likely to be several turning points. These may occur following a holiday or other event which enables the bereaved to get away, for a while, from the reminders of their loss. They may be surprised to find that their appetites and interests have returned. New directions in life begin to have meaning, and the memory of times past can begin to enrich life rather than deplete it.

This sequence of events has given rise to the concept of *phases of grief*, as if grief passes in orderly progression. There is some justification for this concept if it is not taken too literally. Thus Bowlby and Parkes[3] have suggested phases of:

(1)   numbness;

(2)   pining (or yearning);

(3)   disorganization (or despair); and, finally,

(4)   reorganization.

People are permanently changed by grief and there is no clear end-point. What is more, they move back and forth through these phases many times. Even years after bereavement a chance meeting with mutual friends can bring on another pang of grief and the bereaved find themselves back in phase (2) all over again. A more appropriate model for grief may therefore be that of a wave on the sea. Moment to moment fluctuations are the ripples on the surface of a larger swell. At any given moment it may be hard to discern the progress of the larger wave, yet it is none the less real and, with time, its shape and size will become apparent. This means that we should not be too easily influence by single observations when assessing the course of grief. Extreme outbursts of distress are not necessarily ominous, but a consistent lack of progress over many weeks should be taken more seriously.

Risk factors

Given that people vary enormously in the intensity and duration of their grief, it is obviously important to be aware when there may be special risk. Most people will, in fact, come through bereavement without the need for much help from outside the family, but there is a significant minority, around a third of those who suffer a major loss, who will develop psychosocial or psychosomatic problems unless some extra help is given. The risk factors which follow give an indication not only of the situation which lead to problems, but also go some way to explain these problems and contain important implications for prevention and treatment.

Type of bereavement

How a person dies is a factor in determining how the family will grieve. Deaths that are sudden, unexpected, and untimely, particularly if they are especially horrific, as when somebody is murdered, often lead to severe and protracted grief; suicides and other deaths that are thought to be self-motivated commonly present problems, especially if the survivor feels responsible for what has happened.

Although systematic comparisons of different types of bereavement are few, it is generally true that the death of a child and the death of a spouse are more traumatic than deaths of parents and siblings. Sudden Infant Deaths ('SID', 'cot deaths') constitute a special risk because of the legal proceedings and the doubts which many parents feel about their possible contribution to a death, the cause of which seems so uncertain. Stillbirths, especially the birth of a malformed child such as an anencephalic, are much like neonatal deaths and should be taken just as seriously. Even abortions sometimes give rise to severe grief, and the mother's perception of the meaning of such an event determines how she will react to it.

The nature of the attachment

Insecure attachments complicate grief and there is reason to believe that deaths within stormy marriages are more likely to give rise to severe grief than deaths within stable ones. In fact, ambivalence often leads to feelings of self-reproach and anger, which may make it hard for the bereaved to stop grieving. Relationships in which the survivor depended on the partner for emotional support or for reassurance of his or her own strength (e.g. the pseudo-independent partner) are often followed by intense prolonged grieving and a tendency to cling to any person who is willing to take over the caring role.

Personal vulnerability

Personal vulnerability to bereavement, as to other stresses, is reflected in the general style of coping which people adopt. A previous history of mental illness is often an indicator of risk, as are personality factors such as insecurity, general moodiness, anxiety, irritability, or low self-esteem. A tendency to abuse alcohol or other drugs may be aggravated by bereavement.

Social supports

Social supports play an important part in getting people through to the next chapter of their lives. Conversely, the lack of a caring family, or the existence of a family who are seen as unhelpful and who try to distract and discourage a person's attempts to grieve, can be harmful. The existence of a clear set of roles which are available to the bereaved, be it a job of work or domestic responsibility, will often allow people to escape from too much grieving and will help them to find a new identity. On the other hand, such roles can also be used as a distraction from grieving and occasionally interfere with the work of grieving.

Pathological grief

These risk factors seldom occur in isolation. They interact with each other in determining the course of grief. For instance, the sudden death of a spouse may be further complicated by dependence in a person who, because of childhood experiences, is already insecure and lacking in social supports. For this reason we should not expect to find a simple correlation between the type of bereavement and the type of response. Even so, some generalizations are possible. People do run true to type; those who have become depressed in the past are likely to become depressed again following a bereavement; those who have had ambivalent relationships are likely to have further problems in trusting others; those whose self-respect is low are likely to become excessively anxious, and their anxiety may perpetuate itself by leading to psychophysiological disturbance or fears of 'breakdown'.

Unexpected and untimely deaths produce avoidance, disbelief, numbness, and delay in the course of grieving, but this does not prevent the level of anxiety from rising very high. Ambivalent relationships, however, often give rise to very little anxiety at the time of the death; only later does the individual begin to miss the dead person and to suffer delayed, but none the less severe grief. Dependent individuals grieve severely from the start and their grief tends to become chronic.

Clinical depression can arise in the course of any of these reactions and is usually associated with restless anxiety. Only rarely does it follow the typical 'endogenous' or anergic pattern, with diurnal variation of mood, early morning waking, and retardation of thought and movement (see Section 8.4), but when it does it is important to recognize this fact as these patients usually respond well to antidepressant medication. There is an important minority of bereaved people who may become suicidal and it is advisable to ask about suicidal intent if there is the slightest suspicion that this may be the case.

In short, grief may create problems because it is repressed and avoided, because it is misunderstood and aggravated, because it is exaggerated and persistent, because it lights up pre-existing problems, or because it triggers off methods of coping which give rise to fresh problems. Each of these factors must be assessed and understood if we are to help the bereaved towards a healthy outcome.

Helping the bereaved

General practitioners are especially well placed to make valid assessments of bereavement risk. Their knowledge of the previous history gives them a good idea of the personal vulnerability of the bereaved, and they are often in possession of information, gained partly from other members of the primary care team, about relationships within a family. As a trusted person who is likely to become involved when people are dying, the GP is frequently the first person to whom the bereaved turn for help.

Because the members of the PCT are often involved before the death, they are also in a position to help people to prepare themselves for the bereavements that are to come. Adequate warnings should be given, along with the emotional support that will enable the family to take them in and to react. A little sympathy given at the right moment will often unleash feelings that might otherwise be stifled. There will then be less danger that the family will be emotionally unprepared when the death finally takes place.

The moment of death, and the hours that lead up to and follow it, are crucial times for the family and time will be well spent in cherishing them through. 'I'll never forget how that doctor behaved when my husband died', is a reflection of both the importance and the clarity of recall which characterize memories of loss events. This is not the time to start telling people to 'stand on your own feet'. They need all the help they can get, and this means staying close and encouraging whatever words and feelings need to emerge.

We may be asked to explain the reasons for the death as the bereaved struggle to make sense of an outrageous event. 'Why did it happen?' is often a question that is more rhetorical than literal and we should not expect the bereaved to be satisfied with the answers we give. However, they are entitled to honest answers and will only be more disturbed if we evade their questions.

As in other situations where people are distressed, we may find that several explanations are necessary and that the bereaved will need to return more than once to expand and confirm their understanding.

Medical explanations may provide a logical explanation for death, but they will not answer the deeper question of why bad things happen to good people. This is a religious question. Whatever our own beliefs may be it is usually wise to keep them to ourselves and to allow the bereaved to carry out their own search for meaning. We can communicate our faith better by staying close and waiting patiently for rage against God and man to die down, than by forcing our opinions on people whose hurt is too great to enable them to respond to new ideas or complex arguments.

Death certificates are commonly misunderstood. We should always check that the family understand the words which are written on the form. Such terms as 'cerebro-vascular accident' will perplex those to whom 'accidents' are caused by human error. One lady was upset by the word 'sclerosis' because she mistook it for 'cirrhosis' and thought this meant that her husband had died from drink.

If a coroner's inquest is necessary, it is important to explain that nobody is being suspected of murder and to describe the likely sequence of events which will take place. Most people dislike the idea of a post-mortem examination but will accept the importance of adding to our understanding of illness and its consequences. Whatever the reason for the post-mortem, the doctor, usually the GP, needs to be prepared to deal with further questions that arise when the findings are known. Even if nothing new was found, the information that 'the diagnosis was confirmed and it proved that nothing more could have been done' can be most reassuring to family members, whose fears and imaginings tend to colour their assumptions at such times.

During the week leading up to the funeral, the bereaved often feel numb and are likely to be surrounded by family and friends. After the funeral everybody goes away and grief reaches its peak. A visit from a member of the primary care team at this time (10–14 days after the death) will usually be appreciated. Such visits often take a long time as there is much to be talked through; a widow may want to review her entire marriage and to weep over the many implications of her loss. Having done this the intensity of her grief will abate and she will begin to regain control. This may be the first time that she has attempted to talk at length about this major turning point in her life. Often there is nobody else with whom she can share her thoughts and feelings. The family are all too closely involved; they have their own griefs to deal with and are afraid of upsetting each other. Friends are embarrassed, and the bereaved soon learn the truth of the saying 'Laugh and the world laughs with you, weep and you weep alone'. But a concerned GP, nurse, or health visitor who is willing to listen facilitates the work of grieving.

Members of the PCT may be deterred from visiting by the lack of anything positive to say, and it is true that there is nothing we can say which will take

away the need to grieve. We cannot give the bereaved the one thing that the
most want, the dead person. There is no simple answer to the question 'Wha
can you say?' for any formula will sound artificial. The only rule must b
that whatever we do say must be sincere. And, in general, it is best to sa
very little; the bereaved will do the talking.

If someone indicates that they are not ready to talk, we can only show
our understanding and promise to look in again later. They may already hav
all the help that they need, they may need more time to get started, or the
may distrust our intentions. In such cases, it would be wrong to force th
issue and we may have to use our intuition and knowledge of risk factor
to decide whether another visit is needed and, if so, when and from whom
Our own time and feelings are also important and we may have to decid
to draw in another person from the PCT if we are in danger of overloa
or over-involvement. There are now many places where Cruse and othe
organizations are able to offer one-to-one counselling to the bereaved (se
Appendix II). Individual support is most needed in the early stages o
bereavement, when people commonly need permission to express the painfu
mixture of feelings which emerge and reassurance that the physica
accompaniments of grief are quite normal. The time will come when it ma
be more important to help people to emerge from isolation and to engag
with the society to which they now belong. Again, organizations for th
bereaved can be a good first step. As well as providing individual counselling
Cruse runs meetings where widows and other bereaved people can get togethe
and help each other. These reduce the bewilderment and disorientation whicl
causes each bereaved person to feel that he or she is entirely alone, and tha
no one in the world can possibly understand the way they feel. Churches
Age Concern, and many other bodies run similar groups, but it is worth takin,
trouble to ensure that a bereaved person who has agreed to go does follow
up on that intention. There are many bereaved people who are desperatel
lonely, yet too shy to take the step of going to a strange place to meet strang
people. Someone who escorts them to their first meeting and introduces then
to others who will make them welcome will reduce the likelihood that th
bereaved will lose heart at the last minute.

Many GPs keep a 'death book' to help the team remember the firs
anniversary of bereavements. It is notable how many people who have ha
losses come to the doctor with various ailments at this time. If they do not
a death book may help locate those who are perhaps still grieving an
depressed, and may be helped by a visit.

Cultural factors play a large part in determining how people grieve. Thus
in Mediterranean countries and many other parts of the world, grief is ofte
florid and noisy. Such 'uncivilized' behaviour may be disapproved of b
neighbours, and even immigrant members of the same family, who hav
adopted 'Western' mores, may be embarrassed and attempt to force thei
peers to conform to our customs. Yet there is evidence that social sanctio

for mourning is helpful rather than harmful to the bereaved and that people who abandon such traditions may be more liable to pathological grief than those who follow them. By expressing our approval of their mourning, we reduce one source of conflict and may foster more healthy grieving than is usual with our own truncated rituals of mourning.

For those with religious faith funerals can be a great source of comfort, and even the 'silent majority', whose only church attendance is at weddings and funerals, find that the social support, the symbolic or poetic meaning of the ritual, and the opportunity to pay a last tribute to the dead (or 'Say goodbye') are important. Clergy who recognize the psychological value of their roles can contribute a great deal to the process of maturation that is grief.

As time passes it becomes more important to help people to stop grieving than to start. Because grief is a duty to the dead, some people need to be reassured that they have done their duty and can now move on to face the challenges and opportunities which exist; others will need a lot of encouragement if they are to give up the protected 'role' of mourner and take their place in society again.

The treatment of pathological grief

Contrary to the views of some authorities, there is no single method of therapy for all types of pathological grief. This, in our view, explains the mixed results which have arisen from random allocation studies of 'guided grief'.[4] Each patient whose grief is not resolving will need to be individually assessed and the treatment tailored to particular needs.

There are some people who have successfully repressed or avoided grieving. They will most often respond to a therapy which helps them to express their grief. 'Linking objects' (photographs or personal possessions) can be used to 'bring the dead person into the room', and it may help to accompany the bereaved on a much-delayed visit to the grave. Dramatic improvement may follow when locked-up feelings have been expressed for the first time.

Other people have no difficulty in expressing grief. Their problem is in stopping grieving and getting on with life. For them the negotiation of a series of goals which will help them to establish their own autonomy may be required. The withdrawn patient may need us to set up behavioural tasks much as the agoraphobic needs desensitizing.

Antidepressants are sometimes needed, particularly if anergic symptoms predominate, but we should beware of prescribing tranquillizers. It is only too easy for the bereaved to become dependent on these drugs. Some people find that alcohol or other tranquillizers help them to avoid grieving, and it may be difficult to persuade them to stop. Their chances are much improved if we are prepared to offer them alternative sources of support in the form of a counselling relationship.

Vivian S had been dominated as a child by her neurotic, anxious mother. She grew up a timid child who did not begin to thrive until her late teens when her superior sensitivity and intelligence enabled her to get into an art school. It was here that she met her husband, Jim, an enthusiastic idealist, who also tended to dominate her. 'I married him because I could feel safe with him. It was a child–parent relationship', she said. Unfortunately, he developed a depressive illness and, while under treatment in hospital, succeeded in hanging himself. Vivian, who was now 40 years of age and with four children aged between 10 and 15, tried hard to avoid grieving. She spoke to nobody about what had happened for a year, but experienced a chronic sense of guilt and depression. The situation became very much worse three years later when one of her daughters developed a viral meningitis and died, after an illness lasting only nine days. Again, Vivian tried to cope with this loss by putting it out of her mind, but found this increasingly difficult to do and she eventually went to her GP, complaining of uncontrolled episodes of tearfulness and intense feelings of apathy and depression. She had not worked for three years, was blaming herself for both bereavements, and gave the appearance of a little girl who was lost and helpless.

This lady was, therefore, showing signs of both avoidance of grief and of chronic grief, in the sense that her grief was now virtually continual; 'I can't get it out of my mind', she said.

During the next two months she was seen on four occasions. In the course of therapy she was able to face up to, and to grieve, the death of her husband and her child. At the same time she became aware that she had never had an identity of her own. At the second meeting, close to tears she said, 'I've honestly never felt a person.' It was exciting to see this potentially creative woman come alive as she began to channel her discontent into her art. When she did this she became aware that she had been hiding behind other people all her life. 'It's absolutely unbelievable', she said as she described how she now felt that she was 'becoming a person' for the first time in her life.

Although she was very much better at the time of the last session she was appropriately apprehensive and sad. In the course of only five meetings she had become very close to the doctor and was afraid that she would not be able to cope without continued support. But her fears were groundless and two years later she could still report that life was 'fantastic'.

Not all patients with grief problems are as rewarding as this lady. Some people who are 'stuck' may need to turn their attention to some earlier loss before they can begin to tackle the current one. Childhood losses may have set a pattern which is repeated in succeeding bereavements, and it is only when the feelings appropriate to the earlier loss have been expressed that the patient feels safe enough to grieve them anew.

Because turning points in life can enable people to get on with unfinished business of this kind, bereaved people are rewarding to treat. More may be achieved in a few interviews at such times than in years of regular psychotherapy. This makes for a close and fruitful relationship between patient and therapist, but it also sows the seeds of another problem.

When the time comes to end therapy, we may find that the patient has just the same difficulty in grieving for us as for others whom they have lost. It is important to recognize that fact and to allow for the grieving process to begin before the time has come to stop. This can be achieved by making a contract for a set number of further meetings and reminding the patient of the number that remain on each subsequent occasion.

GPs are particularly vulnerable to the patient who cannot stop visiting, and it may be necessary to draw in a partner or colleague to help ease a dependent patient away. Even so, times of loss, like other transitions, are also opportunities for personal growth and development. It is not uncommon to see people emerge from a bereavement stronger, wiser, and more sensitive to the needs of others, than at any time in their lives.

References

1. Parkes, C. M. and Weiss, W. E. (1983). *Recovering from bereavement*. Basic Books, New York.
2. Saunders, C. M. (ed.) (1978). *The management of terminal disease* (2nd edn). Arnold, London.
3. Bowlby, J. and Parkes, C. M. (1970). Separation and loss. In The child in his family, Vol. 1 of *Internat. yearbook of child psychiatry and allied professions*, (ed E. J. Antony and C. Koupernik). John Wiley, New York.
4. Mawson, D., Marks, I. M., Ramm, L., and Stern, L. S. (1981). Guided mourning for morbid grief: a controlled study. *Br. J. Psychiat.* **138**, 185-93.

Further reading

Parkes, C. M. (1975). *Bereavement: studies of grief in adult life* (2nd edn). Penguin, Harmondsworth.
Stedeford, A. (1984). *Facing death*. Heinemann Medical, London.

5.12 OTHER TRANSITIONS

Thus far we have looked at transitions which can be expected to occur at certain stages in the life cycle. But there are other major changes which can occur at any time. These unscheduled transitions are more traumatic because they are seen as unfair and unnatural. The fact that they are often also unexpected means that those who experience them are less well prepared and, as we have already seen, this is likely to increase vulnerability.

It is not possible to list, let alone describe, all the unscheduled events that can occur in the course of a lifetime, but we shall focus on some examples that are likely to come into the orbit of every GP at some time — accidents, assaults, stillbirths, neonatal deaths, birth of a damaged child, and migration. We shall also look at the consequences of communal disasters which, though less common, are so devastating in their consequences that we all need to be prepared for them. Other unscheduled transitions which occur in the course of physical illness will be considered in Chapters 6 and 7.

Accidents

These are the epitome of the unscheduled transition. Occurring without forewarning and with horrific impact, they abruptly dislocate the life of victims, relatives, and all who are involved in them. Even bystanders sometimes find themselves disturbed to an unexpected degree, and severe anxiety and phobic symptoms can be triggered by witnessing a road traffic accident. Likewise, minor accidents sometimes give rise to disproportionate distress with sleep disturbance or 'flashbacks' to the accident, which is repeatedly relived by the victim.

In proportion to the magnitude of the injuries sustained and the degree of personal involvement, the immediate reaction is likely to be one of numbness and incomprehension. Both physical and mental pain are blunted, and severely injured people may take part in rescue operations and fail to recognize their own need for help until they collapse from peripheral vascular failure.

The great need at this time is for reassurance and control, and it is perhaps the acid test of a doctor's training that he or she can remain calm and act promptly and effectively to take control of emergency situations. 'Unflappability' is a personal attribute with which some people are born, but it can also be learned. A good knowledge of what to do, together with experience of coping with similar situations in role play or in real life, can be expected to give most doctors and nurses the confidence to tackle an increasingly wide range of accidents and disasters.

Having achieved control of the physical problems, we must be prepared to 'stay close' in order to give comfort and solace to those most affected by the accident. They may not, at this time, be able to take in much information and it is likely to be non-verbal reassurance that is needed at first. As time passes, however, the need to share feelings and to talk about what has happened will become more evident, and there is then a need to support the expression of grief in much the same way as after major surgery (p. 303) or bereavement (Section 5.11).

The fact that someone is likely to be to blame for an accident adds another dimension to the problem. Unsettled compensation claims often delay recovery, not because people deliberately set out to deceive but more often because the sense of grievance, which is an understandable consequence of an accident, will not be resolved until justice has been seen to be done. Angry feelings easily give rise to *malaise* and a tendency to focus attention on any part of the body that is seen as damaged. Hence, the post-traumatic syndrome that sometimes follows head injuries usually includes persistent headache, and injuries to other parts of the body give rise to other local pains. Obsessive preoccupation with a body part easily augments any pain or discomfort which is present, and it may be difficult to separate functional from organic components.

Not all claims for compensation are financial, and the urge to punish another person for the pain and misery which they have inflicted is a factor in perpetuating that misery. Just as ambivalence towards a dead person complicates the course of grieving, so anger and guilt may complicate the adjustment to accidental injuries. In a paradoxical sense, grief may not be resolved until a grievance has been righted, at the same time it may be hard to give up a grievance until the anger of grief has abated. It follows that neither counselling nor the pursuit of justice is sufficient in itself to quell the fires of angry grief; both are needed.

Sexual and other assaults on the person and assault on property

These are currently becoming increasingly common in our society. The psychological damage which they inflict is often far more serious than any physical damage. Most of us, most of the time, behave as if we are under some special protection. We forget to lock up when we leave the house, we open the door to strangers, and seldom glance over our shoulders when followed in the street. In other words we trust people. But every GP must expect, from time to time, to meet patients who have been assaulted, raped, or subjected to some other outrage to their security.

The psychological reaction to such assaults depends partly on the type of assault, and partly on the personality and previous experience of the person assaulted. A shy, frail, 80-year-old who relies on the security of her home may be devastated by a common burglary. Having little confidence in her ability to defend herself, she may have come to rely on the walls around her as a major source of security. When they have been penetrated she experiences a sense of mutilation which may be almost as severe as that which results from a physical assault on another person. It will be a long time before she begins to feel safe again, and in the meanwhile she may suffer a variety of symptoms reflecting persisting fear.

Other things being equal, it is physical assaults which evoke the greatest distress and, of these, rape is probably the most devastating in its effects. Three factors confound the problem.

(1) The fact that there is nothing to show means that others are less sympathetic than they would be if there was physical evidence of damage.

(2) The sexual character of the assault causes friends to hang back, uncertain whether they should mention what has happened; some may even criticize the sufferer, or infer that the rape was invited.

(3)   The associated police enquiries, medical examination, court appearance, and hostile questioning by the defence counsel (and sometimes disbelieving police officers) adds to the stress which is already present. The victim feels as if the rape is never going to end and may become distrustful of all men. In these circumstances it would be surprising if his/her sex life was not affected and this may create further tension.

The primary care team is sometimes involved as a result of pregnancy or medical conditions arising out of the assault, or members may be consulted for help with sleeplessness, irritability, or other psychological consequences. As far as possible, we should avoid adding to the sense of intrusion which already exists by keeping 'penetrating' questions and examinations to a minimum, and treating the victim in a gentle but matter-of-fact way. Where possible, victims of sexual abuse should be seen by members of their own sex. Their usual partner (if any) will also need support in coming to terms with their anger and confusion.

Victims will sometimes need to be encouraged to take legal action in order to protect themselves and others from the danger of further assault. This is particularly important in cases of incest, or where a person has been assaulted by a marital partner. Sadly, violence is often concealed because of threats of further violence; the victim is cowed into submission. In such cases the anger, which is a natural response to assault, may get turned against the self, and victims (particularly children) may come to believe that they are responsible for the violence which is being perpetrated against them. 'If I wasn't a bad girl he wouldn't keep punishing me' is a common assumption. One result of counselling can be to allow the anger its rightful expression, whereupon the victim may find the courage to take steps to bring the violence to a halt. Often a threat to 'go public' or a call from a lawyer is all that is needed.

Cheryl B, an attractive 23-year-old trainee social worker, was walking home one night when a car drew up and she was forced in at knife point, driven to a secluded place, and raped. After committing the offence the rapist drove off, leaving his victim to walk to the nearest police station, where she arrived, in a state of shock and bewilderment, half an hour later. By now it was late at night and the desk sergeant was inclined to dismiss her story as the incoherent rambling of a drunken girl, but she eventually convinced him of the seriousness of the situation and friends were called to stay with her while further questioning and a medical examination were carried out.

During succeeding weeks she was interviewed again and eventually appeared in court where she faced hostile examination from a defending counsel who tried to discredit her evidence.

The effect of this whole experience was to shatter her confidence both in herself and in others, particularly men. Her sexual attractiveness, which had previously been a source of pride and a boost to her self-confidence, had suddenly become a danger; her confidence in the world as a safe place in which she could move freely in her work as a social worker was undermined, and she found herself anxious and fearful much of the time.

Her GP was a man and, when she visited him requesting a tranquillizer, his questions seemed intrusive, while her reaction to them made him feel that he was raping her over again. She misinterpreted his reluctance to comply with her request for drugs as a rejection, but did accept his suggestion that she should talk things over with a female doctor. Fortunately, this colleague had a special interest in victims of rape and was able to achieve good rapport with the patient. She helped Cheryl to distinguish between the real dangers that she had been forced to acknowledge and the unrealistic fears that had begun to dominate her life and her career as a social worker. Cheryl had lost confidence in her ability to cope with sexual situations and had over-reacted to several bids for friendship from young men whose interest she could later acknowledge as perfectly normal and reasonable.

It required patience, tact, and a fair amount of reassurance before she began to emerge from her shell and to face the world again. She now carries a portable alarm in her pocket when she goes out and will probably never feel safe on her own at night, but in most respects she is happy and well adjusted.

Victim support schemes exist in most areas of the country. These local organizations, with a co-ordinator and a team of volunteers, offer support and advice to victims of personal crime who may be referred by the police or other agencies.

A doctor was called to see Mr X who had been hit on the head with an iron bar by an intruder. Not only had he sustained a serious head injury, but he had also been burgled. After dealing with the head injury, the doctor contacted the local victim support scheme. A volunteer came and talked to Mr X, helping to restore his morale and to put in a claim to the Criminal Injuries Compensation Board. The local Round Table was also contacted by the scheme and changed the locks on the doors of the patient's house.

Sometimes it is the perpetrators of violence who seek our help, either because they have been exposed, or because they have become frightened of the intensity of their own capacity for violence. Since such behaviour is often 'end of tether' behaviour, anything which lowers the level of tension and provides them with greater confidence and control will reduce the likelihood of further violence. Crisis intervention, marital conflict, child abuse, and the management of aggressive persons are discussed elsewhere in this book.

Neonatal deaths

One hundred years ago neonatal deaths were so common that every woman expected half her children to die, hence these deaths could not be regarded as unscheduled. Although we have no direct evidence which allows us to compare the psychological reactions of Victorian women to the reactions of bereaved mothers today, there is indirect evidence from letters and other literature which suggests that women today find the death of a child much more traumatic and outrageous than did their great-grandparents.

During the neonatal period the causes of most deaths are still unknown. The majority of cot deaths are sudden, unexpected, and inexplicable. They have to be reported to the coroner, and the subsequent police enquiries raise suspicions and fears in the minds of the parents which will not be allayed by the eventual indecisive nature of the verdict. 'What did I do wrong?' is a question that can seldom be answered, and it is not surprising that mutual blame, self-reproaches, and blame directed at others often linger and complicate the course of grieving.

Health visitors and other members of the PCT have a most important role to play in such cases, visiting without invitation and providing quite clear and consistent reassurance concerning these suspicions. Police involvement does not mean that the parents are being blamed, and in the vast majority of these cases there is no evidence that the parents have contributed in any way to cause the death of their child. An explanation which is consistent with the evidence currently available can be given. It can include the following points:

- Babies do not breathe in the womb. Their breathing mechanism is 'switched on' by chemical changes in the blood which take place at the time of birth.

- This breathing switch is not completely reliable. Most babies stop breathing again from time to time during the first few weeks of life, but only for short periods of time. The vast majority of babies soon start breathing again and parents seldom even notice the episode.

- Once in a while, however, the episode may go on longer than it should and the baby dies quietly and peacefully in its sleep.

- There is no reason to believe that episodes of this kind are caused by the parents. Hard pillows, soft pillows, pets, and flowers in the bedroom play no appreciable part and, although some of these babies have a snuffly cold, there is no reason to believe that this means that the parents or their GPs have failed to treat a hidden pneumonia or other massive infection.

The Foundation for the Study of Infant Deaths provides a useful leaflet for parents who have lost a child in this way, as well as offering mutual help and a source of education and research in this difficult area (see Appendix II).

Stillbirths

Mothers who suffer a stillbirth are commonly assumed to grieve less than mothers whose baby dies after birth, yet follow-up studies suggest that this it not necessarily the case. For many mothers their unborn child is very much a person and there are some for whom the loss of that baby is a major tragedy. Childless couples who have invested a great deal in this pregnancy, or ambivalent couples who may have wished the child dead, may find the death particularly hard to bear. The fact that many mothers are dissuaded from viewing the body of their child, and others choose not to do so because they are afraid to face the reality of death, further complicates the process of grieving. Fantasy soon takes the place of reality and the mother may become obsessed with horrific imaginings, or distracted by a fruitless search for the image of a child whom she never saw. In most instances it is advisable to encourage the parents to hold the dead body of their child, appropriately wrapped if deformity is present.

Many obstetric departments now take a photograph of the dead baby and either present it to the mother or file it in the records in case she should wish for a print. Members of the PCT may find this useful if they are counselling the parents of stillborn children.

Stillbirths and other accidents of birth inevitably arouse fears that the same will happen in the event of future pregnancies, and it is the obstetrician's responsibility to investigate the risk. It may be the GP who has to communicate this information to the parents, and a close liaison with the obstetrician is important. In most instances parents can be reassured that such risks are small.

A mutual-help group for parents who have suffered a stillbirth exists in the Stillbirths and Neonatal Deaths Association (see Appendix II).

Abortion

Women vary greatly in their response to miscarriage, and there is a great difference between the mother who has lost her only chance of a much-wanted baby and the planned and early termination of an unwanted 'accident'. In general, the reactions to properly planned terminations of pregnancy are less traumatic than would be the consequences of allowing that pregnancy to continue, but there are some cases in which feelings of guilt and recrimination arise. Quarrels may take place between husbands and wives who blame each other for depriving their child of life, and some women conceive again in an attempt to undo the damage.

Both parents will need proper counselling before and after planned terminations and the members of the PCT should not wait to be invited to make contact.

Le Baron *et al.*[1] in a well-conducted study, randomly assigned women who had undergone elective abortions to two groups. Both were treated with warmth and concern, but in one group the patient was recumbent and the physician was more active, telling the patient what to do, making decisions, touching the patient often, and offering only moderate amounts of information. In the second group the patient was sitting up and the physician adopted a more egalitarian role, sharing decision-making with the patient providing much information, giving permission rather than instruction, and seldom touching the patient. All-in-all the patients preferred the former paternalistic approach, perceiving the physician as significantly more warm and supportive and reporting less discomfort and physiological distress. They become more suggestible and may, therefore, have complied better with subsequent care.

While it is hard to know which of several differences (touching, posture paternalism) contributed most to the outcome of this study, it is not unreasonable to conclude that the passive, permissive approaches which are often advocated for the treatment of patients with long-standing emotional problems are not necessarily the best approach when dealing with a threatening life situation or loss.

Unplanned and unexpected miscarriages, particularly those which take place late in pregnancy are a real cause of grief and may resemble the reaction to stillbirths. Again, the parents may wish to view the fetus and should not be dissuaded from doing so. Clergy will be glad to say prayers with the parent and, although there is no formal ceremony of the kind which exists for stillborn children, a ritual can be worked out which will meet the parents individual needs.

Again a mutual-help group, The Miscarriage Association, exists to provide information and support for parents who have problems relating to this kind of loss (see Appendix II).

Birth of a handicapped child

Parents who succeed in giving birth but whose child is subsequently found to be physically or mentally handicapped may need to grieve for the child they haven't got before they can accept the child which they have got. Thus they may reject a new-born baby and demand instant adoption, yet change their mind if given the time and support which they need.

Feelings of disappointment and anger may complicate their relationship with caregivers and spouses. Both marital partners may need the opportunity to express such feelings to a member of the PCT if they are not to antagonize each other.

Having come through the process of grieving, the mother often becomes very attached to the handicapped child. Because the child is damaged the attachment is likely to be insecure and may lead to a very intense and over protective relationship. Some mothers blame themselves for the damage to their child or for wishing their child dead, and their over-mothering may be a means of trying to make restitution. Other children and spouses may be neglected and it is not uncommon for a split to develop in the family, with mother trapped in a bind with the handicapped child and father taking over the care of the healthy children.

Problems of this kind should be approached as family problems whenever possible and treated by means of joint meetings with both partners, aimed at clarifying the salient issues and restoring security and perspective. A variety of mutual-help groups exist to support parents who have children with paraplegia (The Spastic Association), spina bifida (The Spina Bifida Association), and metabolic diseases (The Research Trust for Metabolic Diseases in Children; see Appendix II.

Infertility

Infertile couples are sometimes plagued by chronic grief for the child that they have never had. They, too, may need help if they are to accept the facts of their infertility and open their minds to the possibilities of adoption (if this is a realistic option). Unfortunately, the uncertain outcome of treatments for infertility may feed hope or prolong an agonized and fruitless perseverance or grief. The National Association for the Childless is a mutual-help group for infertile couples with its own journal (see Appendix II). By putting them in contact with each other and keeping them informed of recent research in the field, NAC helps childless couples to come to terms with their situation and reduces the likelihood that they will see themselves as 'freaks'. Members of the PCT may need to discourage infertile couples from becoming obsessed with the problem and 'spectators' of their own sexual activities.

The transition to a new country

Immigrants seem a far cry from infertile couples, yet they, too, may spend much of their lives pining for something that can never be. Grief for the old country may block acceptance of the new, and there are many immigrants who insist that their stay is only temporary, long after there is any practical reason for them to return.

Of course, there are many reasons for immigration and we must expect to find large differences between the reactions of those who have 'run away' and those who have 'run towards' another country. Realistic preparation, the construction of a valid model of the world that is being entered, positive motivation, and good prospects all improve the chances of successful adjustment. Conversely, lack of, or unrealistic, anticipation, forcible or reluctant expulsions from the homeland, persisting ties to aspects of the mother country, and poor prospects in the new militate against successful psychosocial transitions. Sadly, the linguistic and cultural gap that exists between immigrants and their medical attendants often makes it hard for the

PCT to give the understanding and support that is needed. The language of symptoms is not a universal tongue, and it may be difficult to persuade an Indian patient with chest pains that these are caused by disappointed hopes rather than heart disease.

Some immigrants cling to the models of disease common in their parent culture, others reject their parent culture and adopt an idealized and simplistic view of scientific medicine. Witchcraft, curses, and folk cures may be all-pervading, 'all nonsense', or a bewildering mixture. Magical expectations of scientific drugs may enhance their effects, but both patients and doctors are likely to have low expectations of the value of talking about problems when talk is so difficult.

In those areas in which there is a substantial immigrant population the members will have developed their own subculture and systems of support. These can be of great value in providing interpreters of culture as well as of langauge. They may also be the best source of understanding and guidance for the patient. Immigrant doctors, nurses, and social workers can also be valuable, but they are sometimes distrusted by those who have rejected their parent culture.

To members of the PCT who are prepared to take the time to study these transcultural problems, they can be fascinating. In a shrinking world there are real gains for the caregiver as well as the recipient, for, at one level, we are all immigrants to a changing world. Successful mourning consists not in discarding the old in favour of the new, nor in rejecting the new, but in painfully searching out from the past those assumptions and models which can enlighten, enrich, and explain the new life space. Immigrants bring their own special points of view and there is no culture which cannot benefit from them.

Just as we need to be tolerant of the anger and the pain of grief, so we must not expect that immigrants will find it easy to adjust to life in a new world. By the same token, those who are prepared to 'hang in' until the pangs of grief diminish will find their patience rewarded.

Communal disaster

In this book we have accepted the fact that in our society, after family and friends, it is the PCT to whom most people turn when stress becomes intolerable. It follows that the GP has a key place in the community as an agent of support at times of change.

Communal disasters differ from those already considered in their scale, the extent to which they overwhelm and disrupt existing support systems, and in the wide ramifications of the psychological reactions which result. Members of the PCT are key figures in response to disasters, but their close involvement with the community is a mixed blessing. They are, to some degree, victims as well as caregivers. Powerful emotions may impair their judgement, yet there are often no others to whom their fellow victims can turn for help. Rescue teams are solely concerned with emergency care, and there is unlikely to be anybody to hand who understands the special problems of psychosocial care.

Individual reactions to disasters are much the same as those to other unexpected traumata. Numbness, anger, self-reproaches, bewilderment, and intense pining for the world that is lost have been described elsewhere in this book. But in disaster areas they may give rise to group behaviour which compounds the damage. Irrational expressions of anger, major mistakes in judgement, scapegoating, paralysis of decision-making, aimless hyperactivity, rumours, apparently selfish behaviour (the so-called 'illusion of centrality' which causes victims to imagine themselves to be at the centre of the disaster), hypomanic elation, vandalism, paranoid attitudes, and hostility toward potential helpers may complicate attempts to organize and provide emotional support.

Not that all the consequences are negative. Disasters can evoke extraordinary support and self-sacrifice. People who would not normally speak to each other become warm and friendly, and the whole community may develop a solidarity which previously was lacking. Responsible new leaders will emerge to replace those who are lost or disabled, and, in the short run, it is often possible to get things done which, at other times, would have seemed impossible. So a disaster, like other types of loss, is both a time of great stress and a time of opportunity.

Because every disaster is different, there is no one master plan which will suit all situations. But the following guidelines have proved useful:

Impact phase

Promote a calm and supportive network of care. Assess the mental state of those in the forefront of rescue operations and take action to contain, and if possible relieve, any whose behaviour is panicky or over-excited or who are approaching exhaustion. Single doses of diazepam can be used to lower the level of tension in victims or distraught family members, but prescribing excessive quantities of benzodiazepines should be avoided, and requests for amphetamines or other 'pep' pills from rescuers resisted.

Those in positions of responsibility need special care. They will usually deny their need for support but may need to be reminded that they, too, are human beings who need rest and care from time to time if they are to stay in control of the situation.

Recoil

The tide of adrenaline which enables most people to cope well with emergencies will eventually subside, to leave them numb and exhausted. Although rest is needed, there are many who will remain talkative and restless. The process of talking through and making real the events of the disaster will begin with a sense of urgency which contrasts with the fact that there may be nothing to be done. This is, of course, an important part of the process of grieving and should be encouraged. This is the time when the PCT must get together with each other, and with ther caregivers, to take stock of the situation and to make provisional plans for supporting those who are at special risk.

Aftermath

Time spent in planning and liaison is essential if mistakes are to be avoided. The pressure to 'do something' is so great that many potentially useful people get caught up in self-defeating activities, or duplicate the efforts of others. Sometimes there are more caregivers than victims, while at other times the needs of one group of victims may be ignored because of the evident needs of others. Thus, bereaved parents may find it hard to meet the needs of their bereaved children and schools and nurseries may need to provide opportunities for the expression of grief.

Disasters commonly give rise to much guilt, and GPs may be treated as 'confessors' by those who need to share this burden. As in the case of other bereavements, the sharing of grief takes time, and time may be in short supply. One way of coping is to hold group meetings at which those affected by the disaster can come together to share their feelings, and to support each other. Group leaders need to be aware that such groups can easily become a vehicle for the expression of irrational anger. Wherever possible, people who may be in danger of becoming scapegoats should be included in the group and given a chance to share their perception of the situation. Unjust accusations usually melt away in the face of reality, and even just accusations lose some of their bitterness in a group in which everyone can acknowledge some degree of guilt.

A special service to provide support to communities affected by disasters is currently being developed by Cruse (see Appendix II for address), and their expertise can be drawn on by local services. They will not attempt to take away the responsibility of local people to cope with emergent needs, but will focus on providing support to the supporters. This includes training in disaster care, help in the planning of a response, and personal counselling for the front line workers.

Whatever outside support may be drawn in, it is important for the PCT to support each other. Regular meetings at which personal feelings can be expressed, as well as problems with victims and others discussed, are an important part of any disaster plan.

Communities do not 'recover' from disasters, they are permanently changed by them. As the intensity of the feelings of grief begin to diminish, anger and guilt, which cause so many problems in the early stages, may begin to diminish. The 'creative discontent' which may emerge seems to reflect the need of the community to bring something good out of the bad thing that has happened. Given good leadership and appropriate guidance, the cohesive spirit that has arisen may enable real community development to take place. As one woman in Aberfan said, 'This disaster was caused by apathy, it is up to us to show that Aberfan will never become apathetic again.'

References

1. Le Baron, S., Reyher, J. and Stack, J. M. (1985). Paternalistic vs. egalitarian physician styles: the treatment of patients in crisis. *J. Fam. Pract.* **21**, 56–62.

Further reading

Raphael, B. (1986). *When disaster strikes: how individuals and communities can cope with catastrophes.* Basic Books, New York.

6 Mind–body, body–mind

6.1 INTRODUCTION AND CLASSIFICATION

Distinguishing between mind and body is illusory and diminishes our attempts to think in holistic and biopsychosocial terms, but it remains a convenience and enables ideas to be presented more simply. The ideas in this chapter are discussed under the following headings:

- psychosomatic disorders;

- somatoform disorders;

- malingering and factitious disorders;

- psychological reactions to physical illness.

Patients presenting with psychological disorders frequently have physical symptoms—for instance, people with anxiety states may develop overbreathing and tetany. Other patients consult their doctors with physical symptoms such as asthma, but which reflect their psychological state. These are considered under the heading 'psychosomatic disorders', implying that, with our present state of knowledge, there is a potentially identifiable physiological pathway between the psychological state and the physical manifestation. Others have many apparently physical symptoms but cannot be demonstrated, on clinical examination or by laboratory tests, to have any physical or pathological abnormality. These symptoms are thought to result from psychological causes and are considered under 'somatoform disorders'. Others have physical symptoms and signs which are knowingly induced. These are considered in Section 6.4. Lastly, some patients have physical illnesses, such as myocardial infarction, or mutilating surgery, and respond psychologically. They are considered in Section 6.5.

Although the division between these states is far from clear-cut, the mechanisms underlying them, and linking mind and body, can be considered in the context of ordinary emotions (Section 1.2), in the context of symptom detectors (Chapter 2), and in the context of the consultation (Section 4.2).

Emotional states have accompanying neuroendocrine changes which can explain some of the physical symptomatology which patients report. Adrenalin release, associated with anxiety or general arousal, can lead to an increased heart-rate (which is perceived as palpitations), to reduced stomach secretions (leading to nausea and stomach upsets), and to reduced salivation (resulting in difficulty in swallowing). Prolonged or repeated sympathetic arousal may lead to changed physiological functioning, when the patient might present with a psychosomatic disorder such as a gastric ulcer.

Increased muscle tension frequently accompanies anxiety and this may explain some of the various pains people report at times of stress. Thus, pain in the face, head, neck, or back may result from muscle tension. This explanation is supported by evidence that electromyographic (EMG) biofeedback can reduce tension headaches and that other forms of stress management can also be effective.

A type of involuntary behaviour which can lead to particularly distressing symptoms is hyperventilation — fast, shallow breathing which accompanies anxiety states and produces changes in the acid/base balance of the blood due to the loss of carbon dioxide. This may present as breathlessness, parasthesiae, other peculiar sensations, or tetany.

Physical symptoms can arise from more voluntary changes in behaviour. Distressed individuals may change their patterns of eating, sleeping, exercising, taking alcohol and drugs, or smoking, and all of these behaviours are likely to alter their physical state. Symptoms such as tiredness, nausea, and aches and pains may result.

Whether symptoms arise as a result of neuroendocrine changes, muscle tension, hyperventilation, or changes in habits, they are likely to cause distress, and perhaps feed back into the causal pathway. The spiral of anxiety→physical symptoms→anxiety about symptoms→exacerbation of symptoms is a well-known pattern. In its extreme form this spiral may present as a panic attack, where feelings of anxiety and associated bodily symptoms become overwhelming.

If ordinary bodily sensations are interpreted as symptoms of serious illness, leading to anxiety and associated physical changes, and these are then perceived as further symptoms, the same spiral can be entered. This may be the pattern adopted by patients who attract the label 'hypochondriac'.

Recent research suggests that in anxiety disorders patients attend to threatening cues much more than do average individuals.[1] Thus the anxious individual is not only experiencing changes in neuroendocrine, EMG, and behavioural processes, but is also paying more attention to the associated bodily changes. It is hardly surprising, then, that physical symptoms are reported as being associated with the psychological state.

There is ample evidence in laboratory and clinical studies that psychological factors (especially the attention given to bodily sensations and the explanations the individual has for these sensations) can influence the experience of pain. The 'gate-control' theory of pain attempts to account for these phenomena by postulating the presence of descending pathways from higher centres to a gating mechanism in the spinal cord. This controls the access of afferent pain signals to the highest centres, and therefore determines whether the individual experiences pain.

While the physiological mechanisms remain uncertain, these psychological processes do appear to operate, regardless of whether the initial trigger is a symptom of illness or a minor strain of the kind we all experience every day.

General management strategies

Physical symptoms can often be treated by dealing with the psychological state. It is very important to give patients an adequate understanding of the cause of the physical symptoms. Patients may be given simple explanations of the physical changes associated with, for example, anxiety attacks, and these can be incorporated into a set of self-statements which they use to manage their own anxiety; for example, they can be taught to instruct themselves that the feelings they experience are part of a normal fear response, do not signify that something is physically wrong, and will disappear spontaneously if they do not add further frightening thoughts.

While with some patients the psychological source has to be the main focus of treatment, with others it must be the presenting physical symptom. For example, a patient may report pain due to muscle tension, which is in turn due to high anxiety associated with distressing life events. The treatment approach may be to use a stress-management strategy (see Section 3.4) to attempt to resolve some of the problems surrounding the life events, so reducing the anxiety associated with them; or to tackle the muscle tension directly by some form of relaxation training. Similarly, if the symptoms are thought to be associated with changes in the patient's habits, the solution may be in some adjustment of these.

In any management approach, the patient and doctor need a shared understanding of the problem. An explanation of the symptoms as 'psychological' can be unhelpful if the patient understands this to mean

- that the doctor thinks they are imagining the symptoms, when the patient knows only too well that they are real;

- that the patient is malingering, when the patient knows that they are making every effort to overcome the symptoms;

- that the patient is mad, which is an unnecessarily frightening possibility; or

- that they need to 'pull themselves together' when they neither understand how, nor feel capable of doing so.

The explanations suggested above in terms of psychophysiological, behavioural, and attentional processes can bring order to these confusions, minimize worry about the bodily sensations perceived as symptoms, and identify a starting point for efforts to overcome the symptoms.

References

1. Mathews, A. and MacLeod, C. (1986). Discrimination of threat cues without awareness in anxiety states. *J. Abnorm. Psychol.* **95**, 131–8.

Recommended reading

For patients with symptoms attributable to anxiety and stress.

Weekes, C. (1983). *Self help for your nerves.* Angus and Robertson, London.
Wilkinson, G. (1987). *Coping with stress.* BMA Publications, London.

6.2 PSYCHOSOMATIC DISORDERS

In these disorders psychological factors play a significant part in the initiation or exacerbation of conditions in which the resulting physiological disturbance goes far beyond the normal range and justifies the term pathological.

Many people would classify peptic ulceration and irritable bowel syndrome under this heading. Others would spread the net more widely and include myocardial infarction, hypertension, some forms of asthma, and the triggering of rheumatoid arthritis or even sore throats. This lack of agreement reflects the difficulty of assigning the relative importance of physical and psychological factors in the causation of disease, and indeed the futility of trying.

It seems likely that it is the interaction of genetic, familial, stress, behaviour, and environmental factors which determines why one patient develops one condition and one another, or why, when a physical condition is present, symptoms may wax and wane.

The basis of much illness is genetic, but other factors are often necessary to allow a disorder to become apparent. For instance, asthma may not present until triggered by a death in the family. In the same way, environmental factors may exacerbate symptoms.

People with a type A personality which is characterized by aggression, intolerance, demanding behaviour, ambition, dislike of inefficiency, and an expectation of high standards are more prone to myocardial infarction than those of more placid temperament, but apart from this there is not much research evidence to link personality with specific diseases. There is some suggestion[1,2,3] that members of 'enmeshed' families (see Section 4.4) adapt to external stress by developing physical rather than emotional symptoms.

Management

The general approaches were outlined in the introduction. Physical safety should not be sacrificed in the interests of psychological insight. Thus successful symptom relief (e.g. of peptic ulceration by H_2 antagonists, or of the irritable bowel syndrome by antispasmodics), will not only make the patient more comfortable but create trust, which will in turn facilitate psychological insight, particularly if initiated by the same doctor.

Much effort has been spent on formal psychotherapy with patients who have psychosomatic disorders, but there is conflicting evidence about its value. What is agreed is that therapy should aim at supporting the whole person in their environment, and that this may involve appropriate reassurance, help with coping with stressful situations, anxiety management, and behaviour modification, especially in those with type A personality.

References

1. Minuchen, S., Baker, L., Osman, B. L., Liebman, R., Milman, L. and Todd, T. C. (1975). A conceptual model of psychosomatic illness in children. *Archs Gen. Psychiat.* **32**, 1031–8.
2. Wirsching, M. and Stierlin, H. (1985). Psychosomatics 1. Psychosocial characteristics of psychosomatic patients and their families. *Fam. Systems Med.* **3**, 6–15.
3. Wirsching, M. and Stierlin, H. (1985). Psychosomatics 2. Treatment considerations. *Fam. Systems Med.* **3**, 281–98.

6.3   SOMATOFORM DISORDERS

This term refers to a group of conditions in which patients complain of physical symptoms, or induce anxiety about physical symptoms, in the absence of discernible physical disease. They do so for various reasons.

- They think that only somatic symptoms will entitle them to help from doctors.

- They are afraid of the stigma of mental illness, and this attitude can be reinforced by that of doctors; hence, they may emphasize the significance of any somatic symptom.

- They become, for some reason, selectively aware of physiological function such as a fast pulse or borborygmii.

- They have been taught by their families to express distress by bodily symptoms, and are barely conscious of the relationship between the distress and the symptoms.

Somatoform disorders may sometimes be used by patients (at varying levels of consciousness):

● to elicit sympathy and social support;

● to control relatives;

● to avoid intimacy;

● to express anger;

● to avoid anxiety-provoking situations.

For convenience they may be divided into four sub-groups but there is always considerable overlap:

(1)   somatization disorders;

(2)   psychogenic pain disorders;

(3)   hypochondriasis;

(4)   conversion disorders (hysteria).

Somatization disorder or abnormal illness behaviour

This is a newly delineated and named group but all general practitioners will be familiar with patients who fall into it. They are frequent attenders, have fat record-folders and cause frustration by rarely getting better. In anthropological terms the syndrome has been defined as, 'The expression of personal and social distress is an idiom of bodily complaints with medical help seeking.'[1] It is commonest in women, who present, usually before the age of 30, with many symptoms of a recurring nature which cannot be adequately explained by physical disorder or injury. The symptoms cause them to take medicine, alter their lifestyles, and to consult physicians.

Mrs B aged 30, complained of dizziness and frequency of micturition for which no physical cause could be found. She already had a thick folder as, from the age of 20, she had been a regular surgery attender, with a large number of complaints about her body, for few of which any definite diagnosis had been made, but for many of which she had received medication. Her family history revealed that her husband had abused alcohol and that her mother had died when the patient was 14.

Common symptoms include being generally 'sickly'; various pseudo-neurological symptoms such as giddiness and 'tingling'; gastrointestinal symptoms, such as nausea, vague abdominal pains, or continued belching; and reproductive symptoms, such as dysmenorrhoea or sexual dissatisfaction.

Causal factors

Like patients with psychosomatic disorders, such patients seem to have disorders of communication and distinct ways of dealing with emotions. Characteristics of this group are thought to be their inability to articulate their feelings to outsiders or to themselves. They are largely unaware of their emotional state, though they may be demanding and angry.

Many of these patients come from families in which feelings are ignored, so that children have not learned to verbalize them. Any attempt to complain in terms of feelings is disregarded. On the other hand, these children soon learn that if they complain of pain or physical symptoms they get attention. Pain and bodily symptoms thus become the language of distress and they are conditioned to use them. The families of these patients may present similar problems, have depressed members, or present with behavioural problems such as alcohol abuse. A significant number of patients with somatization disorder will have high scores when questionnaires to detect depression, such as the General Health Questionnaire or the Beck Depression Inventory, are used. The possibility of their symptoms being part of a depressive illness always needs to be considered. It may not be clear whether they are depressed because of their incurable somatic symptoms or whether their depression is primary, but it is the experience of many GPs that patients with symptoms such as chronic backache occasionally respond to antidepressants—hence they may be described as suffering from 'masked depression'.

Diagnosis

This should not be made merely on the basis of unexplained symptoms, but should take account of the whole pattern of presentation.

- A history of symptoms which suggest a somatization disorder and not an organic illness.

- A complete physical examination which does not reveal an adequate physical cause.

- Investigations which do not reveal a cause.

- A positive family history of one or more of the following: somatization disorders, alcohol or drug abuse, behaviour problems, unstable relationships, child and sexual abuse, or parasuicide.

- A suggestion in the individual and in the family of difficulty in expressing distress in emotional terms.

- Indications of the presence of anxiety or depression.

It needs to be remembered that some will, with the passage of time, turn out to have bodily illnesses, and some will have somatizing and physical illness present at the same time.

Depressive illness needs to be excluded either by history-taking or by questionnaire.

Management

Once a somatization disorder has been recognized, the doctor needs to scale-down expectations of cure and, in particular, accept the limitations of a biomedical approach.

Some form of understanding needs to be established with the patient, with an acceptance that the symptoms represent an emotional communication. In a group practice it is best for a single person to accept responsibility for continued management, and if, as often happens, these patients present as emergencies when 'their own' doctor is not available, they should be gently but firmly pointed back in his or her direction. It is probably best to arrange regularly spaced appointments to anticipate and deflect these emergency contacts.

The diagnosis and management of these conditions are intermingled. It is important, early in the disorder, to exclude diagnosable organic disease, but it is disastrous to arrange endless investigations and referrals. One must have the courage to ignore minor and irrelevant variations in test results, such as a small rise in the alkaline phosphatase or a duodenal diverticulum. Every new investigation and opinion tends to reinforce the patient's assumption that if only the right test was done the cure would be found.

Table 6.1. *Check-list of conditions which may mimic somatization disorders*

Frontal lobe lesions
Epilepsy
Multiple sclerosis
Head injury
Encephalitis
Myalgic encephalitis or Royal Free Disease
Myasthenia gravis
Klinefelter's syndrome
Alcohol
Diabetes mellitus
Thyroid disorders
Other endocrine disorders
Syphilis
Tuberculosis
AIDS

A check-list (see Table 6.1) of conditions which are great mimics should be kept in mind. It is often difficult for non-sufferers to accept and acknowledge the reality of the patient's symptoms, but unless this is accomplished there will be little rapport and little benefit from the consultation. It is vital to emphasize that the therapist knows that the patient is not imagining symptoms, is not 'putting them on', and that the symptoms do not imply that the patient is mad.

It is traditional to say that the diagnosis of psychological illness must be made positively by finding definite psychopathology and not merely by exclusion of organic disease. However, with the somatization disorders we are in a catch-22 situation, as these patients present with physical-sounding complaints and have no obvious psychiatric disorders. It is seldom appropriate to use tranquillizers or sedatives which will again reinforce the idea that the patient's pain can be removed by the doctor giving treatment, though, as stated before, antidepressants may be helpful.

The basic, but difficult, task is for the therapist to divert the patient's attention from the physical symptoms, and concentrate on their relationships and their general ways of coping with emotions. The genogram (see Section 4.4) may be a useful tool to help bridge this gap, the object being to link events in patients' lives with their feelings, and even to provide a vocabulary for patients to express feelings. Emotional insights, when achieved, need to be acknowledged and applauded.

It may well happen that the therapist's efforts to give the patient an emotional language to express distress in is not successful, and that the patient continues to present somatic symptoms. If the therapist is to avoid frustration he or she needs to realize and accept the likelihood that change will be limited and slow, and that limiting the damage to the patient from unnecessary medical investigations, and to the PCT from overuse of its facilities, may be the only realistic goals.

Psychogenic pain disorders

Mrs A, aged 52, complained of perineal pain. Nothing definite was found on examination but she underwent an anal stretch and a polyp was removed by a general surgeon. The pain remained and she subsequently had a pelvic repair by a gynaecologist, and a urethral prolapse repair by a urologist. Aged 60 she had an unhelpful consultation with a psychiatrist. Aged 62 she had a colectomy, again by a general surgeon. An orthopaedic surgeon performed a sacral block when she was aged 65; and, at the age of 70, she had a stitch removed by a general surgeon. Altogether she had at least nine cystoscopies, four barium enemas, four intravenous pyelograms, and has attended two pain clinics. None of the investigations, operations, medications, or trans-cutaneous nerve stimulations have made any difference to her pain, which has remained the same for over 24 years.

Most practices will have a few patients who come under this heading, complaining of continuing pain confined to one area. No physical cause can be found, and, apart from preoccupation with the pain, there is no overt psychological problem. Common sites for the pain are the head, the face, the abdomen, and the pelvis. These patients are extremely difficult to treat. They do not admit that the symptoms have any relation to emotional disorders or to life events, and if eventually referred to a psychiatrist, often opt out. Analgesics and minor and major tranquillizers seldom seem to help, but antidepressants in high dosage and over a prolonged period sometimes do, and may justifiably be used in this situation without a formal diagnosis of depression being made. Over-investigation and treatment should again be avoided lest iatrogenic problems ensue.

Some of these conditions are undoubtedly forms of conversion disorder as described below. In other cases some real but transient illness seems to have caused a pain which has persisted long after its original cause has gone. The anxious focusing of attention on a pain can magnify and prolong that symptom. When, in addition, some secondary gain arises from the pain as, for instance, in the increased attention and sympathy to which it gives rise, the pain may become perpetual. In such cases, the attention of a doctor is unlikely to satisfy deep-seated needs for love and affection, but it may be sufficient to encourage the patient to persist in seeking medical help. For the doctor two alternatives exist, either to tell the patient gently but firmly that no medical care is going to be of help, or to go to the other extreme and satisfy the patient's need for attention by providing continuous in-patient bed rest with constant care. This paradoxical therapy can be successful but needs to be tied in to a process of rehabilitation which gradually weans the patient off the staff. It is so expensive of staff time and so uncertain in its effects that there are few who feel it worth considering.

Hypochondriasis

Mr A was a relatively frequent attender. About once a year he would express concern about his heart, describing feeling his heart beating when he was in bed and how, as he became more aware of it, it beat more rapidly. He knew that he was probably worrying unnecessarily but his father had died of a heart attack and he couldn't get it out of his mind. Simple examination and explanation reassured him, but his anxiety recurred.

The predominant disturbance in hypochondriasis is an unrealistic interpretation of physical signs or sensations as abnormal, leading to preoccupation with the fear or belief of having a serious disease. Thorough physical evaluation does not support the diagnosis of any physical disorder that can account for the physical signs or sensations or for the individual's unrealistic interpretation of them. The unrealistic fear or belief of having a disease persists despite medical reassurance, and causes impairment of social or occupational functioning.

Some patients will stick to one symptom but others will misinterpret other physiological variants — slight changes in bowel habit, loud borborygmi, hot urine, and so on. These patients, again, do not have a demonstrable psychiatric disorder, often come from health-conscious families, and may have a legitimate reason to be anxious because of their family history.

It is important to ascertain the true nature of their fears so that appropriate reassurance can be given, and, again, over-investigation should be avoided if possible, as should medication. Acceptance by the therapist that the fears are real, reflect the personality of the patient, and are likely to persist unless reassurance is given, gives permission for the patient to consult as and when fears first arise. A relationship between therapist and patient can then develop which allows the patient to come to the therapist when he or she wishes, and allows the doctor to reassure. This satisfies the patient — until the next time

Conversion disorder (hysteria)

Mrs A, aged 35, whispered a complaint of loss of voice. There was no hoarseness and she was referred to an ENT specialist who found no organic disorder. Her elder brother had married recently and moved away. She had stayed at home to look after her mother and father. Her father abused alcohol and her mother was housebound with agoraphobia. Both attempted to involve her in their quarrels. The inability to shout excused her.

Some people find a partial solution to a psychological problem by developing a physical symptom. By losing her voice, Mrs A escaped from involvement in family quarrels. Other patients may faint, become paralysed, or develop a variety of pseudo-neurological symptoms in the face of intolerable stress.

The tendency to 'convert' emotional problems into symptoms has given rise to the term 'conversion disorder' or, as it is sometimes termed 'conversion hysteria'.

This mental process obviously requires sophisticated cerebral activity, yet it apparently takes place without volition, so, by definition, these patients are not malingering, despite the secondary gains which result from the symptoms. In order to explain the mental split which allows the process to take place outside consciousness we need to recognize the phenomenon of 'dissociation'. Dissociation is a normal function which enables us to exert a degree of control over our emotions. Faced with the need to remain apparently calm in the face of an oral examination, we dissociate ourselves from the terror which threatens to erupt and 'put on a brave face'. Similarly when receiving a blow in a public place we 'grin and bear it'. Only later do we burst into tears or give vent to our rage. 'Conversion disorder' appears to be a special case of this kind of defence which explains its third name 'dissociative syndrome'.

Any cerebral function can become dissociated. Thus, dissociation of motor function causes paralyses; of sensory function, anaesthesia, deafness, or blindness; of memory, amnesia, and fugues (i.e. states in which people are found wandering without being able to give any explanation for their whereabouts).

Occasionally, conversion disorders come on following extreme stress. In these cases the prognosis may be quite good, provided the stress has been transient and is unlikely to recur.

A young trainee policeman wandered away from the scene of a hideous traffic pile-up and was found to have lost all memory of the event. He subsequently made a good recovery once he had faced up to the fact that he did not wish to pursue a career in the force.

In other cases, conversion symptoms may occur for little or no apparent reason in people whose capacity for dissociation has been evident for a long time. Here the prognosis is less good.

A woman with a long history of ever-changing symptoms was described by her sister as 'always an actress'. As a child she had kept her family guessing by behaviour which worried her mother and gained her a lot of attention. Her sister never knew if she was 'really hurt' or 'just exaggerating'.

Criteria for diagnosis

● a loss of function for which no physical cause can be found after examination and investigation;

● a history of emotional stress apparently related to the symptom;

● some suggestion of secondary gain;

● a history of somatization disorder in the patient or family.

Conversion disorders are commoner in women, in people with disturbed sexuality, and in those with other psychopathology such as schizophrenia and depression.

'*La belle indifference*' is an unreliable sign. Follow-up of patients diagnosed as having a conversion disorder, usually of a neurological kind, show that between 13 and 30 per cent develop a probably relevant organic illness over the subsequent two years.[2] A salutary statistic!

Management

After the exclusion of physical illness, reassurance as to its absence is seldom helpful and confrontation can alienate the patient. The consultation should be focused on the stresses and strains of the patient's life, while acknowledging the reality of the symptom. A family approach is often helpful.

Patients who have learned to use dissociation as a frequent defence can seldom tolerate the strains of psychotherapy. Faced with problems in their lives they 'switch off' emotionally and the therapist soon gets an uncomfortable feeling that they are acting a part. As R. D. Laing put it, 'The hysteric is acting a part but the part she is acting is true.' Unfortunately, therapy without emotional involvement is seldom successful.

References

1. Kleinman, A. and Kleinman, J. (In press). Somatisation. The interconnections among culture, depressive experiences and the meaning of pain. In *Culture and depression* (ed. A. Kleinman and B. Good).
2. Slater, E. T. O. and Clitheroe, E. (1965). A follow up of patients diagnosed as suffering from "Hysteria". *J. Psychosom. Res.* **9**, 9–13.

Further reading

Eijk, J. van *et al.* (1983). The family doctor and the prevention of somatic fixation. *Fam. Systems Med.* **1**, (2), 5–15.
Lynch, J. (1977). *The broken heart — the medical consequences of loneliness.* Basic Books, New York.
Rosen, G., Kleinman, A. and Katon, W. (1982). Somatisation in family practice — a biopsychosocial approach. *J. Fam. Pract.* **14**, (3), 493–502.
Smith, R. C. (1985). A clinical approach to the somatising patient. *J. Fam. Pract.* **21** (4), 294–301.

6.4   MALINGERING AND FACTITIOUS DISORDERS

Malingerers pretend to have physical symptoms, the goal usually being obvious, given a knowledge of the environmental circumstances. It is important to recognize these patients because failure to do so wastes medical time. Management must be by confrontation, though occasionally this will arouse anger or threats. Prison is the commonest setting for flagrant malingering, although lesser degrees may be presented by the work-shy, or during strikes where obtaining sick-pay may be the objective.

In factitious illnesses, such as dermatitis artifacta, self-induced pyrexia, and varieties of Munchausen's syndrome (after Baron Munchausen, a fictitious character renowned for his tall stories) the goal is less obvious and the management more difficult. Such patients often have disturbed and lonely personalities. The principles of management outlined above and in Section 5.3 again apply.

6.5 PSYCHOLOGICAL REACTIONS TO PHYSICAL ILLNESS

The term 'somatopsychic' (by analogy with 'psychosomatic') disorders has been used to delineate a group of psychological problems which can result from physical illness or accidents affecting the body. These can be broadly divided into threats, losses, and handicaps.

Threats

Threats occur whenever our bodily integrity or survival is at risk. Both specific fears and general anxiety are to be expected along with their physiological accompaniments. These may give rise to secondary fears which can sometimes escalate into panic.

Patients who panic or suffer high levels of anxiety find their judgement impaired and will sometimes run away or act against their own best interests in an attempt to reduce their fear. Thus they may refuse surgery, discharge themselves from hospital, or mislead their doctor about important issues. Most GPs will have come across patients who present with generalized symptoms of anxiety, but fail to mention that they have noticed a breast lump.

Members of the primary care team (PCT) who are aware of what is happening may find it necessary to attempt to reduce the level of anxiety before they confront patients with the need to change. By acting in a reassuring way, boosting self-esteem, drawing in the family, giving people time to talk through their fears, and possibly prescribing a dose or two of a minor tranquillizer, they will usually come to a point where reason will prevail.

Situations of threat or danger seldom last indefinitely, and the time will come when either the danger is past (when somatopsychic symptoms soon disappear) or it becomes clear that some permanent loss must be faced. The commonest opportunity to help a person under threat arises in general practice when a patient comes to the surgery to learn the results of an investigation. High levels of anxiety are found among those awaiting the result of, for example, amniocentesis, cervical smears, and HIV antigen tests. The implications of the results of such tests need to be carefully explained before as well as after the test is carried out, and the patient invited to ask further questions. Even negative results can create further anxiety if they leave the patient with unexplained symptoms.

Losses

The losses caused by accident and illness are many and varied. They range from disablement (e.g. after amputation of a limb) to mutilation (e.g. after loss of a breast). Secondary losses include loss of jobs, roles, and relationships (e.g. with workmates), loss of self-esteem, places, hopes, and expectations. Sometimes the physical environment must change (as when a person has to move into a special home or hospital), sources of income and security may disappear, and people may find themselves pitied or stigmatized. Each of these losses must be recognized and faced if people are to make a satisfactory adjustment to the life that is now open to them. Sometimes the loss extends to include other family members, whose lives must change as a result of the patient's illness.

Difficulties can emerge in accepting the facts of the situation. This is most likely if the progress of the illness is itself ambiguous. Any uncertainty in the doctor's mind, or conflict between doctors about the diagnosis or probable course of the illness, can cause problems for patients and their families. For this reason it is advisable for one person to act as the channel of communication on all important issues and to see those involved sufficiently frequently to monitor their progress towards understanding. Uncertainties need not be concealed but should be explained clearly and supportively. The GP is often the ideal person for this role, since he or she can provide more continuity of support than can hospital doctors, and is often better-acquainted with the family. People can thus be prepared for losses that are to come as well as supported after the event.

Because patients or family members commonly deny the serious implications of an illness, it may be necessary to set up a series of meetings in order to help them, at their own pace, to take in what the doctor has said and to make the implications real. Not one, but a series of griefs may need to be expressed as realization dawns. Some will be overwhelmed with grief, and we may need calmly to 'hold the line' until their distress or rage subsides. (The handling of severe depressive reactions is discussed in Sections 4.7 and 8.4). Others may 'forget' what they have been told, or may need our permission to grieve. We almost feel compelled to do their grieving for them and to share our feelings of sadness as an inducement to them to do the same. 'It must be hard to give up a job that has meant so much to you. I feel so sorry.' This kind of remark may trigger off feelings of sadness that had been avoided.

Having made the expression of grief easier, we can move on to point people towards the process of rehabilitation by which they can now be inducted into a new life. If we do this too soon we may be rejected: 'You'll never get me into a wheelchair.' There are some patients who, having taken a stand on some such issue, will stubbornly refuse to back down. But, in most cases, rehabilitation, despite all the difficulties it entails, is the main hope of a better life, and we can offer real expectations of worthwhile achievement. 'Well I know you don't feel ready for that yet, but let's just suppose, for five minutes, that you did decide to try out a wheelchair, what do you think it would be like?'

To some who cannot see how they could possibly surmount the obstacles along the way, a 'veteran' patient who has come through can provide understanding and example. 'I felt just like you, but now I think I've cracked it.' This may be particularly helpful where patients face mutilating operations, such as laryngectomy or colostomy. Many GPs keep a list of patients who have adapted successfully and are willing to help those facing such problems. There follow some examples from particular types of loss which will clarify these principles.

Reactions to surgery and mutilation

These range from anxiety and depression to frank post-operative psychoses. Minor affective reactions are usually easy to understand, given the circumstances, but post-operative psychoses have been the focus of controversy. Such reactions commonly take the form of acute confusional states. The patient may become deluded, misinterpreting medical interventions as attacks by enemies, removing drips and tubes, and attempting to leave the ward. The organic features of these symptoms (see Section 7.2), and the fact that they are most likely to occur following deep anaesthesia and major physical assault has led many to assume that psychological factors play no part in their causation.

Yet there is evidence that they are more common among people with high levels of pre-operative anxiety, and that the incidence can be reduced by pre-operative guidance and support (see Sections 3.3 and 4.6). The best conclusion would seem to be that both physical and psychological factors interact in such cases, and that anticipatory guidance is needed to reduce the risk of all kinds of post-operative reactions.

Anticipatory guidance

Members of the PCT are often in a position to help people to prepare themselves for major surgery. Three things are needed:

(1)   accurate *information* about the purpose and nature of the operation and about the subsequent course of events that can be expected to follow;

(2)   opportunity for the patient and those family members whose lives are

likely to be affected to *express their fears* and other feelings about th
situation;

(3)   opportunity for them to *ask questions* and to find out what they ca
do to cope with emergent events.

George Smith suffered the loss of his right leg as a result of arterial disease. Whe
he returned home after the operation, a doctor visited and, in the course o
conversation, asked him if he had suffered any pain in his phantom limb. 'Oh yes
I was so pleased.' The doctor expressed surprise, 'Well,' said George, 'I had bee
told before the operation that I would continue to feel as if my leg was present an
that it would hurt for a while, so I knew, when that happened, that it was all goin,
according to plan!' His reaction contrasted with that of other amputees who, havin,
had no such warning, were exceedingly alarmed to find that, having had a leg remove
to relieve pain, the leg was gone, but not the pain.

It does not follow from the above that we should undermine or challeng
those patients who cope with the major stress of surgery by minimizing th
seriousness of their situation and avoiding discussion of the subject
Avoidance can be an effective method of coping in the short term.

Post-operative reaction

Anticipatory guidance not only reduces the risk of post-operative psychose
but also reduces the length of time the patient needs to stay in hospital an
the amount of analgesic drugs required (see Section 4.6).

These findings are less surprising when we examine the common emotiona
reactions to disabling surgery; take, for instance, amputation of a limb
Following this event most patients pass through a period of numbness when
on recovering from the anaesthetic, they feel very little physical or menta
pain; but within a few hours the reality of their loss begins to dawn and the
start to pine — not for the limb itself, but for all the physical functions an
activities which they expect to lose. 'I felt I was done for, on the scrap heap'
said one amputee. Feelings of bitterness and resentment are common ('Why
should this happen to me?') and the patient is upset by any reminder of the
things he has lost.

Clearly, this reaction is a form of grieving which has many parallels ir
the reaction to the loss of a person (see Section 5.10). Even the phanton
limb, that strong sense of the presence of the lost limb which is experience
by most amputees, resembles the sense of presence of the lost person which
is reported by many bereaved people. And just as bereaved people feel bette
when they have the opportunity to cry and rage over what has happened,
so amputees will benefit from expressing their grief.

Unfortunately, a busy surgical ward is not the best place to 'break down
and surgical patients are under considerable pressure to keep a stiff uppe
lip. Consequently, they may wait until they return home before beginning
to share their feelings. 'In hospital we were all heroes. My family visited me

and I was waited on hand and foot. It was only when I got home that it hit me. My wife goes to work and I just sit here with nothing to do.'

Constant anxiety and depression may become severe. Some patients give up, become immobile and sink into a depressive reaction. Others choose the opposite path. They go straight back to work, fill their lives with activities, and refuse to accept that anything must change. This latter response, though it may meet with applause, is likely to fail. Sooner or later the denial of disability breaks down, the patient is forced to accept that they have limitations, and delayed grief emerges in full and disorganizing force.

Counselling after disabling surgery

As in the case of bereavement by death, the post-surgical patient needs permission, opportunity and time to grieve. Because there are no rituals of mourning for a lost part of the body, the first visit to the GP's surgery may take on some of the characteristics of a requiem. Key family members may accompany the patient and all will benefit if they can recount the story of what happened, express their sorrow, and make real the important event that has occurred. Reminiscence should be encouraged and sympathy expressed.

A period of rest and withdrawal will allow the work of grieving to take place, but should not be continued for too long. The struggle to rebuild a life with different assumptions, to discover what it means to be a cripple, to get on and off buses or moving staircases, to deal with children who mimic your disability, these are activities that take courage as much as skill.

The members of the PCT can build up that courage by providing emotional support ('encouragement') to the family as well as the patient. Over-protective wives or husbands can do great harm by worrying excessively about possible falls—having a helpless partner to look after fulfils a need in some spouses. They need to be enrolled as members of the rehabilitation team and rewarded for their own courage in letting go of the patient.

As in the case of bereavement by death, dependence may lead to unnecessary crippledom and chronic grief. Again, a programme of progressive retraining, with continued support being offered on condition that the patient makes the necessary effort, offers the best chance of success.

Mutilation

Similar principles apply in rehabilitation after less disabling types of surgery. Mutilation or removal of sexual organs, be they breasts, ovaries, wombs, or testes, sometimes lead to severe loss of self-esteem. This is aggravated by the difficulties in communication which arise. The fact that a woman may never have intended to use her womb again does not prevent her from feeling that her femininity has been destroyed by hysterectomy. Her surgeon, who is probably male, may not understand how she feels and may try to help her by making light of the whole operation. The patient naturally resents his apparent lack of concern and the situation will be made worse if her own husband shows a similar lack of understanding. The patient may end up feeling both guilty and angry about the situation.

Mastectomy can have a similar effect; women may feel that they have lost their sexual attractiveness along with the breast, and become very sensitive to any uncertainty on the part of their spouse. Some are so embarrassed that they will refuse to look at the scar and will go to great lengths to hide it from their partner. Doctors and nurses who have an excuse to examine the site of the operation can help by making positive comments and inviting the woman to look at and touch the damaged area. Women to whom the breast is particularly important may benefit greatly from restorative surgery.

Burns and other mutilating conditions may have such an inhibiting effect on communication that nobody dares to mention the obvious impact which physical appearance can have. It can be a great step forward when a patient who feels mutilated can be helped to look at him or herself in a mirror for the first time. Caregivers are another kind of mirror, and give much encouragement if we reflect the person rather than the mutilation.

Ileostomies and colostomies are a form of mutilation which constitute a severe blow to self-esteem. Most patients are disgusted by the very thought of an operation which will leave them with an uncontrollable stream of foul-smelling faeces issuing from a hole in their abdomen. They can hardly bear to think of their disability, let alone take an interest in it and learn to control it. A specialist ileostomy nurse or a veteran ileostomy patient can show them how to approach and think about their bodies and to accept the reality of an anus in a different place from normal.

The Dresden China syndrome

It is not only mutilation which is traumatic. Many people who undergo major surgery feel severely damaged and lose the sense of invulnerability which enables most of us to cope with the ordinary run of threats and dangers that beset us. Cardiac surgery, because of the vital function of the heart, commonly arouses excessive fear in patients, family members, and caregivers so that a person may remain psychologically crippled despite normal cardiac function. Rehabilitation must aim to restore *patients'* confidence in their bodies. This will not take place if everyone around continues to treat them as if they are made of Dresden China. In such cases, it is often more important to treat the family than the patient.

Reactions to heart conditions

Myocardial infarction can be one of the most painful and frightening episodes in life. With little or no warning a person is pitched into a state of agony and shock over which they have no control at all. The condition itself is frightening enough, but the fear is made worse by the alarm on the faces of others and often by the nightmarish ride in a clanging ambulance at break-neck speed. Older physicians referred to the '*angor animi*' commonly experienced by the patient, who has every reason to fear the imminence of death.

Although modern emergency medicine has done much to improve the chance of recovery of someone who arrives alive at a hospital, this benefit is largely offset by the dangers of the journey, and some studies,[1] have shown that the overall mortality is no greater if coronary infarction is treated at home.

As in the treatment of the cancer patient, morphine is used for its psychological as well as its physical effects. Given promptly by a doctor who remains calm and attentive to the family as well as the patient, it can help to break the vicious circle of pain and fear, whose escalating effect may well do further damage to the heart.

Support to the family is important whether or not the patient remains at home. The occurrence of an unexpected and untimely event may put relatives at special risk, and excessive optimism about the prognosis is uncalled for. Although the majority of patients will survive their first myocardial infarction, many will have a second, and the prognosis for each succeeding attack becomes worse. A relationship of trust in the GP is an important factor in any such situation. Honesty is fundamental if this is to be established.

The above picture is typical of families who are young or middle-aged. Elderly patients are often less disturbed than younger ones by coronary infarction, and may suffer little or no pain. Their families, too, are less likely to be so severely affected by an unexpected event or bereavement.

Once the acute attack is over, it is important for the patient to co-operate with a programme of rehabilitation. Random allocation studies have shown that appropriate counselling can significantly reduce morbidity.[2] Much research has confirmed the fact that people who plan their lives in such a way that they are always on the go and under pressure (the so-called 'type A' personalities) have higher rates of coronary infarction that others.[3] Stress management programmes which also provide advice about diet, smoking, sex, and exercise are effective in such patients in helping them to reorganize their lives in order to reduce emotional pressure. Regular meetings with a GP or counsellor, and possibly with other post-coronary patients, can do much to reduce anxiety and to foster a more relaxed attitude to life.

Patients and family members may need to change their roles. Thus, retirement of the husband on medical grounds while his wife is still working may lead to inversion of roles between men and women. The man may then feel emasculated and the woman ousted from her proper domains. Frank discussion of these issues may help both parties to revise their assumptions about what is 'proper'.

Reactions to disorders of communication

Because it takes two to communicate, blindness, deafness, and other disorders of communication always affect more than one person. The person who tries to communicate with a deaf person finds out what it is like to be dumb. The dumb render us all deaf. Our reaction to the patient becomes a part of the situation in which the patient lives. Deaf people become aware that people are irritated by them and treat them as stupid. We, too, are disabled by their disability, and experience, in a small way, the frustration that is a part of their daily life.

Disorders of communication (even those due to disparity of language) seldom stop people from communicating altogether, they just slow down the process and complicate the means. Both parties need to change their expectations of the use of time, and to learn new ways of communicating. Such changes are a test of patience and equanimity. The patient, the patient's family, and the PCT all need to set up new and different expectations from those which normally obtain.

The greatest changes of all are faced by the patients, who must accept the reality of loss if they are to learn new ways of communicating. This is less easy than it sounds. Blindness, for instance, is often insidiously progressive and most patients refuse to believe that they are effectively blind as long as they have some glimmer of sight.[4] They commonly refuse to learn the skills that will be needed if they are to cope with their increasing disability. Likewise, the deaf will resist using a hearing-aid, as if to do so would increase the risk of them becoming totally deaf.

Those who deny their disabilities are in need of counselling. This should aim to provide them with the support which they need if they are to feel secure enough to face the losses in their lives. Because counselling in these situations requires even more verbal and non-verbal communication than usual, it will be even more time consuming.

Anger, guilt, and sadness are as much a part of the griefs of the blind and deaf as they are of any other loss; and, just as the bereaved often feel as if the dead person is present, and the amputee feels the lost limb, so those with sensory defects may perceive things that are not truly there. The blind think that they can see and will sometimes describe sights and happenings that they cannot possibly have witnessed, and the deaf will think that they have heard people talking. Such illusions are likely to be coloured by the fear and hopes of the moment. A deaf person who feels frustrated and whose world has become strange and menacing may misinterpret muttered sounds as the voices of people criticizing or plotting behind his back. Blind persons who are desperately seeking for evidence that they can see may incorrectly describe the colour of a dress or continue to 'watch' sport on TV, despite the fact that there is better auditory coverage of the same event on radio.

In the normal course of events it is possible for people to check-out the truth of their misperceptions, but those with perceptual defects find this more difficult and their illusions may become part of mistaken beliefs that may be hard to correct.

Once more, the use of veterans or blind people who can lead the blind through the labyrinth of rehabilitation to a new kind of 'sight' is a useful adjunct to the services of professional workers. 'I know, I've had that kind of feeling myself' is more convincing and more reassuring that doctors' attempts to explain the nature of hypnagoguic hallucinations.

Illusory misperceptions often include strange sensations in the damaged organ. Pain in the eyes in the blind, and tinnitus in the deaf, often have no demonstrable cause and seem to reflect fear and preoccupation with the source of the trouble. Peculiar postures and grimaces may have a personal meaning to the patient, as when blind people screw up their eyes in an attempt to force themselves to see, or deaf persons cock their ear towards a hoped-for sound.

Family and friends easily get caught up and begin to believe the patient's misperceptions ('Whatever you say I *won't* believe that my husband is blind') and it is important for us to support them and, where possible, include them in the rehabilitation team. Just as we must attempt to correct their misperception, so we must guard against our own. It is easy for us to be swayed by patients to carry out needless investigations when none are indicated, and by doing so, to keep alive the unrealistic hope that is obstructing rehabilitation.

Sexual problems and disablement

Fear, shame, and physical incapacity can play havoc with sexual performance. These are discussed in more detail in Section 5.6, but it is worth noting here that impotence and frigidity are common consequences of both mutilating and life-threatening conditions, and of operations. In the former case, patients often believe that they have become unattractive to their partner, and it may be the partner who must come to terms with the situation and convince them that this is not the case.

Genital surgery often leaves both patient and partner fearful of causing damage to a vulnerable area, and reassurance needs to be quite specific. We should ask for details of any problems that have arisen and carry out a physical examination if there are complaints of pain or other local difficulties. The statement 'If I can get two fingers into your vagina without doing you any harm, I'm quite sure that you can have sexual intercourse perfectly safely', may be all the reassurance that is needed.

Heart conditions commonly leave people with the fear that they will drop dead if they have sexual intercourse. This is just as much of a problem to the partner as it is to the patient and leads to much sexual frustration and guilt.

A wife may delay sexual activity so as not to over-exert her husband, and thereby may increase anxiety and enhance the likelihood of impotence.

If sexual intercourse can be included as part of a graded exercise programme which has the function of restoring and exercising the heart along with the rest of the body, then it will come to be viewed in a positive rather than a negative way. Once a patient can climb a flight of stairs without anginal pain or undue breathlessness, sexual intercourse can be regarded as a potentially beneficial form of exercise.

The handicapped child

Handicap may be present at birth or arise in childhood as a lasting result of a physical loss. The effects on the parents of the birth of a handicapped child are described in Section 5.3, and the main types of mental handicap are described in Section 7.1. Children born with a physical handicap seldom suffer from psychological problems until they go to school. At this point they may be teased or made to feel inferior to 'normal' children. This is less likely to constitute a problem at special schools where disablement is 'normal'. On the other hand, special schools do not prepare children fully for exposure to the 'normal world'. Parents are often over-protective of such children and sometimes have unrealistic expectations. Thus, they may insist on their child going to an ordinary school, despite clear evidence that the child is unable to cope. In such cases it is important to help the parents to express their own feelings of disappointment.

Transitions may occur when a handicapped child reaches adolescence. Rejection by members of the opposite sex can bring home the sexual significance of deformity in a painful way, and sometimes leads to depression and withdrawal. Cruel though it may seem, it is probably better to encourage adolescents and their parents to engage in social activities rather than to collude with their wish to withdraw.

Goffman has described the various ways in which people cope with stigma.[5] One is to associate with others who suffer the same or similar stigma. People who are in the same boat can be expected to understand and support each other. Unfortunately, their experience of rejection may cause them to collude with each other in adopting negative attitudes to the rest of the world. Equally, the non-stigmatized remain suspicious and potentially hostile to any minority groups who isolate themselves. Anything which fosters contact and breaks down the barriers between people who are 'different' reduces prejudice and helps to overcome these difficulties.

Handicapped people expect members of the PCT to understand their difficulties. We may be the only unstigmatized people whom they trust, and are in a good position to help them and their families to come to terms with the facts of the situation and to encourage them to take the steps which will enable them to become part of society rather than living a life apart. This is not always easy, and, like other transitions, will take time. We may also have the opportunity, through schools and other educational means, to speak up for those who are disadvantaged and to encourage others to reach out to them and accept them as fellow human beings rather than 'freaks'.

References

1. Mather, H. G., Pearson, N. G. and Read, K. L. Q. (1971). Acute myocardial infarction: home and hospital treatment. *Br. Med. J.* **3**, 334–8
2. Rahe, R. H., Ward, H. W. and Hayes, V. (1979). Brief group therapy in myocardial infarction rehabilitation: 3/4 year follow-up of a controlled trial. *Psychosom. Med.* **413**, (3), 229–42.
3. Rosenman, R. H., Brand, R. J., Jenkins, C. P., Friedman, M. Straus, R., and Wurm, M. (1975). Coronary heart disease in the Western Collaborative Group Study: final follow-up experience of 8½ years. *JAMA* **233**, 872–7.
4. Fitzgerald, R. G. (1970). Reactions to blindness: an exploratory study of adults with recent loss of sight. *Archs. Gen. Psychiat.* **22**, 370.
5. Goffman, E. (1968). *Stigma: notes on the management of spoiled identity.* Penguin Books, Harmondsworth.

Further reading

Egbert, L. D. Battit, G. E. Welsh, C. E., and Bartlett, M. K. (1964). Reduction of postoperative pain by encouragement and instruction of patients: a study of doctor-patient rapport. *New Engl. J. Med.* **270**, 825.
Goffman, E. (1968). *Stigma: notes on the management of spoiled identity.* Penguin Books, Harmondsworth.
Johnston, M. and Wallace, L. M. (1989). *Stress and medical procedures.* Oxford University Press.
Morse, R. M. (1976). Psychiatry and surgical delirium. In *Modern perspectives in the psychiatric aspects of surgery,* (ed. J. G. Howells), Chapter 30. Brunner/Mazel, New York.
Parkes, C. M. (1975). Psycho-social transition: comparison between reactions to loss of a limb and loss of a spouse. *Br. J. Psychiat.* **127**, 204–10.

7 Organic disorders

7.1 DEFECTS IN THE DEVELOPMENT OF THE CNS

Mental handicap

Mental handicap is characterized by limitation in the development of intellectual, social, and adaptive abilities. Precise definitions based on IQ tests are unacceptable because of the imperfections of these tests, and also because poor performance on them is not necessarily accompanied by equivalent lack of social skills. However, IQ scores give a rough approximation which is useful in identifying levels of retardation.

Three per cent of all children have IQs two standard deviations below the average of 100, i.e. less than 70. Mild mental handicap includes those with IQs between 55 and 70, and constitutes 75 per cent of those with a handicap. They develop social and communication skills and their deficits are often unnoticed until early schooling. Normally they go on to be self-supporting and to function adequately in jobs requiring minimal skills, although they are likely to suffer at times of high unemployment. Moderate mental handicap refers to those with IQs in the range of 40–54, and make up 20 per cent of the mentally handicapped population. This group will be able to learn to talk, but will show difficulty in learning normal social conventions and will make little progress in school subjects. Unlike the mildly handicapped, they are likely to continue to need support as adults and to work only in sheltered environments. The remaining 5 per cent, with IQs less than 40, are the severely and profoundly handicapped. At a very early stage they show evidence of poor motor development, are unlikely to learn to talk, and will continue to need supervision as adults. They may have accompanying physical impairments and susceptibility to disease.

Organic causes are thought to account for most cases of severe mental handicap. The causes may be genetic (of which the most common is Down's syndrome), infection *in utero* (such as rubella), metabolic (such as malnutrition), or toxic (e.g. alcohol or drugs). Infections or trauma during or following birth may also result in mental handicap.

Much mental retardation, especially in the mild range, is thought to arise from family, cultural, and environmental factors in general. Most of those affected will have parents or siblings who exhibit some evidence of backwardness, with no sign of brain pathology or physical disorder. This group is concentrated in the lower socio-economic strata, unlike those with organic causes who are distributed fairly evenly.

Presentation and management

Problems associated with mental handicap and with associated physical handicap, can be presented to the general practitioner in many forms. They can arise as questions from a couple contemplating marriage who are concerned about their genetic risk of producing a mentally handicapped child, or from an anxious pregnant woman who is requesting prenatal diagnostic tests. For the pregnant woman complete reassurance is impossible to give, but it may be useful to indicate that the fears are normal. Certainly it is advisable to arrange some follow-up as these fears can persist, and anxiety in pregnancy is sometimes associated with difficult births and/or with postnatal depression. For those who are known to be at special risk of giving birth to an impaired baby, further genetic counselling, including consideration of termination of pregnancy, may be appropriate.

Early detection of mental handicap depends on the recognition of failure to reach milestones at the expected times (see normal milestones listed in Table 5.1). There may be delays in motor development, such as head control, sitting unaided, and learning to walk; in language development, if the child fails to make babbling sounds, to learn words, and to develop grammar; or in social developments, as when the child does not develop eye-contact, play normal peek-a-boo games, or learn social skills and conventions. It may be difficult to reach firm decisions in some cases because of the wide variation in the times at which normal children reach milestones, and also because children may show delays in one area while developing normally in others. Very occasionally a specific developmental disorder may be present.

Parents of mentally handicapped children frequently complain of the manner in which they were given information about their child's condition, even with diagnoses which are clear at birth such as Down's syndrome. This may be an expression of their guilt or anger at having a damaged child, but may also reflect the difficulties of this particular doctor–patient communication. The primary care team (PCT), especially the general practitioner and health visitor, will have to supplement the work done by the paediatrician in giving information, in dealing with emotional responses, and in planning for the future. Initially, it may not be possible to give a clear prognosis for the individual child, only to give sufficient forewarning as one would give for any threatening condition. On the other hand, it should be possible to indicate what resources are available and what the parents themselves can do in the interests of their child. In some areas there are specialist facilities, such as early playgroups, peripatetic instructors, or charities offering baby-sitting or so-called toy libraries (in addition to providing directly for the child, toy libraries offer social support for the parents). Families with a mentally handicapped child often suffer considerable financial and emotional hardship and there is likely to be evidence of emotional and behavioural problems in the siblings of the affected child, and higher rates of marital discord and divorce in the parents. At some stage it may be valuable to see all of the family together to assess how they are coping. Practical forms of help may minimize extra expenses, allow normal wage-earning, and provide more time for ordinary family activities.

The recognition that a child is mentally handicapped faces the parents with a major psychosocial transition. Some attempt to deal with this by refusing to accept the diagnosis. The doctors are wrong, their child is not really slow. They will seize on some long word which the child has repeated as evidence of incipient genius. Others may turn against the child and demand immediate institutional care. It may be necessary to help them to grieve for the perfect child which they have lost before they can accept the imperfect child which exists.

Sooner or later most mothers of handicapped children accept them and they may then develop very close and over-protective attachments. If, subsequently, the child dies, as some will from additional physical impairments, the mother's reaction is likely to be particularly intense.

Unfortunately, these problems in the making and maintaining of attachment to the child often create problems in other attachments. The father and siblings may feel excluded from the 'special' relationship which has developed between the mother and the handicapped child, and angry feelings, though an understandable part of grieving, may spoil relationships and create marital problems.

Additional physical handicaps which may be associated with mental handicap of any degree include; epilepsy, cerebral palsy, hemi- or mono-plegia, congenital heart disease, deafness, visual defects, and dental problems. Any of these may come the way of the GP and the time and skill which he or she is willing to spend in caring for handicapped people may well be a factor in deciding whether or not they can survive in the community.

Secondary handicaps often result from the psychological and social stresses caused by handicap. Thus, many mentally handicapped people experience rejection by the world at large, if not by their own families. In consequence they may feel devalued and feel that they are a disappointment to their parents. This may lead to a state of chronic depressive withdrawal and/or behavioural disturbances.

Like other people, those who are mentally handicapped have sexual feelings, but they are sometimes less tactful and competent at expressing them. This can lead to alarm and to strict curtailment of freedom, which is often quite unjustified. The reader is referred to the books by Ann Craft for a full and balanced discussion of these issues.

It is current policy to close down large institutions for the mentally handicapped and to provide care for them in the community. It is hoped that the provision of special schools and day-centres will enable most to live at home, and those who cannot be cared for at home will be located in small 'core and cluster' dwellings in the community. Although decisions regarding these alternatives are the responsibility of the specialist in mental handicap, it is likely that the PCT will, in future, play a larger part in the care of handicapped individiuals than they have done in the past.

Not only do some children have multiple defects which give rise to health problems, but their resistance to common illnesses is low and many handicapped children die in childhood. Their parents are likely to be aware of this danger and to be correspondingly anxious. It follows that the members of the PCT are very important persons to these children and parents, and need to give special attention to them. Any suggestions that these families are second-class citizens who do not deserve our best efforts will rightly be resented.

Specific developmental difficulties

The child who is mentally handicapped must be differentiated from the child with a specific developmental difficulty. These are rare, and the most clearly identified are autism and specific reading disorder (dyslexia).

Autism

This is characterized by a failure of the young child to develop normal attachments, avoiding cuddles and physical contact, rejecting eye-contact, and generally remaining alone and aloof. Language development may be poor and peculiarities in language use, such as the confusion of 'I' and 'you', can occur. The autistic child reacts particularly badly to changes, even small ones such as rearranging furniture, and may have particular attachments to objects such as toys or pieces of clothing.

The aetiology is unknown. Both psychodynamic and biological theories are current. Psychogenic factors are thought to concern failures of early infant–parent interaction, and biological factors may include disorders of neurotransmission. Evidence for psychogenesis comes from observation of interactions in families with an affected child, where cause and effect are difficult to separate. In favour of the biological theories is evidence of abnormal electroencephalograms in autistic children, and some weak evidence of genetic transmission. The prognosis for the autistic child is poor, especially for those who fail to develop language skills before the age of five. As adults, most are mentally handicapped and less than half of them are likely to lead independent lives. Treatment approaches are limited, but the best results are achieved in structured educational programmes which aim to overcome the child's specific difficulties in a controlled, non-distracting environment. The general practitioner's role is mainly to support the parents in finding the most appropriate educational setting for their child, to enable them to contribute as much as possible to the child's education, and to absolve them from any feelings of guilt.

Specific reading disorder (dyslexia)

Children with dyslexia lag significantly behind the expected level of reading skills for their age and IQ. The presenting problem may be identified as educational or as a behavioural problem in school or at home. These children are likely to have shown earlier problems in language acquisition and are more often boys than girls. Because of the importance of these skills, the children experience difficulties in school, in leisure pursuits, and, later, in finding employment compatible with their intellect. Their problems are probably best dealt with in the educational rather than the health sphere, especially if stigmatizing diagnostic labels are to be avoided. Thus, the general practitioner may recommend that the parents deal with such problems through the child's school, or in consultation with educational psychologists.

Parents who are disappointed with their child's intellectual and scholastic performance may seek the diagnostic label 'dyslexia' in preference to a label implying more global deficits. Enquiries about the child's assets and problems should clarify whether the cognitive deficits are exclusively linguistic, and this may open the way to a more positive evaluation of the child, with a less prominent focus on intellectual achievement.

Further reading

Craft, A. and Craft M. (1985). *Mental handicap*. Baillière Tindall, London.
Davison, G. C. and Neale, J. M. (1982). *Abnormal psychology* (3rd edn). Wiley, New York.
Rimm, D. C. and Somervill, J. W. (1977). *Abnormal psychology*. Academic Press, London.
Rosenham, D. L. and Seligman, M. E. (1984). *Abnormal psychology*. W. W. Norton, New York.
Yule, W. and Carr, J. (ed.) (1980). *Behaviour modification for the mentally handicapped*. Croom Helm, London.

7.2   ORGANIC ILLNESS AND INJURIES TO THE BRAIN

The organic conditions which affect the brain are of two kinds, acute and chronic; the former being rapid in onset, dramatic in effect, and usually transient and recoverable, the latter insidious, undramatic, and usually irreversible.

Acute organic brain syndrome (delirium, confusional states)

Causes

A wide variety of toxic and metabolic substances and conditions which affect the parenchyma of the brain can cause acute brain syndromes. These include

Table 7.1. *Drugs which can cause confusional states*

Alcohol
Sedatives (including sedative antidepressants)
Amphetamines
Digoxin
Diuretics (by reducing serum potassium)
Steroids
L-dopa
Anticholinergics
Benzhexol (Artane)
Hypotensive drugs
Insulin

Table 7.2. *Other causes of confusional states*

Infections (especially pneumonia, cellulitis, or urinary infections)
Cerebral hypoxia (due to atheroma, auricular fibrillation, heart failure, temporal arteritis, etc.)
Malnutrition (especially deficiency of B-group vitamins—often associated with alcoholism)
Dehydration and electrolyte imbalance (especially in the elderly)
Metabolic disorders (especially uraemia and liver failure)
Endocrine disorders (especially diabetic ketosis, hypo- or hyperthyroidism and parathyroid disorders)
Trauma (including all surgical operations, head injuries, subdural haematoma, etc.)
Intracranial lesions (e.g. epilepsy, cerebral tumour, and abcesses)
Hypothermia
Pain in elderly or brain-damaged people (e.g. due to faecal impaction, glaucoma, shingles, toothache)
Other severe psychological stress occurring in elderly or brain-impaired people

drugs, of which the commonest is alcohol (see Table 7.1), infections, acute anoxia, and other disorders affecting the metabolism of the brain (see Table 7.2).

The very old and the very young are more vulnerable than the intermediate age-groups, as are all those whose cerebral function is already impaired from some other cause.

Symptoms

Acute brain syndromes are characterized by confusion and disorientation. Patients lose their bearings and may become alarmed; lacking the ability to know where they are, who the people around them are, and why others are behaving as they are, they often jump to the wrong conclusions.

They may be found at night wandering in the street in search of the lavatory; a nurse or doctor who tries to help them back to bed is thought to be attacking them. Although it is the middle of the night, patients may get the idea that they should be at work, and may even attempt to carry out work tasks in inappropriate places (occupational delirium).

To the confused patient the distinction between dreams and reality is unclear; on the one hand, the patient may relate a dream as if it were true and, on the other hand, events which have occurred may be attributed to dreams. Visual hallucinations and illusions are most likely to occur during darkness, and auditory hallucinations are usually misinterpretations of real sounds.

Emotional responses may be extreme, reflecting in themselves the patient's perceptions. Thus, a delirious patient who wakes in subdued light may believe that a shadow on the wall is the face of a devil, and responds accordingly. But such mistakes are soon forgotten if the light is turned on and reassurance is given. On the other hand, disorientated patients who alarm their families may respond to the family's alarm by becoming more terrified.

Episodes of confusion often fluctuate in severity. One minute a person is totally disorientated, and, a few minutes later, may be behaving quite normally and wondering what all the fuss was about.

Prompt and correct diagnosis of the cause of the delirium is vital since many conditions which cause delirium can, if untreated, progress to coma and death. Increasing drowsiness, rambling incoherence, and weakness or incoordination of motor movement are signs of incipient coma.

Management

If the cause is unknown or the condition worsening, urgent hospital admission is essential even if the patient objects (the doctor's powers under the Mental Health Act are explained in Appendix I).

The immediate treatment of delirium is to remove all ambiguous and alarming stimuli and to present a calm, friendly face to the patient. If it is night-time, lights should be turned on and people should speak clearly, distinctly, and in a matter-of-fact way.

If restraint is necessary, it should be adequate to achieve its aim but relaxed as soon as this has been done. Struggling, screaming patients will sometimes stop struggling if those who are holding them down are asked to step back (but it may be wise to make sure that they don't go too far away!).

Chemical restraint is a last, rather than a first, resort and should only be used if the diagnosis is clear and the patient's general condition good. In essence, one is administering an anaesthetic dose of medication on top of whatever drug or toxic substance may already be in the patient, and this requires one to be very careful. The dosage level should take into account the patient's age, size, and general fitness. Thus, it may take a very much larger dose of medication to 'knock out' a tough 30-year-old alcoholic labourer than a frail old lady of 83. A typical regime for the labourer would by 100 mg of chlorpromazine by deep intramuscular injection, repeated 20 minutes later if necessary, while the old lady would probably respond to 25 mg.

The longer term treatment of acute confusional states is the treatment of the underlying cause. Some of these are discussed elsewhere in this volume.

Chronic organic brain syndrome (dementia)

The poor prognosis associated with this condition arises from the fact that, once adult brain cells have been destroyed, they cannot be replaced. Lasting damage to the brain gives rise to fundamental changes in the personality of the individual and produces profound disruption of the dynamics of the family.

Causes (see Table 7.3)

Senile dementias are most commonly caused by Alzheimer's disease, a gradually progressive condition, but they may also result from multiple

Table 7.3. *Causes of dementia*
(after Copeland 1986[1] by permission of the author and publisher)

Mainly in elderly patients
Alzheimer-type or senile dementia
Multi-infarct
Creutzfeldt–Jakob (rare)

Mainly in younger patients
Alzheimer
Pick's disease
Huntington's chorea
Punch-drunk syndrome
Renal dialysis

Must consider and exclude
Neurosyphilis
Tumour
Subdural haematoma
Communicating hydrocephalus
Myxoedema
Vitamin B_{12} deficiency
Chronic alcoholism
Cranial arteritis
Disseminated lupus erythematosus
Hypocalcaemia
Chronic drug intoxication
Acquired immune deficiency syndrome (AIDS)

cerebral infarcts which tend to occur intermittently and to produce rather more rapid deterioration occurring in fits and starts. Presenile dementias are less common, but no different in symptomatology.

Other organic conditions which can cause chronic brain syndromes are much less common. They include cerebral tumours and myxoedema, whose presence is usually detectable from their effects on other parts of the body, though tumours may be difficult to diagnose if in a 'silent' part of the brain. A careful physical and neurological examination is advisable along with a full blood-count, B_{12}, thyroid-function test, alkaline phosphatase, and referral for EEG and brain scan.

Symptoms

It is surprising how often the onset of dementia is ignored by the family and missed by physicians. This arises from the fact that although the patient's memory for recent events is lost, the memory for remote events is retained until a late stage of the illness. This causes the family to disregard mistakes or to dismiss them as normal for an elderly person. It may take some dramatic error, such as a car accident, because the patient has forgotten to put the brake on when parking, or a succession of burnt-out saucepans, to bring home the fact that something is out of the ordinary.

Because the brain is so vital an organ, it might be thought that dementia would cause great distress to the patient, but, in fact, reactions are very variable. Many patients do not worry because they forget what to worry about. They fill in gaps in their memory by making up a story which satisfies them even if it fools nobody else. On the other hand, they may become extremely distressed if forced to acknowledge their inability to think or remember obvious things. This so-called 'catastrophic reaction' may give rise to impulsive or aggressive outbursts which only make a bad situation worse. Organic lesions in the midbrain can bring about emotional lability with floods of tears, or laughter, triggered by the least stimulus. Patients may be aware that their reaction is disproportionate to its cause, and may explain that they do not feel as miserable or as fractious as they look. Having got hold of an idea, some dementing patients seem unable to let go of it. This perseveration of thought and speech, together with the general slowness of all thought processes, results in impairment of the rhythms of communication. To family and friends the dementing patient speaks too slowly, to the patient everybody else speaks too fast. As with sensory defects, the result is a breakdown in communication which leaves the patient isolated from those who would normally stimulate thought and action. Like other functions, cerebral function atrophies with disuse, and a mild dementia may soon become severe if patients are not stimulated to use those grey-cells that they have. The situation may be aggravated by other defects, such as deafness or the presence of aphasia, both of which are not uncommon in brain-impaired elderly patients.

Patients with chronic brain syndromes are also vulnerable to superadded acute brain syndromes. Thus, a dementing patient may become acutely confused if sedated, or a change from a familiar to an unfamiliar environment may trigger off confusion, panic, and all the acute symptoms described above. Conversely, there are some severely demented patients who cope surprisingly well so long as they remain with familiar people in a familiar environment.

All change is difficult for the demented, even change for what may seem to be the better, and there is evidence of an increase in mortality rate among brain-impaired patients who are relocated.[2]

Depression, because of the difficulty in concentration and slowing down of thought and movement which accompany it, commonly resembles early dementia. If it arises in an elderly person who already has some loss of memory, the resemblance is all the greater and may reinforce any fears which the patient has that he is 'going ga-ga'. This further increases the depression and may cause a 'pseudo-dementia'.

Depression is a common feature of early dementia, and the differential diagnosis between this and pseudo-dementia is not always easy. The situation is further complicated by the fact that tricyclic antidepressants sometimes cause confusion in old people, whereas in others they reduce confusion by relieving depression.

Reactions of relatives

'He looks like my husband, he sounds like my husband, but he isn't the man I've been married to for 40 years'. The wife whose sensitive, intelligent, caring husband has become insensitive, stupid, and self-centred can be forgiven for feeling outraged. Some refuse to accept the evidence of their senses. They persist in believing that behind the child-like behaviour there is a normal person trying to get out, and they may agonize over how the clever husband must be suffering as a result of being imprisoned within the stupid one; others are constantly trying to bully their partner to stop him from behaving so stupidly. Attempts to persuade them that their partner is not suffering because he is no longer capable of intelligent awareness, or to convince them that his stupidity is not his fault, evoke anger and rejection. 'You don't understand, you don't live with him'.

When it is a widowed parent who is dementing, it is usually a daughter who is expected to cope. The upheaval in her own life may be enormous and it is hardly surprising that she, too, may have difficulty in taking a balanced view of the situation. Rather than accepting the necessity of changing her own life plan to enable her to look after a boring impaired parent, she may either refuse to take seriously the evidence of dementia or go to the other extreme of insisting that the patient is so sick that hospital admission is urgently necessary. It is easy to blame such daughters for their lack of care, but, in fact, the competing pressures of children, husbands, and job can make it very difficult for them to take on the added responsibility of an elderly relative.

Management

The fact that there is no curative treatment for senile and presenile dementias does not mean that there is nothing which can be done to help these patients and their families. Any activity which prevents stagnation will help to preserve whatever cerebral function is possible. Attendance at a day-centre, regular conversations, walks in the park, the performance of simple household or gardening tasks, drawing, colouring, or simply sitting at a window with a view of passers-by will all make a difference. But they place a considerable burden on the relatives who may find it much quicker to peel the potatoes themselves and who worry about possible disasters that may occur if they are not constantly watchful. 'Will he set the bed on fire if he smokes in bed?', 'Can he be trusted to boil a kettle or fry an egg?', 'Can he be left alone in the house, and if so for how long?', 'Will he get lost if he goes out alone?' These are valid questions for which there are no easy answers. Some risks can be reduced (by hiding the matches, turning off the electricity when the caregiver leaves the house, and so on), but other risks may have to be accepted if the dementing patient is to remain at home.

The caregiver may need more psychological support than the patient. She (and it is usually a woman) may need permission and time to grieve for the person she has lost before she can relate to the person she has got. Members of the primary care team (PCT) can help her to do this by encouraging the expression of sadness, anger, and/or fears, either through individual counselling, or the provision of carers' groups. Sensible discussion of the probable course of the illness, and assurance of our continued support will often enable the grief to be worked through, and relatives who, at one time, are demanding instant admission and 'treatment' for the patient may change their minds.

Anxiety and depression in the patient will often respond to tricyclic antidepressants, such as amitriptyline (10–15 mg tds) which has the advantage of a sedative effect. Side-effects are common and all drugs need to be closely supervised when they are first introduced. Patients with minimal loss of memory for names will often respond very positively to reassurance that they are not dementing.

The decision to admit a patient for institutional care is a difficult one which will be influenced by the availability of suitable care as well as the facilities available in the community. Dementing patients can, of course, be compelled to accept admission under the Mental Health Act (see Appendix I), but we need to weigh up the possible deterioration which may result from leaving a familiar environment against the benefits to the family who may be paying a high price for the patient's presence at home. Occasionally a brief period of respite (or holiday) care will relieve an intolerable burden on the family and enable them to cope better when the patient returns. Early involvement of the local psychogeriatric team and social services will help the PCT to arrange these alternatives.

Careful attention to the physical health of dementing patients and elderly caregivers is important, and the provision of spectacles, hearing-aids, or a good chiropodist can make all the difference between contentment and misery. It also helps to reassure the family that we are genuinely mindful of their needs and appreciate the burdens which they carry. Provision of meals-on-wheels, home helps, or the offer of a lunch club or a day hospital place on two days a week may relieve some of this burden.

Home care often fails because the caregiver is unable to cope at night. Some dementing patients are restless and the situation is not helped if they have a tendency to incontinence. The former problem may be solved by the prescription of a hypnotic such as dichloralphenazone or nitrazepam, but these may make a confused patient more so, and aggravate the risk of wet beds. A laundry service and the provision of incontinence pads, plus restriction of bedtime drinks, may need to be considered, as may the provision of night-sitters, paid for from an attendance allowance, which a social worker or health visitor can help the relatives to obtain.

The Alzheimer's Society and social service departments run meetings in many areas at which family caregivers can find understanding and practical advice. Similar support can also be obtained from Age Concern (see Appendix II) and other local sources.

Head injury

Both functional and organic factors may contribute to the psychological effects of head injuries. The severity of the organic damage can usually be gauged from the duration of unconsciousness. People who have been 'knocked out' for a few minutes to an hour are unlikely to have suffered lasting damage to the brain although they may suffer transient concussion, with headache and acute confusion on recovering consciousness. More severe damage, however, can give rise to lasting impairment and to a chronic brain syndrome. Patients who appear to recover well may yet have problems, perhaps on returning to work, resulting from the persisting effects of brain damage. The patient may find these problems difficult to describe, but a full cognitive assessment can reveal defecits in memory, word-finding, etc.

The psychological effects of head injury are likely to be coloured by the circumstances in which the injury takes place, and the possibility of compensation. Naturally enough, people often worry about the possibility of brain damage and they may be alarmed by the headache which commonly occurs after any head injury. This may cause the headache to persist and give rise to a post-traumatic neurosis.

Epilepsy

The psychological effects of epilepsy are many and various and it is beyond the scope of this volume to cover the numerous forms which these may take. Common problems are anxiety and depression which may result from the secondary stresses associated with the condition (unemployment, social isolation, etc.), or may be a direct effect of the organic changes which occurred in the pre-ictal period. These may be associated with deep-seated effects on the personality. Blunting of sensitivity and slowing down of thought-processes may result from frequent fits or from the medication used to control them. Peculiar sensations are experienced in certain types of temporal-lobe epilepsy and may, at times, resemble brief attacks of psychoses.

The situation is further complicated if the epilepsy is symptomatic of a brain tumour, encephalitis, or withdrawal of alcohol or other drug.

Children are more susceptible to fits, but less likely to suffer lasting damage. Thus parents may need to be assured that a single short convulsion in the course of a feverish illness is not likely to lead to epilepsy. In those children who do become epileptic, frequent fits and medication can interfere with school work. Parental anxiety and restrictions on swimming and other sports and games further affect the child.

Management

The proper investigation of epilepsy and control of fits is a matter for consultation with the neurologist, but the PCT has important roles to play in monitoring progress and providing the psychological support which is needed. Fits are frightening events for patient and family, who need a full explanation of what has happened. Family members need clear advice on how to handle an attack. Myths about epilepsy (e.g. that it causes madness or is a fatal disease) are not uncommon and epileptics often feel stigmatized. The Epilepsy Association provides a forum where mutual help can be obtained (see Appendix II).

Strokes

The PCT also plays a crucial role in the rehabilitation of the victims of cerebral vascular accidents. The sudden onset of hemiplegia, with or without aphasia, often gives rise to depression in the patient and the immediate family. A person who has previously been able to cope suddenly becomes dependent on others. Spouses and daughters give up work to nurse them, or, if they decide to continue working, may leave a crippled person alone at home all day. Depression amongst the carers needs to be watched for.

The patient, who may have been waited on 'hand and foot' in hospital, easily slips into a passive, depressed state on returning home, giving up any hope of recovery. Fearful of accidents, the relatives often take over total care, and the patient is made to feel redundant and a burden.

This sorry situation can be improved if the relatives can be enrolled as members of the rehabilitation team. They need to know what symptoms are likely to improve and what lasting disability will remain. They need to know how the patient can be helped to live with the disability and remain as independent as possible. It is often difficult for the patient and relatives to understand the complexities of cognitive dysfunction.

A woman was perplexed that after her husband had had a stroke, he could not find his way around the bungalow that they had lived in for many years, though he was fully mobile. He would get lost, urinate in the larder and if he went outside, could not find his way home. A sympathetic explanation of the visuo-spatial difficulties resulting from right hemisphere impairment was helpful in giving the wife a rational understanding of what had appeared to be wilful behaviour.

When patients have dysphasic problems, relatives consistently over-estimate the patient's ability to understand language, tending to assume that the problems are related to the motor side of speech. Even when they have grasped the nature of dysphasia, they are faced with the enormous problem of communicating and may need some guidance towards non-verbal communication and methods of relating and spending time together which do not depend on words.

One couple's favourite shared pastime had been Scrabble; after the husband's stroke this was impossible, but Dominoes, which involves visual matching rather than language, was a possible alternative.

Domiciliary physiotherapy and occupational therapists can be enrolled. Relatives will need permission to grieve for the very real losses that they are suffering as a consequence of the patient's illness, and to know that they are entitled to our time and sympathy. If they feel bitter and angry, it is better for them to take it out on us than to blame the patient. Both patient and family may need the help and support of such organizations as a Stroke Association or Age Concern (see Appendix II).

References

1. Copeland, J. (1986). The diagnosis of dementia. *Pract. Rev. Psychiat.* **6**, 7.

2. Aldritch, C. K. and Mendkoff, E. (1963). Relocation of aged and disabled: a mortality study. *J. Am. Geriatrics Soc.* **11**, 185.

Further reading

Sacks, O. (1985). *The man who mistook his wife for a hat.* Picador, London.

8 The functional disorders

8.1 INTRODUCTION

Throughout this book we have focused on the life changes and situations that impinge upon a person at different points in the life cycle and on the effects that these can produce.

This model, however, has its limitations. There are some psychiatric problems which are determined more by the personality and other predispositions of the patient than by the particular circumstances that trigger them off. For these disorders the more traditional classification used by psychiatrists provides us with a useful frame of reference. In using it, however, we need to be aware of its limitations.

The greatest danger arising from the use of these diagnostic attributions is that they imply a stability to a situation which may be unjustified. To label a grieving person as suffering from 'reactive depression' is a fundamental attributional error which may have very harmful consequences for both griever and family. Attributions based on the disposition of a person rather than the nature of a situation satisfy our own need for clarity but run the risk of ignoring the complexities of a life situation. If we see our main role as the making of a diagnosis, we may imagine that the problem has been solved once the diagnosis has been made. And since some of these labels imply that a stable attribute cannot be changed, there is a danger that we shall dismiss as 'intractable' a person who is embedded in a situation which is not entirely frozen.

Of course, the opposite may also hold true. There are some people whose lasting predispositions will dominate any life situation in which they find themselves, and for this group dispositional attributions do have some value.

Most textbooks of psychiatry begin by defining neuroses and psychoses. The term 'neurosis' is reserved for those disorders of thought, feeling, and behaviour which are comprehensible in terms of the situation in which they arise, but whose features (or 'symptoms') are excessive in *quantity* by comparison with what is regarded as 'normal'. 'Psychoses', by contrast, are not comprehensible in terms of the situation in which they arise, and their features are different in *quality* from 'normal'. Furthermore, psychotic patients are said to lack any insight, whereas neurotic patients have at least some understanding of their condition. The psychoses are further subdivided into organic and functional, according to the presence or absence of demonstrable damage to the brain. The dividing line alters with advances in scientific knowledge.

By classifying the functional disorders according to the predominant presenting emotion, which is itself assumed to reflect lasting traits in the personality* of the patient, we end up with a system of classification into which most psychiatric patients can be neatly slotted. Anxious patients have anxious personalities and suffer from anxiety states (or reactions), depressed patients have depressive personalities and suffer from depressive states (or reactive depression), and so on.

The system breaks down when we come to seek for the emotion behind obsessive–compulsive disorders, although 'disgust' has been postulated as a possible contender. Conversion disorder (hysteria) runs into similar difficulties, the problem here being not so much the type of emotion expressed, but the absence or inauthenticity of the emotion (see p. 298).

Table 8.1. *Classification of moods, personality, and functional disorder*

Mood	Personality	Mental disorder
Unhappiness/sadness	Gloomy/depressive/pessimist	Depressive illness
Happiness	Optimist/cheerful	Mania or hypomania
	Cyclothymic	Manic-depressive (bimodal)
Anxiety (general)	Worrier/over-anxious	Anxiety state/reaction
Fear (specific)	Specific situational sensitivity (e.g. shyness)	Phobias
?Disgust/disdain and anxiety	Perfectionist/obsessional	Obsessive–compulsive neurosis
?Detached	Histrionic/hysterical	Conversion disorder (hysteria)

The essential components of this system of classification are illustrated in Table 8.1. Missing from this table are the so-called 'personality disorders'. So great is the importance of personality that some psychiatrists regard all neuroses as falling within this category. Others reserve the term 'personality disorder' for the group of disorders which were formerly termed 'psychopathy', i.e. disorders of behaviour in which lasting behavioural tendencies lead people to commit acts which are regarded as antisocial.

The strength and weakness of this type of classification is its comprehensiveness. Almost anybody who seeks, or is referred for, help from a doctor can be fitted into one or other of the available slots. Many doctors work on the assumption that everybody who consults them must be sick, but there are many people whose reaction to a particular life event may be

*Personality can be defined as the sum of those traits of thinking, feeling, and behaviour which last and which distinguish one person from another.

well within the limits of normality. None the less, they seek help from their doctor—perhaps they are not familiar with intense emotional distress and fear that they may be sick, or perhaps they want to take advantage of the doctor's power to excuse them from work, prescribe drugs, etc. Having arrived in the consulting room, they may find themselves diagnosed as 'neurotic' or suffering from a 'personality disorder'.

The fact that a diagnostic system is often misused does not, of course, invalidate the entire system. But it does reduce the credibility of particular attributions and warns us to be careful in making and authenticating such diagnoses.

Personality disorders

These have been classified in a variety of ways. The simplest is as good as any and subdivides patients into two groups:

(1)   insecure personalities;

(2)   aggressive personalities.

Insecure personalities

These comprise a large group of people who lack confidence in themselves (e.g. they lack 'basic trust', see p. 7). If their lack of self-confidence causes them to cling to other people, they are likely to be seen as 'dependent personalities', but if they also lack trust in others, they may simply be seen as anxious people. Many become socially withdrawn and isolated. They are termed 'schizoid' because of a resemblance to, and an occasional association with, the negative symptoms of schizophrenia (see Section 8.6). Others who seek to escape from their problems by depending on drugs may be termed 'addictive personalities' (see Section 8.5).

Aggressive personalities

People with aggressive personalities have a low tolerance of frustration. Some are consistently irritable and aggressive, while others may become so at times of frustration or stress. They often blame others for their own inadequacies (paranoid personality), or become abnormally jealous (pathological jealousy).

In general, people with personality disorders are their own worst enemies. Lacking confidence in the chance of any long-term plans being realized, they tend to settle for short-term gains. This leads some of them into criminal or other antisocial activities which, in the end, are likely to prove self-defeating. As patients, they are unlikely to comply with treatment programmes which require any commitment on their part. They either become over-reliant on the doctor or give up too easily. Many are avid tablet-takers, but they cannot be relied upon to stick to the prescribed dose and easily become as dependent on drugs as they do on the doctors who prescribe them.

Doctors, on the whole, fight shy of patients with personality disorders, although there are a few psychiatrists who have developed 'therapeutic communities' aimed at meeting their needs. The most notable of these, Maxwell Jones, formerly of the Henderson Hospital, pioneered the development of residential programmes aimed at increasing self-confidence and a sense of personal responsibility. This was done by eliminating many of the features of mental hospitals which tended to encourage passivity and dependence in patients. 'Therapy' was seen as a collaborative relationship between people with problems, in which professional staff did their best to break down the hierarchical 'them and us' division which is found in most hospital settings. Staff uniforms were abandoned and 'bad' behaviour in patients dealt with by the patients' own peers rather than the staff alone.

Because the implications of the 'therapeutic community' affect so many psychiatric patients and offenders, some of the principles espoused by Maxwell Jones have been taken up and applied in other institutions. But few have dared to take these to the point which Jones did at the Henderson Hospital during the sixties and seventies, and few have accepted aggressive and other antisocial patients, whose ability to confound even the most benign system of care may eventually lead to disillusionment among the staff.

Jones recognized that an institution should be geared to be therapeutic 24 hours a day, but there is no way in which the primary care team (PCT) can provide this amount of care. Yet the PCT is obliged to look after patients with personality disorders.

In a paradoxical sense, the fact that patients are registered with a particular practice 'for life', or at least for relatively long periods of their lives, provides an opportunity which is lacking in hospitals, which can only admit people for short periods of time. The successful treatment of personality disorders takes time and patience, and it is important to recognize this fact from the outset. Members of the PCT who put too much time and effort into providing intensive therapy will soon 'burn out' and be disappointed when the patient relapses. Yet a limited commitment over a long period of time, which provides the patient with someone to fall back on in a crisis and a consistent 'parent' who is not afraid to set limits, will often contribute to increased maturity. This is most obvious in young people who often go through periods of insecurity and antisocial behaviour before they 'settle down'.

Because many personality disorders are caused by inadequate parenting, it is common for such patients to lack any parent-figure whom they can trust. The GP may not feel like being a parent to his or her patients, but is often the best they are going to get. If others can be drawn in to share the responsibility and support the patient's family or social network, the results may be surprisingly effective.

MB was the son of an alcoholic mother and an insecure father. He developed asthma at the age of 13 and, while being treated for this, built up a relationship with his GP which allowed him later to discuss problems which he was having at home and with his peers. At 17 he got his girlfriend pregnant, at 19 he was convicted of driving while drunk, and he subsequently became severely depressed. He usually came to his GP when a crisis developed and was encouraged to persevere, to recognize the good parts of himself, and generally to build-up his self-esteem. He gradually settled down, got married aged 27 and has now been happily married and in a stable job for six years. He rarely consults, has no symptoms of asthma, and greets his GP warmly when they meet in the street.

One of the problems with the term 'personality disorder' is that it is a label which is easy to attach, but difficult to get rid of. Once a person has been branded in this way, he may find that people who would normally be optimistic and supportive withdraw or reject him. This increases the insecurity which is at the root of the problem. Another difficulty is that it is not always easy to distinguish between a lasting personality disorder and the types of insecurity which arise out of particular life situations. It is not unreasonable for people to lack trust of others if they live in a criminal subculture; antisocial behaviour is a necessary means of survival in some places. People whose ideas and principles differ from social 'norms' are easily dismissed as 'cranks, freaks, or psychopaths' and, while we condemn the possible treatment of political dissidents as an abuse of psychiatry, we should not assume that our own hands are clean.

Further reading

Jones, M. (1952). *Social psychiatry*. Penguin Books, Harmondsworth.

8.2 FEARS AND PHOBIAS

Fear is a normal response to danger or threat. Its physiological and psychological effects have been discussed in Section 1.2. The degree of fear differs in different situations and in different people. Most people will experience more fear hanging from a high cliff face than looking from a second floor window, but the keen mountain-climber is likely to experience less fear than the average person, who will, in turn, be less frightened than the person who is afraid of heights.

Phobias are persistent fear reactions that are out of proportion to the objective danger. For example, it is unlikely that spiders can be as dangerous as might be implied by the behaviour of a spider phobic, who refused to enter several rooms in her house because she thought there might be spiders there. The commonest phobias are agoraphobia and social phobia. Specific phobias of animals, inanimate objects, and illness are less common.

The development of phobias in an individual appears to owe something to predisposing characteristics and something to learning from experience. Fears are normal and have to be learned if the child is to survive, and it is usually the parents who teach the child what to fear. Parents with abnormal fears can easily pass these on to their children. The critical learning experience may occur when the vulnerable child or adult comes to associate some frightening or painful experience with a previously unfeared object or situation, and, as a result, avoids it in future. It may also be possible to acquire phobias by imitating other phobic individuals. It would appear that certain objects, animals, and situations are more likely to elicit phobic reactions than others, and it has been suggested that these have biological significances which we are born predisposed to fear.

Agoraphobia

By far the most common phobia to present in general practice is agoraphobia, the name coming from the Greek words '*agora*', market place, and '*phobia*', fear. It is used to describe an extreme fear of leaving a safe home-base. It is more common in women than in men and typically starts in early adult life. The presenting symptoms may be fearfulness or feelings of panic, and the patient may not have observed that the fears depend on where she is; it may, therefore, be necessary to enquire in some detail as to whether the fears are associated with specific places, such as supermarkets or buses. Alternatively, she may present with anxiety-related physical symptoms, such as dizzy feelings, pains in the chest, and breathlessness, which are in themselves quite frightening sensations and which can maintain the level of anxiety. Again, careful questioning will reveal that these symptoms are associated with locations outside the home. Patients frequently comment that the symptoms disappear when they return to their homes. Sometimes the physical symptoms can be very severe and the patient experiences a panic attack; the tendency to hyperventilate increases these alarming experiences. Finally, some agoraphobics refuse to go to particular places, such as shops or cinemas, and the patient's family may initiate the consultation. A patient whom the doctor has seen a number of times for anxiety symptoms and who stops coming to the surgery may not have been cured but have become totally housebound. When managing patients with anxiety it is always worth remembering the possibility of agoraphobia in the background.

Social phobia

Social phobia is an exaggeration of the anxiety normally felt in social situations. It is a common experience in adolescence, which is the typical age of onset for persistent social phobias, and is more equally distributed between men and women than is agoraphobia. People with social phobias fear being observed. Their presentation may be very similar to that of those with agoraphobia, but the situations they fear or avoid always involve the presence of other people. While the person with agoraphobia may be comforted by the presence of others, the social phobic is threatened. Thus, they have difficulties eating in public places, such as restaurants, or when they may have to interact with other people, for instance in theatres, at concerts, shopping, queing, or giving any kind of public performance. They may find difficulty signing cheques in shops or banks, where the assistant may observe their activity. On the other hand, they are unlikely to complain of difficulty in deserted places far from home. Simple questions can discriminate between agoraphobia and social phobia and this can be helpful in management.

Animal phobias

These phobias, usually connected with fear of spiders, cats, rats, or birds, are most common in childhood and normally reduce to manageable proportions in adulthood. Persistent animal phobias are more common in women. Most of us have some irrational fear of these animals and such fears can readily be elicited, a fact exploited by producers of horror films. These phobias often present in a global picture of high anxiety and general nervousness. They may also present after some traumatic experience, e.g. when a bird falls down the chimney and flies around the room, or when the need to avoid a commonly met animal interferes with everyday life.

A four-year-old boy was brought to his general practitioner because his fear of spiders was preventing him from playing happily with other children, and because it made it very difficult for him to go to bed at night. He had been teased by the boy next door, who had taunted him with a spider, and he was now resisting any suggestion by his mother that he should have a bath, or use the toilet, until his parents had thoroughly searched the bathroom for the possible lurking spider. Similarly, he insisted on them searching the bedroom for the spider that might be hiding in the curtains or under the bed.

Other phobias

Amongst the inanimate objects that are feared are storms, heights, and enclosed spaces. These phobias are equally common in men and women.

Like the animal phobias, they are likely to present with global anxiety, after a traumatic experience, or when they interfere with normal functioning.

Mr X presented when his fear of thunderstorms became so great that much of his waking time was preoccupied with checking weather forecasts, reading the barometer, and observing the sky. At the least sign of clouds or impending rain he became unable to go out, and if there was more than the briefest shower, he hid himself in the cupboard under the stairs for safety.

Mrs Y was claustrophobic and could not cope with any form of restricted space, or anything which covered her face. She presented as unable to wear garments which had to be put on over her head, because she was terrified that they would get stuck over her face. She also felt very restricted with her children, being unable to play peek-a-boo, enter their tent in the garden, or take them to see the dungeons in a castle while on holiday.

Phobias of illness or injury are equally common in men and women, and typically begin in middle age. The most common phobias are of cancer or heart disease, and the phobic frequently knows someone who has the disease. More recently, fear of AIDS has become common. Very often there are other accompanying psychological problems. The phobia is characterized by extreme vigilance about the disease and can be very disruptive. It most commonly occurs in healthy people but, as in the case below, can be associated with other illness.

Mr Z was 45 when mild diabetes was diagnosed and controlled successfully by diet. He read about the complications of the disease and became convinced that he would develop heart disease. His normal pattern of behaviour was quickly overtaken by his need to avoid unnecessary exercise and to check his cardiac function. At the time of presentation he had given up exercising, had to be able to park his car within 100 yards of his destination, and was taking his pulse 15–20 times per day.

In this, as in many other cases, excessive fears of illness resulted from misunderstanding. In all cases it is important to explore the patient's view of the illness and to give information and reassurance where appropriate.

Management

Phobias have been very successfully treated by behavioural methods, and it is, therefore, important that they are satisfactorily diagnosed.[1] The general principle of all effective treatment is that it should involve exposure to the phobic object or situation, so that the sufferer can discover that the feared event is not as threatening as had been imagined, and that techniques for dealing with the situation can be learned. It is critical that avoidance should not be encouraged and that an approach akin to getting back on the horse after a fall should be adopted. Anything which makes it possible for the person to re-engage in the situation will be helpful.

Perhaps the best approach is one which encourages a graded, desensitizing strategy. The man who is frightened of having a meal in a restaurant might be encouraged to try a cup of tea in a cafe, and the woman who cannot go to the shops might be able to go to the end of her road as a first step. Starting with something that the patient can just manage, the steps are gradually increased in difficulty until the target is reached.[2] Manuals describing this approach to agoraphobia have already been referred to.[3]

It may also be useful to offer a cognitive strategy, a way of thinking that interferes with the doom-ridden thoughts of the phobic. For example, the person who interprets an increased heart rate as a sign of an impending heart attack might find it useful to remember that it is part of a normal fear response. A self-help booklet by Gillian Butler called *Managing anxiety*, available from the Warneford Hospital, Oxford (price at going to press £1.50) is excellent, with a particularly good section dealing with avoidance and loss of confidence.

In extremely fearful patients it may be helpful to prescribe an anxiolytic or beta-blocker for use when undertaking specific tasks as an adjunct to desensitization, and taken just before entering the phobic situation.

Some phobic patients present with significantly depressed mood or with high levels of generalized anxiety. These can lift as the phobia is treated or may require more specific attention (see Section 4.7).

Cynthia Jones had never been a very secure person. After the birth of her first baby she had a panic attack in a crowded supermarket and thereafter found herself unable to leave the house unless accompanied by another person. This made her very dependent on her mother who lived nearby.

The GP saw her with her mother and suggested a programme of progressive desensitization. At first her mother would accompany her to the shops, but would walk 10 yards behind her all the way home. Once she had got used to this the distance would be increased a little each day.

A week later things were already starting to improve and the GP was able to express his delight at the patient's progress. This boosted her confidence and she was soon able to get to and from the shops without difficulty, although she still needed her mother to be with her at the supermarket check-out counter.

A set-back occurred when, on one occasion, she thought she had lost her mother in the store, and she returned, for a while, to a more close contact. She eventually overcame the difficulty in checking out by visiting the store at a time when she knew there would be few customers and buying only one item. It was a great day for her and her mother when eventually she made the whole trip and made general purchases entirely on her own.

References

1. Marks, I. and Horder, J. (1987). Phobias and their management. *Br. Med. J.* **295**, 589–91.

2. Johnston, M. (1977). The treatment of agoraphobics in general practice. *Behav. psychopath.* **5**, 103–9.
3. Mathews, A. M., Gelder, M. G., and Johnston, D. W. (1981). *Agoraphobia: nature and treatment*. Guildford, London.

Further reading

France, R. and Robson, M. (1986). *Behaviour therapy in primary care: a practical guide*. Croom Helm, London.
Davison, D. G. and Neale, J. M. (1982). *Abnormal psychology* (3rd edn).

8.3   OBSESSIONS AND COMPULSIONS

Like phobias, obsessions and compulsions are exaggerated forms of normal experience. We have all experienced the persistent intrusive thought which keeps coming back into mind, or the repeated need to check that the door has been locked or the gas switched off. Children frequently develop obsessive–compulsive rituals such as avoiding stepping on cracks in the pavement or having to repeat protective rhymes, but these usually remain manageable and do not interfere with normal activities. Although irrational, obsessions and compulsions differ from psychotic symptoms in that patients have insight into the irrationality of their thoughts and behaviours. They are often ashamed and regard their behaviour as 'silly'. Therapy aimed at uncovering possible unconscious mechanisms has not proved very productive.

Obsessions

These are repetitive thoughts that cannot be ignored or dismissed. They often have a threatening or repulsive component and are therefore both distressing and disabling. The thoughts may be doubts, such as 'Have I put something poisonous in the pie I have just baked?', or impulses to action, such as 'Am I going to drive my car on the wrong side of the road?' Obsessional images can have equally distressing aspects, for instance the repeated or persistent image of a loved one dying.

Compulsions

Compulsions are repetitive, irresistible acts which are distressing to the performer. The most common forms of compulsive behaviour are habitual collecting, repeated checking, and repeated cleaning rituals such as hand-washing. In each case the same type of behaviour is repeated over and over again, and can reach exhausting proportions.

One woman collected so many paper bags, boxes, tin cans, and old clothes that her flat became virtually uninhabitable; she was so busy collecting that she had little time to care for herself.

It is not uncommon for an obsessional hand-washer to have red, damaged hands from spending hours each day trying to free them of germs.

A 30-year-old woman had a compulsive routine which prevented her from getting dressed and out of the house each day. She would start the routine by boiling the kettle to get water to wash in, washing, getting dressed, doing her hair, and putting on her make-up, but would have to stop and return to the beginning every time she heard a noise. She lived in a bed-sit in a multi-occupancy house which was very noisy. Frequently she would persevere in trying to accomplish this task for 7 or 8 hours, until completely exhausted by her efforts.

In each case the compulsive behaviour is driven by anxiety, the need being to perform the behaviour to fend off some ill-defined but dreaded consequence of neglect. Performance of the ritual reduces anxiety and the patient experiences considerable anxiety when it is prevented.

Obsessional thoughts often coexist with anxiety states. Because patients are ashamed of them they may not be revealed unless the patient is asked 'Do you have thoughts which go round and round in your head?'

Management

People with obsessions and compulsions usually have an obsessional personality. Abnormally careful, clean or tidy, inclined to check everything, they make excellent book-keepers and function well in jobs where meticulous care and patience are needed. At times of stress, however, their obsessional tendencies become exorbitant and they may take so long over simple tasks that they cease to be able to function effectively.

One approach which is often effective is to ignore the obsession and to seek for ways of helping the patient to manage stress.

Margot James, aged 16, was a devout Christian. She lived at home with her parents and had never had a boyfriend. Always a perfectionist she found it hard to cope with the increasing attention of a young man in her church group who had tried to persuade her to sleep with him. She came to the GP for help with a problem of compulsive praying. She knew it was pointless to spend much of her life in prayer but felt compelled to do this. The GP suggested to her that the endless praying was itself a reflection of the wider conflicts with which she was faced at a difficult time her life. He suggested that she spent some time talking to the community psychiatric nurse at the practice, who was a young Christian woman with a good understanding of sex education and adolescence. Given the support, the compulsive praying soon ceased to be a problem and the patient found a new and more secure identity within the community of young people who attended her church.

In other cases, referral to a psychologist will be helpful. Behavioural treatments by habituation or thought-stopping may be used with obsessions, and response prevention with compulsions (see Chapter 3).

It is sometimes possible to limit the obsessions or compulsive behaviour, perhaps with the co-operation of a friend or spouse. The instruction to 'stop doing it' can be surprisingly effective, as the patient may then discover that the dreaded consequence does not occur. In the case of the 30-year-old woman above, progress was made in the first instance by limiting her rituals to five hours per day — after that time she had to give up and stop trying to get out. Considerable success was achieved, and gradually the time allowed was cut back.

The self-help booklet by Gillian Butler (see p. 335) may also be helpful in patients with compulsions.

Further reading

France, R. and Robson, M. (1986). *Behaviour therapy in primary care: a practical guide.* Croom Helm, London.
Weinman, J. (1987). *An outline of psychology as applied to medicine.* Wright, London.

8.4   DEPRESSION AND MANIA

Depression

'To the person in the bell jar, blank and stopped as a dead baby, the world itself is a bad dream.'[1] Depression is a continuum — there is no clear-cut distinction between 'sadness', being 'depressed', and having a 'clinical depression'. Aubrey Lewis'[2] often quoted definition that 'anyone can be said to be suffering from a depressive disorder if they are in a state of sadness and unhappiness of such degree that they can be justifiably regarded as sick' evades the question of what is a depressive illness by not indicating who decides that a person is sick. Dorothy Rowe writes from a different perspective —

Depression is as old as the human race, and rare is the person who has not felt its touch. Sometimes, suddenly, without apparent reason, we feel unbearably sad. The world turns grey and we taste a bitterness in our mouth. We hear an echo of the bell that tolls our passing, and we reach out for a comforting hand, but find ourselves alone. For some of us this experience is no more than a fleeting moment, or something we can dispel with common-sense thoughts and practical actions. But for some of us this experience becomes a ghost whose unbidden presence mars every feast, or, worse, a prison whose walls, though invisible, are quite often impenetrable. What is the difference between being depressed and being unhappy? There is a difference, and when you have experienced both you know what this difference is.

When people are unhappy, even if they have suffered the most grievous blow, they are able to seek comfort and let that ease the pain. They can seek out and obtain others' sympathy and loving concern; they can comfort themselves. But in depression neither the sympathy and concern of others nor the gentle love of oneself is available. Other people may be there, offering all the love, sympathy and concern any person could want, but none of this compassion can pierce the wall that separates the sufferer from them. Inside the wall there is not only the refusal of the smallest ease and comfort but also punishment by words and deeds. Depression is a prison in which the person is both the suffering prisoner and the cruel jailer.[3]

It is this peculiar isolation which distinguishes depression from common unhappiness. In depression a central feature is the inability to feel pleasure coupled with a sense of hopelessness and helplessness.

Classification of depression into reactive, endogenous, bipolar, and psychotic is useful only because these terms give some indication of the likely prognosis and response to treatment, but involved in the aetiology of all types is a variable mixture of causes — genetic, past experience, current experience, family, environmental, and physical.

Patients with severe, maybe psychotic, symptoms need to be identified. Though rare, these patients are likely to need urgent treatment, probably with drugs or ECT, usually in hospital, and may even need to be sectioned for their own safety.

A depressed family member will usually be part of a family system, so other family members will be both involved in the maintenance of the symptom and recipients of its effects. Not uncommonly, depressed patients choose not to consult their GPs, or if they do, not to present the illness as recognizable depression but in the guise of a physical illness. Other family members may then come and discuss the depressed patient, or may present symptoms as part of the family's distress. Depression should be particularly remembered when children present with a recurrent illness such as abdominal pain, or with behaviour problems (particularly insomnia), and when spouses present with non-specific illnesses such as alcohol problems and insomnia; also when relationship problems are in evidence.

Aetiology

Depression is the product of the interaction of the individual's constitution and the environment. There is no doubt that depressive illnesses run in families, but there is good evidence that both nature and nurture play their part in causation.

Past experience

The ability to cope with the world arises from a childhood which has allowed the development of reasonable autonomy and trust, and a satisfactory differentiation from one's parents. The early experience of death and loss, particularly of a mother, is correlated with an increased risk of depression in later life.[4] Brown's work showed not only that losses in childhood predispose to depression in later life, but that the type of loss influences the type of depression. Thus, the insecurities which result from a childhood which has been disturbed by intermittent separation, in which the parents are separated or divorced or where there are frequent quarrels between them, leave the child predisposed to reactive depressions in later life. But the effect of the death of a parent, particularly the mother, is to produce a tendency towards what Seligman[5] calls 'learned helplessness', which is deeper and more hopeless than the foregoing and which is likely to be associated with the anergic or 'endogenous' type of depression in later life.

Other factors which contribute to a depressive tendency are likely to reflect the quality of parenting. While the physical loss of a parent is easy to describe and understand, the experience of having been in great need of a close relationship which was unrequited, and having no control over this situation, creates a feeling of helplessness which in many people leads to a state of hopelessness and depression. This pattern of reacting becomes learned and may be reactivated whenever people find themselves in similar circumstances. Thus, children who are repeatedly prevented from playing with their peers by being locked in their home may become depressed. Later in life when they are trapped in a situation, or are unable to do what they want, they may respond by depression, rather than by attempting to solve the problem.

Current experience

The commonest trigger for depression is some form of loss, whether of a person (by death, divorce, absence, or emotional withdrawal) or of work, house, limb, or other object.[6] The loss may revive echoes of earlier losses following which similar difficulties may have arisen. Hence depression may complicate and prolong the work of grieving.

While change may be equated with loss, other psychosocial transitions, particularly those involving changes of role, may create the same sense of helplessness and hopelessness which leads to depression.[5]

Interpersonal difficulties or conflicts may also create a feeling of powerlessness from which an escape may be depression, as in the case of a patient who believed she had a good marriage, but when her husband had an affair she became depressed, rather than face this issue.

A realization of inadequacies, or intrapersonal deficits, which may be true or imagined, can be destructive of hope and optimism.

Mr A, an accountant, aged 50, worked for a company which was taken over by another which subsequently instituted computerization. He found it difficult to learn the new skills and more difficult to acknowledge this difficulty. He felt trapped and became depressed.

Beck and other 'cognitive theorists' have suggested that it is not the losses *per se* that lead to depression but the individual's tendency to take a negative view of themselves, the world, and their future. Beck has identified systematic biases and distortions (see Section 1.3), which he suggests increase vulnerability to depression. His 'cognitive therapy' is designed to interrupt these dysfunctional thought-patterns (see p. 72).[7]

Physical and psychological factors in current life contribute to the development of depressive illnesses. Physical illness may trigger a depression. Brown's work showed that in working-class women in London, lack of employment outside the house, presence of young children at home, and lack of an adult in whom one can confide all increase vulnerability to depression.[4] It may be possible to ameliorate these difficulties by steering people towards sources of practical help—crèches, employment schemes, etc.

The family may create, if not maintain, depression. The helplessness of one member may reassure another member of his or her own competence. When the depressed patient gets better, the other family member may get depressed—a see-saw situation.

Endogenous

Although there is often a life event which triggers the onset of a depressive illness—physical or psychological—some depressions descend on the individual like a black cloud from nowhere. Patients who have recurring depressions of this kind have been labelled as suffering from 'unipolar' depression. When periods of manic elation intersperse the depressive episodes, the illness is termed 'bipolar' or 'manic depressive'. These people may be normal in mood for long periods and become quite unaccountably and suddenly depressed. They often benefit greatly from the use of antidepressants, and lithium may prevent recurrence.

Symptoms

The individual symptoms may be grouped under four headings.

1. Cognitive

The person thinks that they are not working effectively, or are defective in some way, and have thoughts of worthlessness, uselessness, helplessness, hopelessness, guilt, and loss of interest. This may be accompanied by slowness of thinking, poor memory, and suicidal ideas.

Those who usually believe in God may complain that they have been abandoned and that they have lost their faith. Unbelievers will talk of the meaninglessness of life.

In the psychotic variant it may be evident that thoughts are unrelated to reality, or frankly delusional. Often the delusions are of infamy and constipation. Sufferers believe themselves to be the wickedest persons in the world and to be literally 'full of shit'.

2. *Vegetative and physiological*

The autonomic system is involved in the depressive state. This may be expressed by weight change (usually loss and anorexia, but sometimes gain resulting from compulsive eating), constipation, dry mouth, and palpitations. There may also be sleep disturbance characterized by early morning waking, with a tendency to be most depressed early in the morning Some, however, experience hypersomnia. Mood swings, with alternating periods of lack of energy followed by agitation, restlessness, and irritability are not uncommon.

Not infrequently patients complain of a variety of pains. The presentation of headache, backache, abdominal pain, and constipation occasionally mimics organic disease. The unwary physician who does not enquire about, and give credence to, the other symptoms of depression, may embark on lengthy and fruitless investigations which reinforce the patient's belief in an organic basis for these symptoms. In this way the development of a somatoform disorder may be encouraged (see Chapter 6).

3. *Affective*

It would be difficult to make a diagnosis of depression without some evidence of sadness, depression, and gloom being elicited. It is not uncommon, also, to find feelings of irritability and anger, directed at the self, at others, or at the world.

4. *Behaviour*

The picture of a person lying in bed unable to make the decision to get up is seldom seen in general practice today, but one of the commonest difficulties for patients is to make decisions. This makes therapy difficult as the patient will find it hard to act on any suggestion which is made. The inability of patients to make decisions and to motivate themselves into activity is manifested by a restricted way of living. They may not go to work, may have little social life, and may be dependent on their family or friends for nurture. The affairs of life may be neglected. GPs may be asked to visit such patients at home by relatives who have been trying to get them to come to the doctor for a long time, but have been unable to persuade them to go out.

Diagnosis

It is still difficult for many people to go to the doctor and talk about psychological problems. Doctors themselves are just as reluctant, if not more so, to consult other general practitioners or psychiatrists about their own mental symptoms. Patients may be preoccupied with the physical manifestations of their psychological problems, having little insight into their mood or thought-processes, but the failure to recognize the depression may be as much due to the reluctance of the doctor as of the patient. Thus, the fact that a high proportion of people are not recognized as depressed by their general practitioner is not surprising.[8] A cheerful, but sometimes brittle, exterior can hide a very depressed and even suicidal interior. If there are any clues, depression should be considered and the GP must have the willingness and skill to ask the appropriate questions, of which the following may be crucial.

'Has your appetite or weight changed?'

'Has your pattern of sleep changed?'

'Do you feel you lack energy or drive?'

'Do you feel agitated or slowed down?'

'Do you feel self-reproachful or guilty?'

'Are you unable to concentrate or make decisions?'

'Do you have recurrent thoughts of death or suicide?'

Five positive answers combined with two weeks of depressed moods suggest a fair degree of depression.

If there is a suggestion that the patient is depressed, the depth and severity of the depression needs to be ascertained and a questionnaire much as the Beck Inventory may be used.[9]

Assessment of suicidal risk

Many people have fleeting suicidal thoughts without any serious intent, but any suggestion that the method has been thought out, or that suicide has become a preoccupation must be taken seriously. It is not true that those who talk of suicide do not do it. Many people who attempt suicide will have mentioned the idea, either directly or indirectly, to family or friends, or will have consulted their doctor with non-specific symptoms, in the weeks before,[10] and may use prescribed drugs to carry out their threat.[11]

Difficulties in diagnosis

While classical depression may be easy to recognize, depression presenting as physical illness is underdiagnosed, as is the depression that accompanies much physical illness. The implication of this failure, which has been recognized in all practices which have been adequately researched,[8] is that general practitioners need to increase their index of suspicion, and possibly screen patients. Screening questionnaires seem seldom to be used in general practice, yet research suggests that tools such as the General Health Questionnaire have good specificity and sensitivity for anxiety and depression.[12] It can be a useful tactic to offer a patient in whom the

Table 8.2.   *Screening investigations which may be helpful in defining a physical cause for depression*

Full blood count
Virology
Vit. B_{12}
Red cell folate
Screen for collagen disease
Electrolytes and urea
Urate
Blood sugar
Thyroid function tests
Liver function tests
Calcium studies
Serological tests for syphilis and HIV infection

diagnosis is uncertain a questionnaire, which takes little time to complete. The act of filling this in may also help patients to crystallize their thoughts about the problems they are bringing to the doctor.

We have acknowledged that depression may present with physical symptoms, but depression may also be caused by drugs, of which alcohol is the most important.

So many drugs can cause depressive symptoms that it is worth bearing this possibility in mind whenever a depressed patient is on any form of drug therapy. In addition, many organic disorders are associated with depression, either as part of their own symptomatology or as a psychological reaction to the disease. Sometimes physical disease presents with depressive symptoms and Table 8.2 lists a number of investigations which may help diagnose a physical cause for depression. Research in general practice is needed to ascertain the value of screening by such tests.

The correct differentiation of a major depressive illness from a primarily physical disease is important because it allows the condition to be appropriately treated and relieves patients and their families of great misery, as well as being rewarding for the doctor.

There can also be less obvious disadvantages. The communication of a diagnosis of 'depressive illness' to patient and family can do harm when minor depression arises out of a situation in which a psychiatric label will further undermine the patient's self-respect and encourage the family and others to reject or over-protect. In such cases it may be more helpful to define the problem as a 'family problem', a 'work problem', or some other kind of 'problem', in order to draw in the support that is needed and ensure that the sufferers' views are treated with respect.

Depression in young people
Children and adolescents also have a range of behaviours, thoughts, and

feelings for which the label 'depression' seems appropriate. Whether a label is given or not, it is important to recognize the distress of such young people and to remember that suicide is one of the commonest causes of death in adolescents. Children seldom present with a mood disorder, and indeed may not be able to understand the term depression, and parents seldom recognize the problem as depression. As in adults, it is common in the presence of chronic illness, and in situations of loss, such as death or separation of a parent, and may be triggered by academic, sporting, or social failures. The presentation is often somatic, particularly loss of energy, headache, abdominal pain or fatigue. An alternative presentation may be behavioural, including deterioration of school performance, social withdrawal, unexplained violence, and other acting-out behaviour.

Clues as to the misery are often non-verbal; neglect of self-appearance, slow speech, gaze avoidance, and a slumped posture. Asking about depression may be unrewarding, but the following phrases may be useful: 'John, I have the feeling that things are not going too well for you' and if there is a positive response, perhaps by eye-contact, continuing with 'Tell me about it.' Or 'Everyone gets low sometimes. I am wondering if there is anything that is getting you down'. Having broken the ice it may help to enquire about feelings of low esteem, loss of interest, and feelings of being unloved, unworthy, guilty, hopeless, or helpless. If there is confirmation of a degree of depression, it is vital to enquire about thoughts of suicide. Suicidal intentions, and probably even thoughts, need to be taken seriously.

Management

The art of treating depression in general practice is to remember that all these facets may be points where the system can be helped to change. Patients may need antidepressant drugs, but it is usually also important to explore the losses and the difficulties, to question the assumptions, to involve the family, and to suggest changes of behaviour.

It is only for convenience that this section is subdivided into separate headings. Different approaches may be used concurrently in the same patient.

Antidepressants

The use of antidepressant drugs has been fully considered in Section 4.7. The small space alloted to these drugs in this chapter does not reflect their usefulness and importance in managing depressive illness. They are particularly helpful in patients with severe mood disturbance, with anergic, 'endogenous', or psychotic depression, with sleep problems, with lack of ability to make decisions, and in those who have recurrent depressive episodes without obvious triggers. Their disadvantage is their delay in action, and though they are not always effective, toxicity is not a problem in normal dosage, nor are they habit-forming like benzodiazepines.

Although physical treatments do not get to the root of the problems which may underlie depression, and should not, therefore, be given without full assessment of these, they do temporarily alter the enzyme systems in the brain which, in many instances, are thought to play a part in causing clinical depression. Even though most depressions will eventually improve without therapy, anything which shortens the duration of one of the most unpleasant conditions from which man can suffer deserves consideration.

Psychotherapy

A depressive illness is often triggered by a loss. Helping the patient to face up to the loss and to bear the painful emotions which are aroused can be helpful. In acute situations, crisis intervention may be needed, but for more deep-seated problems other forms of uncovering therapies may be more appropriate (see Section 3.5). If depression is so severe that the patient is mute or retarded, then talking will be of little use, but this need not prevent the patient from being given emotional support.

One of the main reasons that general practitioners can be effective in helping people who are depressed is that they provide the confiding relationship that many people do not have in their everyday lives. This may also explain why so many patients value contact with the doctor, but fail to become fully well and independent. Understanding that their role carries the risk of dependence may help doctors to avoid or change the situation. Finding a surrogate, such as a good neighbour, priest, or self-help group may be one of our tasks.

Changing behaviour

Depressed patients tend to withdraw from social and work activities, and this withdrawal reinforces their helplessness. It also separates them from normal sources of support and self-esteem and distraction from depressing thoughts. Encouragement, perhaps by involving friends, relations, good neighbours, and members of self-help groups helps patients to become involved again in the outer world. This may be painful for patients, especially at first, but eventually they will come to realize that they have actually started to enjoy themselves.

Cognitive therapy

The theory behind Beck's work on cognitive therapy, which was originally concerned with its use in depression, is described in Section 3.4.[7] Controlled trials in general practice on patients with major depression have demonstrated that cognitive therapy is initially more effective than treatment with imipramine, but after three months there is little difference in outcome between the two methods.[13] Individual cognitive therapy was assessed by Ross and Scott and found in general practice to be more effective than no treatment.[14] It is perhaps too early to make dogmatic suggestions about the

use of cognitive therapy, except to say it is worth exploring if a su
psychologist is available, but its cost in professional time needs to be l
in mind. Simple cognitive therapy carried out by general practitione
patients with less severe depressions may be helpful, especially if combined
with other manoeuvres.

Family therapy

Whatever initiates depression, it is frequently influenced and maintained by
the patient's family.

Mrs A had been depressed for some years. She had responded to amitriptyline briefly
on at least two occasions but had relapsed. Psychotherapy by her general practitioner
and a psychiatrist had neither ameliorated the depression nor prevented relapse. During
a session with the family (Mr and Mrs A and children aged 14 and 11), it became obvious
that Mr A regarded himself as more competent than his wife in all activities, including
cooking and managing the house. He needed to feel competent because of his own
insecurities, and this left no room for his wife to be anything but hopeless and helpless.

Surprisingly, this one session enabled the family dynamics to change so much that
Mrs A no longer had to be depressed to get sympathy, and her husband no longer
had to show himself competent to feel secure. Family therapy had changed their
perceptions.

Attempting to treat depression without attempting to assess the dynamics
of the family and its resistance to change may be frustrating and short-sighted.
One session with the family, or with just the marital partner, or even one
session with the individual constructing a genogram (see p. 125) may enable
change to occur, and the identified patient to improve. However, as stated
above, ripple effects among other members of the family may ensue, and
may need treating.

Manipulating the environment

No amount of individual, couple, or family therapy will be sufficient if there
are serious deficits in the patient's housing, employment, etc. Anything which
improves the patient's sense of being in control of the environment will help.

Initially, this may mean ensuring that patients are getting all the state
benefits they are entitled to,[15] writing letters to housing authorities, pointing
out the availability of a suitable crèche, or giving permission to go out to
work — if it is available. Citizens' Advice Bureaux are often helpful, as are
other members of the primary care team, e.g. social workers.

Some doctors will feel compelled to campaign at national level for
improvements in the lot of their patients.[16]

ECT

Most patients whose depression has been severe enough for ECT to be
considered will already have been referred to a psychiatrist. The GP needs

to know the potential benefits and disadvantages of this method of treatment in order to discuss these with patients and their relatives, and occasionally to suggest a second opinion if there is uncertainty as to whether ECT should be used.

The advantages of ECT are that it works quickly—often within a few days, that it sometimes works with patients who have been resistant to other treatments, and that it is safer than drugs for suicidal patients. On the other hand, it is felt by many to be a drastic form of treatment, which causes temporary loss of memory, and which does not address any of the basic causes of the depressive illness.

Its use is now mostly restricted to patients who are actively suicidal, grossly retarded, resistant to other forms of treatment, or who express delusions, excessive feelings of guilt, and ruminate about their misery. It may be used to gain a remission which may make the patient more amenable to other therapies.

Mania and hypomania

On hearing that an exam has been passed, after a successful interview, on winning the pools, or completing a difficult task, most people become elated. They will celebrate with exuberant behaviour and do things which they would not do under normal circumstances. After a serious bout of depression some people also go 'over the top' and instead of settling down they, too, become elated and behave inappropriately. Behaviour of this kind is labelled 'manic'.

Depression and mania are linked together because they often occur sequentially in the same person, and because mania often seems to be a defence against the admission of underlying depressive problems.

Definition

Mania, which is in many ways the antithesis of depression, can occur in isolation. The term describes a state of unusual excitement during which the sufferer is out of touch with reality. It is rare in general practice, but its minor form, hypomania, is not uncommon and its recognition is vital. Without being psychotic, patients may be so over-confident, so uncritical, so energetic that they squander money, exhaust their family, or destroy their business.

Symptoms

Cognitive

Irrational optimism, grandiose delusions with blind faith in the ability to succeed, and assumptions that people will co-operate and favour them characterize manic persons, who may think they are God, or specially chosen by Him to save the world. Thought and speech are rapid, but are often jumbled and inaccurate. There may be flights of ideas which separately may make sense, but, put together, are irrational. In acute mania the thought processes may become so disorganized that it is difficult to differentiate this disorder from schizophrenia. In extreme cases a loosely connected word salad may emerge, and the patient may become confused and hallucinated.

Vegetative and physiological
The whole body tends to be over-active. The patient hardly eats or sleeps and may present in a state of exhaustion, denying any such situation. Increased tension, tachycardia, and, in chronic cases, loss of weight may occur.

Affective
The mood is usually of excitement, elation, over-optimism and unjustified confidence, but impatience, irritability, and anger can also occur.

Behavioural
Patients may be over-active, restless, agitated, sleep little, and have unbounded energy. Sometimes they will complain of sleep loss but often they will regard this as an advantage, to give them more time and opportunity to complete their tasks. Because of this confidence, wild schemes may be entered into, through which resources may be squandered and family life sacrificed.

Diagnosis

Acute mania often presents as a crisis when there may be little difficulty in recognizing that the patient is seriously disturbed and in need of help. The differential diagnosis of schizophrenia can be difficult and, though irrelevant in the crisis, important for long-term management and the prevention of further episodes.

Other causes of hypomania are drugs—particularly the amphetamine group, and tertiary syphilis. Occasionally antidepressants may convert depression to mania.

Hypomania may be much more difficult to recognize than full-blown mania, and families will often alert the doctor to differences in behaviour. Patients seldom recognize that seeing a doctor is necessary, and rarely complain of any abnormality. Criticism, or the suggestion of illness, may be greeted with anger or dismissal.

The diagnosis is important because of the destructive nature of the condition in which irrevocable decisions about marriage, money, or work may be made.

Management

Management and diagnosis are linked problems. Both will usually involve working with the family. It is often impossible on the first occasion to offer help before a crisis develops, when a Mental Health Order may need to be invoked (see Appendix I). Subsequently, it may be possible to make a contract with the patient and the family, who should be educated to recognize the early signs of recurrence—particularly sleeplessness, restlessness, and agitation. If this can be done, the contract may also include giving a power of attorney to a trusted friend, or having the money in a shared bank account which can be frozen by the spouse. If people have experienced a previous severe and disastrous episode, early help may be more acceptable.

While the background and source of the mania will need to be investigated, most GPs will initially wish to use sedation because of the potential dangers. The use of drugs is discussed in Section 4.7.

References

1. Plath, S. (1963). *The bell jar*. William Heinemann, London.
2. Lewis, A. J. (1983). States of depression; their clinical and aetiological differentiation. *Br. Med. J.* **287**, 875.
3. Rowe, D. (1983). *Depression. The way out of your prison*. Routledge and Kegan Paul, London.
4. Brown, G. W. and Harris, T. (1978). *The social origins of depression*. Tavistock, London.
5. Seligman, M. E. P. (1975). *Helplessness: On depression, development and death*. Freeman, San Francisco.
6. Paykel, E. S., Myers, J. K., Dienelt, M. N., Kierman, G. L., Linpenthal, J. J., and Pepper, M. P. (1969). *Archs Gen. Psychiat.* **21**, 753-60.
7. Beck, A. T., Rush, A. J., Shaw, B. F., and Emery, G. (1981). Cognitive therapy in depression. John Wiley, Chichester.
8. Freeling, P., Rao, B., Paykel, E. S., Sireling, L. I., and Burton, R. M. (1985). Unrecognised depression in general practice. *Br. Med. J.* **290**, 1880-3.
9. Beck, A. J. (1961). An inventory for measuring depression. *Archs Gen. Psychiat.* **4**, 561-71.
10. Hawton, K. and Blackstock, E. (1976). General practice aspects of self poisoning and self injury. *Psychol. Med.* **6**, 571-5.
11. Prescott, L. F. and Highley, M. S. (1985). Drugs for self poisoners. *Br. Med. J.* **240**, 1633-5.
12. Goldberg, D. P. and Blackwell, B. (1970). Psychiatric illness in general practice—a detailed study using a new method of case identification. *Br. Med. J.* **2**, 439-43.
13. Teasdale, J. D., Fennell, M. J. V., Hibbert, G. E., and Amies, P. L. (1984). Cognitive therapy for major depressive disorder in primary care. *Br. J. Psychiat.* **144**, 400-6.
14. Ross, M. and Scott, M. (1985). An evaluation of the effectiveness of individual and group cognitive therapy in the treatment of depressed patients in an inner city health centre. *J. R. Coll. Gen. Pract.* **35**, 239-42.

15. Jarman, B. (1985). Giving advice about welfare benefits in general practice. *Br. Med. J.* **290**, 522–6.
16. Townsend, P. and Davidson, N. (1982). *Inequalities in health: the Black report.* Penguin, Harmondsworth.

Further reading

Davis, T. C., Hunter, R. J., Nathan, M. M., and Bairnsfather, L. E. (1987). Childhood depression: an overlooked problem in family practice. *J. Fam. Pract.* **25**, 451–7.
Freeling, P., Downey, L. J., and Malkin, J. (1987). *The presentation of depression — current approaches.* Royal Coll. of GPs, Occasional paper, No. 36.
Gotlib, I. H. and Colby, C. A. (1987). *Treatment of depression. An interpersonal systems approach.* Pergamon Press, Oxford.

Recommended reading for patients

Ffrench-Beytagh, G. (1978). *Facing depression.* SLG Press, Fairacres, Oxford.
Rowe, D. (1983). *Depression — the way out of your prison.* Routledge and Kegan Paul, London.

8.5 ABUSE—ALCOHOL, TOBACCO, AND OTHER DRUGS

Our attitudes to the drugs available to us are determined by cultural, social, and economic factors which are rooted in history, and often seem to have little relationship to the real value and dangers of the drugs in question. Alcohol is approved by Europeans but forbidden by Moslems, cannabis is approved by Rastafarians but forbidden by Europeans, hallucinogenic drugs are used in religious ceremonies by South American Indians but even doctors are not permitted to prescribe them in much of the rest of the world.

Within Western society there are wide divergences in attitudes towards drugs. There are few doctors (in the U.K.) who smoke tobacco but many nurses do. Diazepam is regarded as relatively harmless by most doctors but many patients see 'Valium' as the most dangerous drug on the market. The truth seems to be that most drugs can be harmless or even helpful if used sensibly, but all physiologically active drugs are dangerous if abused, and there are a few people who will become habituated to quite innocuous substances.

Abuse can arise either because the abuser is not aware of the danger or because the danger is known but ignored. In the former case the solution is one of public education. If people are made aware of dangers, and believe what they are told, it is assumed that they will take heed. Unfortunately, not all people accept the information that they are given, and those who do may choose to continue to run risks because of the short-term benefits which result. Thus, a person who relies on tobacco for tension relief may prefer to run the risk of heart disease at some time in the future, rather than suffer continuing nervous tension now.

This issue of a trade-off of short-term benefits against long-term risks accounts for a lot of drug abuse, and is most likely to occur in people who have little faith in the value of long-term planning. Those people who have grown up in a world in which they have learned to postpone gratification in the interests of long-term benefits, and whose parents rewarded them consistently for self-controlled behaviour, find it easier to resist the temptation to abuse drugs than do people who have never learned to control or influence their future welfare.

Looked at in this way, the tendency to abuse drugs can be seen as a form of personality disorder and it is certainly true that many, but not all, drug abusers are inadequate people who cling to their drugs for support, in much the same way that dependent persons cling to their fellows. In such cases it follows that anything which improves people's confidence in their ability to cope with problems and to influence their own future will increase their chances of getting by without drugs. Conversely, punitive attitudes or control exerted from outside will further undermine confidence and perpetuate the problems.

In the chapter which follows we shall take alcohol abuse as our prime example, but most of the lessons which we can learn from treating alcohol abuse are applicable to the abuse of other drugs.

Alcohol

Alcohol abuse is presented to general practitioners either because it is seen by patients as a problem or because of the damage it has caused to them or their families. Abuse of alcohol, tobacco, drugs, and food is accepted by patients as being within the province of general practice, though for all of these problems there are other sources of help, both lay and professional, which may be as effective, if not more so. About one-third of people seriously abusing alcohol 'recover' without any professional intervention, often consequent on forming a new relationship, changes at work, or adopting a faith.[1]

For many years doctors have been pessimistic about the outcome of trying to help people with lifestyle problems, but Russell's recent research with smokers[2] and Scottish work on alcohol abuse[3] encourages a more optimistic view. The RCGP Report on Alcohol[4] suggests that offering help to alcohol abusers in the form of education and support early in their careers may constitute a more effective use of the doctor's time than attempts at treatment later on.

Factors that influence alcohol consumption

Alcohol gives pleasure to many people, and small quantities of alcohol may even be beneficial by reducing the incidence of cardiovascular deaths,[5] though this has been questioned recently.[6] In general, however, the more we drink the greater the risk of harming ourselves.

The following are some of the factors that influence the use of alcohol:

Genetic

Twin studies suggest that there is a genetic factor, though it is not clear whether this is associated with an increased desire to drink, or an increased susceptibility to its effects. Some Orientals drink less because of an inherited tendency to an unpleasant flushing sensation when drinking alcohol.

Family

The family is a most potent influence, and it is not uncommon to find several members of the same family misusing alcohol.

Culture

Alcohol is culturally acceptable in most of British society and most adults have at least tasted it. People usually learn to drink in company, and their level of drinking is influenced by their peer group—the gang, the 'medical rugger club', the 'miners' club', the pub, and so on. Culture determines not only the quantity of alcohol drunk (by tradition Jews are moderate in the use of alcohol and Mormons drink little or none), it also determines the pattern of consumption. Mediterranean races drink a lot with meals, rarely get drunk, but develop cirrhosis of the liver, while people in Ireland and Scandinavia tend to binge drink but suffer less from cirrhosis.

Cost and occupation

On a general level, the cheaper alcohol is, the more it will be consumed and the more it will be abused. But alcohol is always cheap to the rich, and to certain groups such as sailors and the armed forces abroad. It is easily available to publicans and people in catering, and is drunk more by those whose flexible timetables allow more drinking time, such as journalists, travellers, doctors, and printers. Within our national culture there are subcultures in which heavy consumption in alcohol is acceptable—medical schools, demolition gangs, dockers, miners, etc.

Choice

Alcohol misuse can be thought of as a learned behaviour which can be at least partly relearned. Everyone who drinks is on a continuum from harmless to harmful drinking, and the individual moves along this continuum. At any time the position (the drinking behaviour) will be determined by what are seen as the advantages and disadvantages, and the pleasures and discomforts, of drinking. It is difficult to remember that even someone who is seriously misusing alcohol may choose to continue in this vein because it seems less painful than attempting to reduce consumption. The role of the doctor is both to help patients to clarify their perspective of the benefits and harms, and to shift the balance towards drinking less, especially since alcohol itself may impair the ability to make choices.

Balance sheet

Address to the legislature by a Mississippi state senator in 1958:

You ask me how I feel about whisky; all right, here is just how I stand on this question:

If, when you say whisky, you mean the devil's brew, the poison scourge, the bloody monster that defiles innocence, yes, literally takes the bread from the mouths of little children; if you mean the evil drink that topples the Christian man and woman from the pinnacles of righteous gracious living into the bottomless pit of degradation and despair, shame and helplessness and hopelessness, then certainly I am against it with all my power.

But, if when you say whisky, you mean the oil of conversation, the philosophic wine, the stuff that is consumed when good fellows get together, that puts a song in their hearts and laughter on their lips and the warm glow of contentment in their eyes; if you mean Christmas cheer; if you mean the stimulating drink that puts the spring in the old gentleman's step on a frosty morning; if you mean the drink that enables a man to magnify his job, and his happiness, and to forget, if only for a little while, life's great tragedies and heartbreaks and sorrows, if you mean that drink, the sale of which pours into our treasuries untold millions of dollars, which are used to provide tender care for our little crippled children, our blind, our deaf, our dumb, our pitiful aged and infirm, to build highways, hospitals and schools, then certainly I am in favour of of it.

This is my stand, I will not retreat from it; I will not compromise.

Benefits and incentives

Alcohol can help people in many ways, for instance by relieving stress or boredom, or by helping them to relax in company. It goes well with meals, picks us up when we feel tired, and helps us to go to sleep. It tastes good, is socially acceptable, breaks down inhibitions, and helps us to have a good laugh. In moderation it helps with sexual performance.

The doctor might look for deeper reasons which are not so easily recognized or expressed: it may be used to reduce feelings of inadequacy or to relieve dependency conflicts; its use can serve as an expression of rebellion against parents or others in authority, or to help a person to achieve peer status. It may relieve sex-role conflict, or role-strain in a person's job, and it may enhance fantasies of personal power. It may serve as self-reward or as self-punishment.

Additional pressures to drink arise from social conditioning and habit. People become psychologically conditioned to drinking by the sight of their favourite pub, the armchair in the evening, or the smell of alcohol, and because of secondhand thoughts and assumptions; 'What I need now is a good drink', 'If I were a real man, I could hold my drink', 'People who do not drink are dull and boring'.

Disincentives and harms

On the other side of the balance sheet are the disincentives to drinking, and the harms of alcohol misuse. Whereas the benefits of drinking are, generally speaking, incentives to drink because of an awareness of what those benefits are, it is important to distinguish between disincentives and harms: many drinkers are ignorant of the harmful consequences of alcohol misuse.

Disincentives

Some people are not interested in alcohol, some dislike the psychological response, some abstain for religious or philosophical reasons, because of the cost, or because they are too busy. Incipient awareness that alcohol is harming

Table 8.3. *Problems relating to intoxication*

Social problems	Psychological problems	Physical problems
Family arguments	Insomnia	Hepatitis
Domestic violence	Depression	Gastritis
Child neglect/abuse	Anxiety	Pancreatitis
Domestic accidents	Amnesia	Gout
Absenteeism from work	Attempted suicide	Cardiac arrythmias
Accidents at work	Suicide	Accidents
Inefficient work		Trauma
Public drunkeness		Strokes
Public aggression		Alcohol poisoning
Football hooliganism		Failure to take
Criminal damage		prescribed medication
		Impotence
Burglary		Fetal damage
Assault		
Homicide		
Drinking and driving		
Taking and driving away		
Sexually deviant acts		
Unwanted pregnancy		

This list of problems is also an indication of the ways in which alcohol presents to the practitioner.

them and is affecting their work, family life, or sporting prowess are other disincentives.

Harms

The harms of alcohol are best divided into those that relate to intoxication and those that relate to regular heavy drinking, though there is some overlap.

Acute intoxication (see Table 8.3)   These effects are usually obvious and correspond to those of an acute confusional state (see Section 7.2). Mood may vary from aggressiveness to acute depression. Activity varies from restless hyperactivity to drowsiness and eventually coma.

Motor co-ordination becomes seriously impaired when blood levels of 80 mg/dl are reached (after *c.* 4 units of alcohol have been consumed) and

Table 8.4.   *Problems relating to regular heavy drinking*

Social problems	Psychological problems	Physical problems
Family problems	Insomnia	Fatty liver
Divorce	Depression	Hepatitis
Homelessness	Anxiety	Cirrhosis
Work difficulties	Attempted suicide	Liver cancer
Unemployment	Suicide	Gastritis
Financial difficulties	Changes in personality	Pancreatitis
Fraud	Amnesia	Cancer of mouth,
Debt	Delirium tremens	pharynx, larynx,
Vagrancy	Withdrawal fits	oesophagus
Habitual convictions	Hallucinosis	Cancer of breast (?)
for drunkenness	Dementia	Cancer of colon (?)
	Gambling	Nutritional deficiencies
	Misuse of other drugs	Obesity
		Diabetes
		Cardiomyopathy
		Raised blood pressure
		Strokes
		Brain damage
		Neuropathy
		Myopathy
		Sexual dysfunction
		Infertility
		Fetal damage
		Haemopoietic toxicity
		Reactions with other drugs

This list of problems is also an indication of the ways in which alcohol problems present to the practitioner.

it may be dangerous to drive a motor vehicle or operate machinery at levels considerably below this point (for definition of the term unit see p. 359).

It is tempting to assume that everyone who smells of alcohol and is confused must be intoxicated, but we need to remember that confusion may also be caused by head injury (e.g. following a road traffic accident), drugs (which are often taken with alcohol in attempts at suicide), or any of the other physical causes of acute organic brain syndromes listed in Section 7.2).

Estimation of the blood alcohol level, together with drug screening and other relevant tests, may need to be carried out.

Chronic alcoholism (see Table 8.4)   Regular drinkers find their tolerance for alcohol increasing steadily until a threshold is reached beyond which tolerance falls off. When they pass this point people whose drinking was not seriously affecting their life may go rapidly downhill, memory lapses become frequent, intoxication obvious, work is seriously affected, concentration and judgement impaired. If drinking continues, gradual deterioration into a chronic organic dementia (see Section 7.2) may occur. Some permanent damage to the brain is likely.

If drinking is stopped abruptly, as when an acute illness prevents a heavy drinker from getting to the pub, the patient will suffer acute withdrawal symptoms. In minor form these consist of nausea, restlessness, and tremor ('the shakes') but severe acute delirium (delirium tremens — the 'DTs') may result and the patient may suffer from terrifying hallucinations. The condition is a serious one and can end in circulatory collapse and death. All such cases require treatment in hospital as a matter of urgency. *Grand mal* fits can also follow withdrawal of alcohol.

Alcoholic hallucinosis may be the presenting symptom in a person who has no other impairment of mental functioning. Auditory hallucinations in which voices are heard talking about the patient, often in obscene language, are the most common, although tactile hallucinations may occur and should lead us to suspect the presence of alcoholic neuritis.

Hallucinations may be accompanied by paranoid delusions, though these can also occur on their own. Most typically these are delusions of jealousy, and unjust accusations may be made against the patient's spouse. Serious physical abuse is not uncommon.

The neurological effects of alcoholism include nystagmus, incoordination, memory loss, paraesthesiae, numbness in the extremities, squints, and a variety of other symptoms, details of which will be found in textbooks of neurology. Like the other signs of organic damage, their effects are often permanent. So, too, is alcoholic cirrhosis of the liver. Fortunately, abnormal liver-function tests which precede this are usually reversible and can be used to convince the patient of the importance of abstinence.

The role of the general practitioner

Alcohol as a risk factor

If the problems relating to alcohol misuse are to be grasped in general practice, the consumption of alcohol needs to be regarded as a risk factor in the same way as we already regard smoking, raised blood pressure, and raised serum cholesterol. This implies that GPs need to know about the alcohol consumption of all their adult patients, and this can be helped by having an identified space on every patient's summary card for dated entries regarding alcohol consumption so that prevention can be included in our management. Contributing factors, such as those mentioned at the start of the chapter, can help to identify those most at risk. Conditions such as pregnancy, epilepsy, diabetes, and hypertension increase the patient's physical vulnerability and make it all the more important for members of the primary care team to enquire into the patient's consumption of alcohol.

At this point it may be helpful to re-read the section on 'Helping people to change' (p. 111).

Education and treatment

As already suggested, once an alcohol problem is identified, one of the main roles of general practitioners is educational: many patients are not aware that they have a problem; others are aware, but see no advantage in drinking less. By explaining the balance sheet to patients, doctors can demonstrate the need for change. Where patients can see an advantage in drinking less, but think it looks too difficult, GPs will need to stress the negative side of the balance sheet and also to suggest ways in which the patient can cut down consumption.

Patients are often convinced that tranquillizers will help save them from drinking, but they need to be told that one of the main actions of tranquillizers is to dampen down critical thought and reduce self-reliance. The result is that if they take them, they are more, not less, likely to drink.

Eliciting information

A vital part of educating patients about alcohol is the process of eliciting information about drinking behaviour. It is important to emphasize that history-taking and clinical investigation are better at case-finding than blood tests. Taking a history and asking questions provides information for the doctor, but, more important, clarifies patients' thoughts about themselves, their family, and their social milieu.

Patients may be identified as being heavy drinkers by the use of screening questions such as those suggested by Wiseman.[7]

'How often do you drink?'

'How many drinks do you have in a day when you drink?'

'How many drinks per week do you have?'

'How often do you drink any of the following or more in one day?
   seven pints of beer or cider
   two bottles of wine
   one bottle of sherry, port, or martini; or half a bottle of gin, whisky, rum,
      brandy, or vodka.'

The figures in the last question are set deliberately high, but can be lowered progressively as required. This approach has the effect of reassuring the patient and encouraging frankness.

Questionnaires such as the 'CAGE' (Table 8.5) will also identify a high proportion of patients misusing alcohol.

Table 8.5.   *CAGE.*

1. Have you ever felt you should CUT down on your drinking?
2. Have you ever been ANNOYED about and critical of your drinking?
3. Have you ever felt GUILTY about your drinking?
4. Do you drink in the morning? (EYE opener)

The quantity drunk is usually measured in units, where one unit equals ½ pint normal beer; ¼ pint strong beer; one measure of spirit; one measure of sherry, port, or martini; one glass of wine (seven glasses equals one bottle).

Men who drink more than 21 units/wk and women who drink more than 14 units/wk (or who give two or more positive answers to 'CAGE') deserve further history-taking, examination, and investigation. Filling-in a questionnaire, or keeping a drinking diary for a week, provides the patient with some objective evidence of their use of alcohol.

History-taking should then seek to establish where, and how, alcohol misuse was learnt. The pattern of drinking in the patient's family of origin may be significant, together with the drinking pattern and frequency in the current family. An enquiry should be made into the possible harms that alcohol may be causing the patient and their family. It helps if the patient can be induced to ask about these; a lecture from the doctor may simply lower the patient's self-esteem.

Finally, the patient should be encouraged to examine the reasons for continuing to misuse alcohol and to discuss solutions so far attempted.

It is traditionally believed that people who abuse alcohol have a tendency to lie, but this has not been confirmed by research. Most people underestimate their consumption of alcohol, but thorough history-taking, together with good doctor–patient interaction, can usually overcome this tendency. If patients seem to underestimate the effects of alcohol on their lives, it may be counter-productive to confront them directly. It is better to use such statements as 'I am worried even if you are not', 'I am sorry, I can't share your views'. At all times it is best to avoid condemnation or threat, however disguised.

It is helpful to take stock often, and summarize what has been discussed to date. The doctor may restate the position, using the patient's words where possible. 'You were concerned about the effect of drinking on your wife' . . . 'You were worried about your gamma GTs' . . . 'You said you really wanted to change' . . . . If the patient has expressed negative thoughts these should be included and acknowledged.

In this way the doctors may be able to reassure patients, and increase their self-esteem and awareness of the situation. Only then will it be appropriate to discuss the direction of change: 'What do you think you can do?'

Whatever the doctor's preferred route, it is helpful to discuss several alternatives. Many drinkers will know that abstention would be the best solution. Some will prefer to try a period of abstention followed by controlled drinking; some will opt for a trial period of controlled drinking. Different solutions will tend to suit different groups. For instance, the most successful route for young, male, unmarried, and less severely dependent drinkers is likely to be controlled drinking.

Goals

Controlled drinking
Patients should set themselves feasible goals.

Mr A is a widower, aged 70, with no children or family nearby. His only social occupation or contact with people is the pub, where he has been drinking about eight pints of beer a day. His liver is damaged and so probably is his brain, so abstinence might be a recommended medical solution. However, he and his GP agree that there would be nothing left for him to live for without the pub. A few months later, he drinks eight pints of shandy a day and is a little fitter. The doctor sees him regularly to encourage him to keep to this regime.

It is best to aim for specific short-term goals at first rather than general long-term ones, as this allows the patient to concentrate on the short term and gain positive reinforcement from a sense of achievement. Under pressure, it may be necessary to focus on one day or even one hour at a time. A short-term goal could be a week's abstinence, a night at the pub taking soft drinks only, or simply having the ability to say 'no' to one offered drink.

The diary may have indicated risky circumstances to the patient which have, in the past, led him into trouble, such as particular pubs, bars, clubs, particular times of day or days of the week, particular companions, or certain states of mind.

Relapse often occurs because patients take unnecessary risks by placing themselves in situations regularly associated with heavy drinking in the past.

Patients need to learn to avoid these situations, especially early on, and to confine their drinking to places where it is easier to practise moderation. If difficult situations are unavoidable, the risk needs to be recognized and extra care taken.

Advice on how to consume less alcohol can often be helpful. The following can be adopted as personal rules:

- Dilute alcoholic drinks.

- Take smaller sips.

- Take less into the mouth and less often.

- Occupy yourself. Do something else enjoyable while drinking, as this will help distract attention from the drink, for example listen to music, watch darts, make conversation.

- Change the drink. Changing the type of drink can help break old habits and reduce the amount of alcohol.

- Drink for the taste. Drink more slowly and enjoy the flavour.

- Imitate the slow drinker. Try and identify someone in the group who is drinking slowly, and become their shadow, not picking up the glass until they do.

- Avoid rounds. This can be done by buying your own drink, or by buying one round and then going solo. It is possible not to buy for oneself, or to buy a non-alcoholic drink, when one's turn comes.

- Eating. Drinking with a meal slows down the absorption of alcohol, and may reduce the amount drunk. Have a separate glass and a jug of water on the table.

- Days of rest. Try to abstain from alcohol for at least one or two days a week.

- Start later in the day.

- Learn to refuse drinks. 'No thanks, I'm cutting down', or 'not tonight'.

Total abstinence

The temptation of friends in the club or pub, or the strength of conditioning in some situations, may mean that if the patient has decided on abstinence, then life needs to be reshaped. Perhaps the most difficult problem is to find alternative uses for time, and to find alternative sources of pleasure and enjoyment. Some will restructure their lives around Alcoholics Anonymous and, indeed, involvement in AA can become as addictive as alcohol. Most will need encouragement and a supply of imaginative ideas to fill the gap. Using counsellors from community alcohol teams or alcohol community services may be helpful. In dealing with alcohol problems, it is vital to encourage the patient's autonomy and self-esteem. Dependence on alcohol must be replaced by a greater degree of self-reliance.

Follow-up

Whatever the route chosen by the patient, offers of follow-up are not only helpful, but also express the interest of the doctor. Some doctors find a contract helpful at this stage. Agreement may be reached about follow-up, including positive recall, continuing the alcohol diary, and regular investigations such as gamma GTs, MCVs and blood alcohol levels, or breathalysing the patient at every consultation. The breathalyser is a useful piece of equipment in any GPs surgery. The aura of optimism, positivism, and enthusiasm by the doctor is catching and effective.

Relapse

If the doctor can accept relapse as natural and not as failure, it will help the patient. If it can be seen as a chance for the patient to learn something which can be used to change the balance, it will be even more helpful. It is wise to pre-empt the feelings of loss of self-efficacy and to concentrate on achievements made before the relapse.

The family

The family may be the most important determinant in maintaining the drinking habit.

Mr B had learnt to drink with 'the boys' before he got married. He occasionally called into the pub on his way home. During his wife's first pregnancy, Mrs B became absorbed with the baby inside her and gave less time and love to Mr B, who spent more time at the pub. When he arrived home she nagged him, so he began to delay coming home and drank a little more on the way.

Many spouses collude and alternate between the role of rescuer and victim.

Mrs C often phoned her husband's office when he had a hangover, saying that the car wouldn't start, or that he had flu, when, in fact, the hangover was being treated with early morning brandies.

Suffering and abuse borne by the family as a result of alcohol misuse and depression may be alleviated by individual support. However, the closer and more complex the family system, the harder it is to unlock the harmful cycles of behaviour without seeing the family as a whole. Members of the family can be involved to clarify the extent of the harms, to help them understand their role in the 'system', and to recruit their support for the abuser.

Patient literature

The written word is of value in reinforcing advice, and informing the patient more fully. Self-help manuals for some may be an alternative to professional advice. The Health Education Council's *That's the limit* booklet and the Scottish Health Education Group's *Drams Pack* are particularly good in supplementing the consultation. There are other books for further reading by patients, and examples are listed at the end of this section.

Tobacco

Given agreement that all tobacco-smoking is undesirable, it should be easier to help people to stop smoking than to wean them off alcohol, especially as the benefits of smoking are less obvious. But is it?

Learning to smoke

The mean age of starting to smoke is 12. It is a learnt behaviour, and the majority of first cigarettes induce nausea. It requires practice to develop tolerance and to acquire taste. Rewards seem to be the emulation of adulthood, the joy of risk-taking, and appearing to be tough and sophisticated. The smoking habits of parents and peers are the most important determinants of whether young people learn and continue to smoke. It is best never to start!

Maintenance of the habit

Cost

Any abrupt increase in cost, usually through taxation, does decrease the total consumption of cigarettes for a while and encourages some smokers to quit, although a considerable number of these will recommence.

Social and cultural

There is an association between smoking and drinking alcohol. There is also an association with sexual activity. In a sample of teenagers in 1985, 90 per cent of teenage girls who smoked more than 20 cigarettes a day had had sexual intercourse, as against 16 per cent of the rest of the sample.[1]

Personality—vulnerability to psychiatric disorder

Although extroverts tend to smoke more than introverts, there is no other demonstrable association with personality.

Patients diagnosed as having schizophrenia are said to smoke more than others, but the reasons for this association are not clear.[2]

The balance sheet

Benefits and incentives

Once the habit is established, smoking is used to change mood and to relieve withdrawal symptoms. Nicotine can both stimulate and depress mental function, depending on the person, the situation, and the timing. It can be used to relieve anxiety and depression and to stimulate thought and alertness. The effect on the brain is rapid—probably within 30 seconds—and is biphasic.

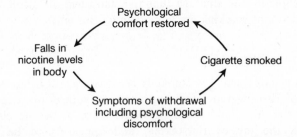

Fig. 8.1.   The regulation of blood nicotine level in the smoker.

There is evidence that tobacco is smoked to keep the nicotine level in the blood reasonably constant (Fig. 8.1). If the tobacco is altered so that it gives less nicotine, people either inhale more or smoke more cigarettes to achieve the same effect.[3] Withdrawal symptoms, which include anxiety, restlessness, agitation, irritability, sweating, and insomnia, are maximal between 24 and 48 hours after the last cigarette and may continue for up to a year. However, some people stop smoking and have no apparent withdrawal symptoms even after a lifetime's habit.

Apart from the more conscious 'pleasures' of smoking, people continue to smoke for less obvious reasons. The process of getting a cigarette, filling up a pipe, and lighting up, are often conditioned by circumstances and events, so that people find themselves with a cigarette in their mouth without any conscious awareness of having made a decision to smoke. The act also provides occupation for the hands, and, for some people, is an adult form of thumb-sucking.

Harms and disincentives

For young people, most of the harm of smoking is seen to be in the distant future; fear is not always a good disincentive—it may even be counter-productive, causing anxiety which increases the desire for a cigarette. Many people, because of the withdrawal symptoms, do not immediately feel fitter if they stop smoking. Moreover, for some smokers, coughing may be more troublesome for a while after stopping, and initially weight may be gained.

Helping people to stop smoking

Most people who continue to smoke have been told of the dangers and cost of continuing, but, to reduce cognitive dissonance, they erect defences against admitting the danger (see p. 23). Questionnaires and research suggest that they have modified their beliefs, and selectively remember information which supports the argument on the side of continuing to smoke.[4] While there is increasing knowledge in the population as a whole about the dangers of smoking, smokers find it harder than non-smokers to believe that giving up can improve their health. A major difficulty is that the chief reward, better health and increased longevity, may be 40 years away, while the pleasure is immediate. The fact that smokers are now in a minority may help to tip the scales away from smoking.

The doctor's role

The pathway to stopping smoking is similar to that leading to drinking less alcohol:

- awareness that there is a problem;
- deciding to act;
- implementing the decision.

The awareness that there is a problem and deciding to act

The patient alone can make the decision to stop smoking. The doctor's role is to ask questions that focus attention on the dangers and provide knowledge and education. This education is important to counteract the effects of cognitive dissonance. It may be helpful to calculate the possible financial savings of stopping smoking, and to fantasize about how the money could otherwise be used. Objective feedback can be given to the patient in primary care by using a peak expiratory flow meter, or breath carbon monoxide analyser.

Implementing the decision

Stopping smoking will enhance self-esteem, be rewarded by the approval of friends and relations, and will save money. These gains need to be balanced against the patient's perception of the efficacy of their own willpower in the battle to give up.

The majority who succeed in stopping do so abruptly. A tobacco-related illness, such as a chest infection, or the development of ischaemic heart disease will often act as a spur. Those who cannot stop abruptly may be helped by structuring a slower withdrawal plan.

- Stopping for one day a week, increasing to two days a week, and so on.

- Reducing the daily consumption on a fixed and written plan.

- Creating no-smoking zones and times for themselves, and gradually extending these.

It is helpful to counter the difficulties that may be met during withdrawal.

- The symptoms may be modified by the use of nicotine-containing chewing-gum.

- Relaxation techniques may help some people, and may be taught individually, in a group, or by using an audio-cassette.

- Adopting a positive emphasis on health by giving advice on increasing the amount of exercise.

- Warning of the possibility of weight gain (which does happen to some people over the first few months) and giving advice about a healthy diet.

- Discussing the inappropriateness of drinking more alcohol.

- Discussing cues for smoking which need to be avoided, such as smoking areas in public places, and places associated with smoking, e.g. pubs.

It is easier to stop at the same time as a consort and with the aid of the family. Patients may make contracts with themselves about rewards, and sponsorships seem helpful, at least in the short term. Offers of follow-up by the doctor can be an added incentive.[6]

Drugs
The provision of tranquillizers only substitutes one habit for another. Similarly, antidepressants should be used to treat depression but not to treat smoking. Nicotine (as in Nicorette chewing-gum) seems, on balance, to be helpful to some people.[7]

Evaluation of success in smoking prevention

About a third of people who have ever smoked have stopped, although some have relapsed. Eighty to ninety per cent of smokers say that they would like to quit and consider their doctor as an appropriate person to help them. In their pioneer research, Russell *et al.*[8] demonstrated that general practitioners using brief advice (two minutes) helped one in five of their patients to stop smoking in a year. Richmond and co-workers helped smokers to stop by using a more intensive initial programme and offering five follow-up visits over six months. They evaluated the effect at three years and found that one in three had stopped.[9]

Other drugs

By comparison with alcohol and tobacco, abuse of other drugs is relatively rare. Even so, abuse of proscribed, as opposed to prescribed, drugs looms large in the public imagination and many parents live in fear that their rebellious adolescents will become 'junkies'. Part of the reason for this fear arises from the widespread use of cannabis among young people. Although relatively harmless (but see Anderssen *et al.*[1]), this drug is illegal, and youngsters who are inducted into its use may not see it as very different from more seriously addictive drugs which are likely to be purveyed by the same network of pushers. Young people who are experimenting with drugs commonly find themselves offered cannabis, cocaine, and heroin, but only a small proportion become seriously addicted. Even so, the number of addicts has been growing in recent years and there are no grounds for complacency.

Non-prescribed drugs

Cannabis ('pot', 'grass', 'marijuanha', 'ganja', 'kif', 'dagga', or 'hashish') Cannabis is the raw form of tetrahydrocannabinol. It is usually taken by inhalation from cigarettes, but can also be absorbed from the intestine if taken by mouth.

Reactions vary greatly and are influenced by the circumstances in which the drug is taken. Some people become euphoric and giggly, others detached and abstracted. Perceptual changes include increased vividness and intensity of colours, and distortions of size and time similar to, but less intense than, those evoked by LSD. Some people have feelings of inspiration, as if they had discovered an important truth, although they may have difficulty in describing just what this is. Memory and concentration may be impaired, and this makes it dangerous to drive or operate machinery while under the influence of cannabis. 'Bad trips' may occur, unpleasant experiences which occasionally become terrifying, but these are not as common as with LSD.

There is sometimes reddening of conjunctivae, unsteadiness, and tachycardia, and habitual users may get a smoker's cough or become lethargic and ineffective.

Withdrawal of the drug may give rise to depression, anxiety, tremor, and insomnia, but these do not amount to physical dependence or reach the severity seen after withdrawal of 'hard' drugs.

Although it is likely that cannabis does no more harm than alcohol or tobacco, this is no reason to encourage its use. Patients may need to be warned of its possible damaging effects if taken habitually, and those who get the habit should be persuaded to give it up. Emotional support will help them to tolerate withdrawal.

Lysergic acid diethylamide (LSD, 'acid')

LSD is similar in many respects to cannabis, but its effects on perception are much more pronounced and associated with a greater risk of psychosis. Given by mouth or by injection, it may produce hallucinatory experiences or delusions. Although these symptoms usually disappear within 12 hours, they occasionally persist or may return in 'flashbacks' at some future date— particularly under the influence of cannabis. 'Bad trips' occasionally give rise to suicide attempts and, although some take the drug for its supposed 'inspirational' effects, most do not find the experience particularly pleasant. Consequently, although young people may experiment with LSD or with hallucinogenic mushrooms, if available to them, few make it a habit.

Cocaine ('smack' is a mixture of cocaine and sodium bicarbonate)

Cocaine has become fashionable in recent years in certain circles, and is a drug of addiction. It can be sniffed, smoked, swallowed, or injected, when it produces a euphoric mood and stimulation of the central nervous system which sometimes leads to panic. Depression and fatigue follow as the drug wears off. Restlessness and paranoid irritability may follow regular use. Its only clinical use is for topical local anaesthesia. It adds nothing to morphine and diamorphine as a treatment for chronic cancer pain and can be omitted from the 'Brompton Cocktail'.

Inhalants

Glue-sniffing is a popular form of intoxication in some youngsters. It is usually harmless, but accidents can happen, e.g. when a child inhales the glue with a plastic bag over the head. Most solvents such as carbon tetrachloride and methyl chloroform (Thawpit) are toxic to the liver, and butane gas can cause cardiac arrest.

Morphine and diamorphine (heroin, 'snow')

These are the most dangerous of opiate drugs. Given by mouth or by intravenous injection, they produce states of euphoria and detachment which last for up to six hours. Tolerance of these drugs soon develops and addicts then require larger and larger doses in order to maintain the effects. Physical pain is relieved and this makes them extremely valuable in the treatment of advanced cancer and transient medical and surgical conditions which cause severe pain. Cancer patients for whom these drugs are sometimes prescribed regularly, and at high dosage, rarely show the antisocial behaviour and physical dependence which is often associated with addiction. This suggests that it is the interaction of the drug with other factors which explains many of the worst features of opiate abuse.

A main cause of opiate dependence is the severe symptoms which may occur when the drug is withdrawn. Intense craving for the drug, along with restlessness, streaming nose, salivation, vomiting, and stomach cramps are common and may continue for several days.

Because the effects of the drug are more intense when it is given by intravenous injection (main-lining), addicts are at risk for venous thrombosis, hepatitis B, AIDS, and pyaemia. The risk is greater if, as is usually the case, the drug itself is impure (cut).

Any competent importer can transform morphine to heroin and, since the latter is more powerful, most illegal opiate is sold as heroin. It is very expensive and since few addicts have either a steady job or a private income, they are likely to engage in criminal activities in order to maintain their addiction. Thieving, prostitution, and drug pedalling are the most common methods, and these further complicate the life of the addict.

Quite apart from the dangers of sharing needles for injections, many addicts neglect their health. Because opiates dull the appetite, addicts may choose to use their income on drugs rather than food. They become susceptible to a wide range of minor infections and other ailments. They tend to lie and to cheat their family and friends in order to obtain money for drugs. Sooner or later this leaves them without emotional support.

Most addicts are vulnerable people and this drives them further into the drug trap. Lacking any hope of a worthwhile life without drugs, they settle for a twilight existence. If they find themselves without supplies, they may commit suicide or engage in other reckless or dangerous activities.

Members of the primary care team (PCT) have important roles to play in the prevention of opiate abuse. They can reduce the risk of people becoming addicts by not using opiates in people with non-fatal conditions which produce chronic pain. People with post-herpetic neuralgia or arthritic conditions are at special risk. Addicts commonly complain to doctors of bodily pain and it is not always easy to know whether they are malingering or not. Some become addicts as a result of injudicious treatments.

Young people should be warned of the dangers of 'experimenting' with hard drugs, but such injunctions lose credibility and are likely to be dismissed as the hypocritical mouthings of a killjoy older generation if they become part of a blanket condemnation of all drugs, hard or soft.

Abuse of prescribed drugs

Much drug abuse is iatrogenic. Even people who abuse hard drugs often take other drugs as well, and many of these are obtained on medical prescription, forged or real, or are stolen from chemists' shops.

Almost anything can be abused, but the most common are the commonly prescribed psychotropic drugs.

Benzodiazepines

The withdrawal effects of benzodiazepines (anxiety, tremor, sweating, and other sympathomimetic symptoms) are often the same as the symptoms for which the drug was taken in the first place, and this leads many patients to continue to take these drugs long after their clinical indication is past (see Section 4.7).

Two groups of drugs which are now seldom prescribed, but which remain popular among drug abusers, are the amphetamines and the barbiturates.

Amphetamines ('speed', 'uppers')

Amphetamines are taken for their euphoriant effect. They produce hyper-alertness and enable people to keep awake through the night, hence their popularity among all-night musicians. A generation of doctors who grew up using amphetamines to get them through their exams or to reduce weight (because of their effects on appetite) tend to dismiss their dangers. But, like harder drugs, their abuse by vulnerable individuals, and the uncontrolled circumstances under which they are often taken, makes them a menace.

Given by mouth, amphetamines can cause delirium or paranoid psychosis, but the risk is very much greater when they are sniffed up the nose or dissolved and injected by 'speed-freaks'. It is now generally agreed that the dangers of amphetamines outweigh their clinical usefulness, and their only indication today is in the treatment of narcolepsy and (for short periods only) in the management of hyperactive children.

Barbiturates

The benzodiazepines have replaced the barbiturates as the favoured hypnotic and minor tranquillizer because of their relative safety. Barbiturates have a depressant effect on the respiratory centres which makes them dangerous in overdose, and for many years they were a common cause of death. Because they are potentiated by alcohol and because the borderline between therapeutic and toxic effects is not very wide, accidental overdosage can easily occur.

They are still widely used by drug abusers in an uncontrolled way with a hotchpotch of other drugs, many of which are likely to interact with barbiturates.

Abrupt withdrawal of barbiturates can trigger *grand mal* attacks, along with the anxiety, tremor, insomnia, dizziness, and nausea which are the more usual withdrawal symptoms. Their only acceptable indications today are for anaesthetic use, epilepsy, or occasional severe insomnia.

Other drugs which are addictive and have become widely abused in recent years are dipipanone (Diconal), methadone, pethidine, phenazocine (Narphen), buprenorphine (Temgesic), and dextromoramide (Palfium). All of these, except buprenorphine, are narcotic analgesics which, like morphine, diamorphine, and cocaine, are Class A drugs under the Misuse of Drugs Act 1977. GPs are required by law to notify the Chief Medical Officer about any patient whom they suspect to be addicted to one of these drugs. Less addictive, but none the less subject to abuse, are codeine, pholcodine, methylphenidate (Ritalin), and dexamphetamine (Dexedrine) alone or with amphetamine (Durophet).

Drug-induced psychoses

The symptoms of the psychoses induced by drugs are varied and are sometimes indistinguishable from acute schizophrenia and manic-depressive psychosis. More often, however, they cause acute confusional states (see Section 7.2). These tend to be florid and associated with acute emotional outbursts. The prognosis is usually good if the drug is discontinued, although this is not invariably the case, and occasionally a drug may trigger a true schizophrenic or manic illness.

Amphetamine abuse seems most prone to cause paranoid psychoses, and cocaine abuse may cause cuaneous hallucinations (e.g. of insects crawling under the skin). These may reflect paraesthesiae and other direct effects upon the peripheral nerves.

The treatment of drug abuse

This stands or falls on the motivation of the patient and this, in turn, may depend on the confidence and trust which he or she feels towards the PCT. It is a good sign if patients initiate contact by asking us to help them to get off the drug. More often we learn of the addiction indirectly — because they seek help for the treatment of side-effects, or because a friend or relative calls us in.

In general, the same principles apply to the management of the abuse of other drugs as to alcohol and tobacco.

Careful analysis of the underlying causes of the drug abuse is crucial. If the drug is being taken for social reasons, or is part of the expected behaviour of a group of friends, then it will be wise for the patient to cut off links with this group. If the drug is used to treat depression or some other psychiatric problem, then attention should be directed to alternative methods of treatment. If it is an escape from intolerable life circumstances, then the circumstances may need to change if the drug is to be stopped.

If the patient has a personality disorder, complete abstinence is unlikely to be achieved, but it may be possible to persuade the patient to cut down or to switch to some less harmful type of escape.

In some cases the original cause of the addiction has ceased, but the abuse has become habitual and self-perpetuating. Such cases hold out the least hope of cure, and complete abstinence should be the aim.

Martin[2] has recently outlined the approach of his practice to managing long-term dependence in general practice and has defined the aims as follows:

● to enable dependent patients to develop some social stability by withdrawing from the chaotic street market for drugs;

● to enable these patients immediately to withdraw from illegal activities such as drug-dealing to pay for their own drugs;

● to develop a secure and trusting relationship with their family doctor where they accept that the only reason they will be rejected from the list is for overt aggression towards the doctor, staff, or other patients;

● to make considered plans for the major changes in their social life needed if they are to attempt narcotic withdrawal;

● to reduce drug-taking;

● to accept that many patients have several dry runs before they manage to withdraw from dependency (if this occurs, the whole process starts again; the patient is not rejected);

● to recruit what social service help is available to support these patients in a major life upheaval.

This article makes helpful reading to anyone facing this problem in general practice. In particular, Martin emphasizes the support partners need to give each other if one of them is involved in treating a drug addict, and the importance of operating an agreed policy within the practice, whereby one partner is responsible for the management of any individual patient.

In instituting treatment we have five alternatives:

(1) stop the drug and provide close social and emotional support through the period of withdrawal;

(2) rapidly taper the drug and stop it over 2–3 days, using other drugs to ameliorate withdrawal symptoms;

(3) switch from the drug of abuse to another less dangerous alternative as a first step in stopping all drugs;

(4) withdraw the drug gradually;

(5) maintain the patient without a formally agreed time limit on a prescribed dose of a drug, usually methadone.

Every effort should be made to wean the patient off all addictive drugs permanently. How to achieve the goal of getting such patients completely off their drugs will depend partly on the drug being used, and partly on the patient.

If hard drugs are being used and the patient is willing to co-operate, alternatives (2) and (3) are the best choice, especially if a regional drug unit is available to give support. Withdrawal effects of opiates can be reduced by regular sedation with diazepam. Having said this, we need to be realistic in our approach, bearing in mind that many drug addicts will not attend a drug unit and that the PCT may be the only group of professionals that the addict is prepared to trust, and hence to negotiate with.

The fifth alternative, that of maintaining the patient permanently on a prescribed dose of the drug, on the grounds that it is wiser for the doctor to accept less than the optimum but retain a measure of control over the dosage level, has disadvantages and advantages. The control may be spurious, patients obtaining additional prescriptions elsewhere, and some will sell the drug which has been prescribed, either for cash, or to obtain a more harmful alternative. However, some patients who are not motivated to give up may do well on this regime. They will not have to steal to maintain their habit and they will not have to be in contact with the street scene. Such patients can keep a full-time job, avoid contact with the law, and do not seem to need to increase their dose. Initially they are best seen by the same doctor twice weekly for supervision and prescriptions, but as trust grows they need to be seen less often. Relapses can be seen as learning events and, with time, lifestyle issues can be tackled and drug reduction begun.

Social support for patients is all important and most patients should be advised to join a support group. Some of these are run by local psychiatric services, others by voluntary bodies such as Narcotics Anonymous (for hard-drug abusers) and Tranx (for those who need help in getting off tranquillizers). The Standing Conference on Drug Abuse (SCODA), provide details about local services. Further information about these organizations are given in Appendix II.

Families, too, need our support, and there are some organizations which enable the wives and parents of addicts to support each other (e.g. Families Anonymous).

The PCT may find it advisable to discourage the family from financially sponsoring the addiction. If the addict then transgresses the law, it is his or her responsibility, not theirs. Addicts usually know the probable outcome of their actions, but it is sometimes possible to take advantage of some intercurrent illness or event (such as a frightening encounter with the law)

374 *The functional disorders*

to bring home to them the dangers of their current course. Since most drugs impair the ability to drive or operate machinery, patients should be warned and informed that the law demands that they return their driving licence.

The advisability and implications of having a blood test for AIDS, other venereal infections, hepatitis B, and for other drugs should be discussed with the addict, especially if the intravenous route is being used to administer the drug.

References

Alcohol

1. Vaillant, G. (1983). *The natural history of alcoholism*. Harvard University Press, London.
2. Russell, M. A. H., Wilson, C., Taylor, C., and Baker, C. D. (1979). Effect of general practitioners' advice against smoking. *Br. Med. J.* **2**, 231-5
3. Heather, N., Campion, P. R., Neville, R. G., and Maccade, D. (1982). Evaluation of a controlled drinking minimal interventions for problem drinkers in general practice (the Drams Scheme). *J. R. Coll. Gen. Pract.* **37**, 358-63.
4. Royal College of General Practitioners (1984). *Alcohol—a balanced view*. Report from General Practice, No. 24.
5. Marmot, M. G., Rose, G., and Shipley, M. S. (1981). Alcohol and mortality. U-shaped curve. *Lancet* **1**, 580-3.
6. Shaper, A. G., Phillips, A. N., Pocock, S. J., and Walker, M. (1987). Alcohol and ischaemic heart disease in middle-aged British men. *Br. Med. J.* **294**, 733-8.
7. Wiseman, S. M., McCarthy, S. N., and Mitcheson, M. S. (1986). Assessment of drinking patterns in general practice. *J. R. Coll. Gen. Pract.* **279**.

Tobacco

1. Russell, M. A. H. (1971). Cigarette smoking: natural history of a dependence disorder. *Br. J. Med. Psychol.* **44**, 1-16.
2. Cherry, N. and Kiernan, K. (1976). Personality scores and smoking behaviour. *Br. J. Prevent. Soc. Med.* **30**, 123-31.
3. Stepney, R. (1980). Cigarette consumption and nicotine delivery. *Br. J. Add.* **75**, (1), 1181-8.
4. Spelman, M. S. and Ley, P. (1960). Knowledge of lung cancer and smoking habits. *Br. J. Soc. Clin. Psychol.* **5**, 207-10.
5. Eiser, J. R., Sutton, S. R., and Wober, M. (1977). Smokers, non smokers and the attribution of addiction. *Br. J. Soc. Clin. Psychol.* **16**, 329-36.
6. Marshall, A. and Raw, M. (1985). Nicotine chewing gum in general practice: effect of follow up appointments. *Br. Med. J.* **290**, 1397-8.
7. Russell, M. A. H. Merriman, R., Stapleton, J., and Taylor, W. (1983). Effect of nicotine chewing gum as an adjunct to general practitioners' advice against smoking. *Br. Med. J.* **287**, 1782-5.
8. Russell, M. A. H., Wilson, C., Taylor, C., and Baker, C. D. (1979). Effect of general practitiones' advice against smoking. *Br. Med. J.* **279** (2), 231-5.

9. Richmond, R. L., Austin, A., and Webster, I. W. (1986). Three-year evaluation of a programme by general practioners to help patients to stop smoking. *Br. Med. J.* **292**, 803–6.

Other drugs

1. Andreassen S., Allebeck, P., Engström, A., and Rydberg, U. (1987). Cannabis and schizophrenia. *Lancet* **2**, 1483–6.
2. Martin, E. (1980). Managing drug addiction in general practice — the reality behind the guidelines. *J. R. Soc. Med.* **80**, 305–7.

Further reading

Alcohol

British Medical Journal (1982). Alcohol problems. *Br. Med. J.*, London.
Heather, N. and Robertson, I. (1985). *Problem drinking.* Penguin, Harmondsworth.
Royal College of General Practitioners (1958). *Alcohol — a balanced view.* R. Coll. Gen. Pract., London.

Reading list for patients

Chick, J. and Chick, J. (1984). *Drinking problems (patient handbook).* Churchill Livingstone, London.
Grant, M. (1984). *Same again (a guide to safer drinking).* Penguin, Harmondsworth.
Royal College of Psychiatrists (1986). *Alcohol — our favourite drug.* Tavistock, London.

Smoking

Ashton, H. and Sterney, R. (1982). *Psychology and pharmacology.* Tavistock, London.
Taylor, P. (1984). *Smoke rings. The politics of tobacco.* Bodley Head, London.

8.6 THE SCHIZOPHRENIAS

It is with deliberate intent that schizophrenia, the epitome of true madness, has been left to the end of this book for, whatever its prominence in mental hospitals, schizophrenia is an uncommon problem in general practice. Even so, most primary care teams (PCTs) will have a number of former or actively schizophrenic patients on their register (in ACM's practice the prevalence is 1.6/1000 patients) and the increasing trend towards community care is likely to lead to the discharge from hospital of more schizophrenics in the years to come. Even a few such patients can make a lot of work in any practice.

Despite much research, the root causes of schizophrenia remain obscure. Studies of identical twins, reared apart, indicate that genetic factors play an important role, but this accounts for only half of the variance found and there are good grounds for seeking elsewhere for other factors.

Life events undoubtedly play a part in triggering acute episodes, but the studies of Brown and Harris[1] suggest that most of these episodes would have occurred sooner or later. More lasting circumstances which are thought to contribute to the onset or recurrence of the condition are to be found in the family or home environment. Homes characterized by high 'expressed emotion' (intense expressions of anger, anxiety, criticism, or intrusive emotional pressure) are inimical to those vulnerable to schizophrenia.[2] Other family influences which have been thought to play a part in sowing the seeds of schizophrenia include parents who face the child with repeated mystifying or confusing 'double binds'; for instance, a mother who is constantly telling her child to grow up while punishing any expression of autonomy. Ronald Laing sees schizophrenia as 'a way of living in an unlivable situation'.[3,4] His accounts of the tortuous and mystifying communication patterns in the families of schizophrenics make fascinating reading, but most other psychiatrists find his attempts to explain schizophrenic symptoms unconvincing. Unfortunately, the public attention given to his writings has evoked reactions of anger and guilt among many parents of schizophrenic patients, which only adds to the burden of having a mentally ill son or daughter.

Diagnosis

The onset of schizophrenia commonly occurs in young adult life. There is often a history of the patient having become increasingly socially withdrawn ('schizoid') throughout adolescence and few have close friends of either sex. Although the abrupt onset of bizarre symptoms may be alarming to the family, this type of onset carries a better prognosis than the insidious loss of motivation and emotion which is sometimes termed 'schizophrenia simplex'.

Diagnostic symptoms to look for are:

● ideas of influence or reference (delusions that people are influencing the patient's actions or referring to the patient behind his or her back);

● passivity feelings (unseen persons or forces are controlling or removing the patient's thoughts and behaviour, others can read the patient's thoughts);

- thought-stopping or blocking (sudden interruptions in the train of thought or speech, followed by silence, or the unexpected and illogical intrusion of a new train of thought—the so-called 'knight's move');

- incongruity of affect (the patient's non-verbal communication of mood—happiness, sadness, fear, etc. is out of keeping with the context of what is being said); this leads to lack of empathy between patient and doctor such that the doctor may feel that he or she is being laughed at;

- auditory hallucinations in the third person (patients hear voices speaking about them rather than to them);

- delusional perceptions in which a patient makes a false interpretation of a normal perception (e.g. the sun's rays reflected in a puddle mean that the end of the world has come).

Although there is a wide variety of bizarre and dramatic hallucinations and delusions which may occur in schizophrenia, the diagnosis is likely to be in doubt unless one or more of the above symptoms is present for more than a short period of time. Because of these diagnostic difficulties, and because of the serious implications of the diagnosis, it is wise to seek the opinion of a psychiatrist whenever this disorder is suspected.

Introspective adolescents sometimes worry about their thoughts and may fear that they are going mad. Obsessional thoughts and feelings, and recurrent mental images of sex or violence, may bear some superficial resemblance to schizophrenic thought disorders but lack the above features and can usually be dispelled by explanation and reassurance.

Other conditions which may resemble schizophrenia, and which need to be seriously considered in all cases, are mania, (see p. 348), drug abuse (see Section 8.5), and other organic conditions (see Section 7.2). Of these, the most difficult to distinguish are the psychoses caused by amphetamines and hallucinogenic drugs, which may have all the features of schizophrenia except that they usually resolve when the drug is discontinued. Affective and organic disorders seldom show the diagnostic features listed above, and have their own distinctive characters.

Following the initial episode, approximately 40 per cent of patients will recover completely and have no further attacks in the next five years, 40 per cent will remain permanently damaged, and the remaining 20 per cent will improve but suffer further episodes. Less than about 10 per cent require long-term residential care. Most practices will have on their books a few middle-aged patients who have had a well-documented schizophrenic episode in their youth, and have had no problems since.

Late-onset schizophrenia tends to be of the paranoid type. Delusions of persecution predominate and may be quite circumscribed. That is to say, patients may appear quite sane until the topic of their delusional beliefs is touched upon. If such people can be persuaded to keep unacceptable ideas to themselves, they may be able to work and survive quite well in the community. Thus, one patient, while denying that he was mentally ill, could accept that other people would think he was mad if he told them about the accusing voices in his head. By taking his doctor's advice to keep his voices secret from others, he escaped the dangers of being stigmatized by his family and friends.

Contrary to popular belief, most schizophrenics are not a danger to themselves or to other people, but there is a small minority whose unpredictable or threatening behaviour gives just cause for anxiety. Compulsory treatment may be needed since most such patients do not accept that they are sick (see Appendix I).

Management

Although it is not always essential to admit schizophrenic patients to hospital for assessment, it is usually easier to get the acute condition controlled on a psychiatric ward, and this should always be done if there is thought to be any danger. Phenothiazines (see p. 163) are usually the treatment of choice and will control many of the acute symptoms, but they have little effect on the loss of motivation and drive which often accompanies schizophrenia. In large dosage they may slow the patient down and further impair ability to cope with jobs and other responsibilities.

Unfortunately, schizophrenic patients are seldom reliable tablet-takers, and those whose symptoms have been well controlled in hospital commonly relapse when they leave, because they discontinue or change the dosage of their medication. Long-acting drugs, such as fluphenazine and flupenthixol as the decanoates (Modecate and Depixol, respectively), have been developed to overcome this problem. They are administered by injection once every 2–3 weeks, and this makes it possible for the medical team to ensure that the drug has been taken. If the patient fails to turn up for the injection, it is most important for someone to make contact to find out what has gone wrong. It follows that practices who take on responsibility for the day-to-day management of the medication of schizophrenic patients must have a water-tight system for checking compliance. With this condition the responsibility for follow-up rests with the health professionals *not* the patient. Unfortunately, many patients elect to discontinue treatment, either because they feel so well that they 'don't need it', or because of side-effects.

Side-effects of long-term phenothiazines are not uncommon and can be serious. When the drug is first started, acute muscular spasms, most often in the neck muscles ('oculogyric crises'), may be dangerous and require the intramuscular or intravenous injection of 5–10 mg of procyclidine.

Subsequent regular oral anticholinergic medication will prevent recurrence and can also reduce motor restlessness (akathesia) and parkinsonian types of tremor and rigidity.

Patients who have been taking these drugs in high dosage over a period of years occasionally develop tardive dyskinesia, champing of the jaw and 'fly-catching' movements of the tongue, which are often resistant to treatment and may persist after the phenothiazine has been stopped. For this reason long-term medication should be kept to a minimum. In practice, it is usually possible to reduce the dosage level of medication once the acute attack is over and it may be wiser to allow minor symptoms to persist, rather than to control them with long-term drugs. The decision to discontinue medication is a difficult one and should not be considered until a person has been free of major symptoms for some months (except in the presence of dangerous side-effects from the drugs). This does not mean that people who have had an attack of schizophrenia should take phenothiazines for the rest of their lives. The dangers of long-term medication are such that it is wise to periodically consider reducing and then stopping drugs in all patients to see whether it is possible to get by without them.

Intolerance of 'expressed emotion' means that some people will be less likely to relapse if they live in lodgings rather than in their own home. However, this does not mean they do not need any sort of human contact. A relative or friendly landlady who will make sure that the former patient gets to work on time in the morning and who treats them with respect is invaluable. Too little contact with people may lessen contact with reality and allow the patient to become a recluse.

Work is often a problem. Many employers are reluctant to take on 'mental patients', and there are some patients who are unpunctual and unreliable, the illness having left them with little confidence or motivation. Attendance at a sheltered workshop or other rehabilitation centre may accustom them to the work environment and increase their chances of obtaining employment. It may help to get them registered as disabled, since large firms are compelled by law to employ a proportion of disabled persons.

In many places community psychiatric nurses are very willing to take responsibility for administering medication and providing support to families after a person has left hospital, but they cannot always offer the continuity of care that is possible in general practice, and there is no reason why complete care should not be given by the PCT. The fact that the family are likely to know and trust the PCT is an advantage and may help to make continued medication more acceptable. Many schizophrenics have difficulty in trusting people, so it is important that they have a continuing relationship with one or two members of the practice team. It is sometimes necessary to override the normal rota systems of partnerships to ensure this. Although formal psychotherapy is contraindicated (and may do more harm than good), occasional contact with a trusted health visitor, nurse, or doctor can act as a safety valve and enable an eye to be kept open for further trouble.

Communicating with patients with schizophrenia

Schizophrenia has no effect on intelligence but it can have a profound effect upon verbal and non-verbal communication. If the patient's thoughts are disordered, many of the clues which we take for granted in our day-to-day interactions will be absent, and we may find it difficult to know how the patient is reacting to our approaches. Sometimes it may feel as if the patient is laughing at us behind our backs, at other times the patient may seem completely indifferent. Strange mannerisms or postures make us uncomfortable and it is tempting to assume that the patient is stupid or childish (unlike with most patients, it may be wiser to believe the verbal rather than the non-verbal communication). Yet this is not the case, and these patients have the same need for our care and the same need for our advice as other adults. If we disregard their peculiarities and treat them in a matter-of-fact way, they will eventually come to accept us.

The difficulty we have in understanding schizophrenics is nothing to their difficulty in understanding us. Paranoid projections may lead some patients to expect hostility, others are fearful of eye-contact, or physical contact, as if these were invasions of privacy. It is important to respect such fears, as long as they do not prevent the patient from receiving the help that is needed. Thus, there is no harm in allowing the patient to stand by the door with his back to the doctor throughout an interview, but this does not mean that we should curtail the interview. In fact we may need to spend longer, and to repeat our advice in unambiguous language in order to ensure that the patient has understood it, and maybe even accepted it.

Hints, allusions, jokes, and ambiguous remarks are likely to be misunderstood and are best avoided. We need to have a clear idea of what it is important to achieve and to take care not to be deflected from this agenda. If the patient is in danger of losing his job because he cannot get up in the morning, it may be more important to work out with him how to adjust his medication than to listen to another long account of what the voices are telling him. At the same time, we should not completely disregard the irrational components in the illness. Hallucinatory voices, like dreams, are a reflection of the patient's thoughts and fears and may help us to understand what is needed.

A young man was plagued by voices who made derogatory comments about him, referring to him as a 'black failure' and a 'disgrace'. He came to Britain some years ago in the hope of taking a university degree but had to settle for a job as a laboratory technician. Part of the therapy was to reassure him of his real worth as a human being who had managed to keep working and to support his wife and child despite great difficulties.

Many schizophrenics are sufficiently in touch with reality to know that they are mentally ill, and also to know the diagnostic label which has been attached to them. Such patients will be helped by having this acknowledged and discussed. It may help to explain the nature of the illness to them and their family, including its prognosis and its management, so that concepts such as limiting expressed emotion can be explained, signs of relapse can be recognized, and the need for medication made as rational as possible. It may also be possible for patients to be helped to understand, at least partly, that their 'voices' or 'hallucinations' are the result of 'crossed wires' in their brain, and to accept that these are part of themselves and so be enabled to mitigate their effect. The therapist should not accept as true the patients' misperceptions and misrepresentations, as patients need to be helped to be reality-oriented. Remaining firm in such situations requires tact, as direct confrontation may damage the relationship.

Because schizophrenia often follows a fluctuating course, both the PCT and the patient's relatives need to be on the look out for evidence of relapse, of which insomnia may be the first symptom. Stressful events, or the appearance of new symptoms, may suggest the need for extra support and a temporary increase in medication. Given this help, repeated admissions to hospital (with all the attendant dangers of stigmatization, loss of employment, etc.) can be minimized. Not that hospital admission is always a mistake. There are many patients who will have to return to hospital from time to time, either for their own sake or to give their families a rest. Here, too, it is important to ensure continuity of care whenever possible and to return the patient to the care of familiar staff on a familiar ward.

The ability of a person to live out of hospital often stands or falls on the ability of the family to tolerate difficult behaviour. There are many chronically disturbed or 'burnt out' schizophrenic patients who would spend the rest of their lives in the back wards of mental hospitals were it not for the devotion of parents or spouses. Negative symptoms which sometimes persist include social withdrawal, lack of motivation and drive, emotional blunting, poverty of speech, and self-neglect. The burden on the family can be considerable. They may need to initiate and encourage activities which others take for granted—getting the patient up in the morning, insisting on personal cleanliness, and so on.

This makes it all the more important that these people receive all the help and emotional support which we can offer. As in other kinds of stressful life situations, family carers will benefit from talking to others who are 'in the same boat', and there are many areas where mutual support is available from 'relative groups' run by MIND, the Schizophrenia Association, or the local psychiatric services (see Appendix II). The members of the PCT are also an important source of information and support to the family, explaining the nature of the illness to them, reassuring them of the value of their own contribution to care, and acting promptly if the situation at home becomes intolerable. It is a standing reproach to our society that so many of those who are permanently damaged by schizophrenia are to be found in prisons, living rough, or 'dumped' in common lodging houses, where conditions are far worse than the old 'asylums'. Members of the PCT can do much to ensure that community care lives up to its name.

References

1. Brown, G. W. and Harris, T. (1978). *Social origin of depression: a study of psychiatric disorder in women.* Tavistock, London.
2. Vaughan, C. E. and Leff, J. P. (1976). The measurement of expressed emotion in the families of psychiatric patients. *Br. J. Soc. Clin. Psychol.* **15**, 157–65.
3. Laing, R. D. (1960). *The divided self: a study in sanity and madness.* Tavistock, London.
4. Laing, R. D. (1971). *Knots.* Penguin, Harmondsworth.

Further reading

Green, H. (1972). *I never promised you a rose garden.* Pan Book, London.
Laing, R. D. (1971). *Knots.* Penguin, Harmondsworth.
Scher, M., Wilson, L., and Mason, J. (1980). The management of chronic schizophrenia. *J. Fam. Pract.* **II**, 407–13.

9 Postscript

Readers who have read this far may feel that if they attempt only a fraction of what is possible in the field of psychological medicine from general practice, they will not have time for anything else. Nevertheless, our conviction, supported by the evidence outlined in Chapter 2 on the high levels of psychological symptoms present in the community, is that the effort is both necessary and worthwhile. If some of the preventive and therapeutic strategies outlined in this book are followed, it is likely that our patients will be spared much distress. Moreover, our work-load may actually be reduced.

Whether dealing with physical or psychological problems, our first task is to make an assessment, and then to promote change towards well-being, if we can. Although this may involve complex skills, much in the psychological area resembles what we try to do when friends come to us to share worries or ask for help. Indeed, living in a community, as many GPs do, and meeting our patients in various roles, the relationship with them approaches that of friendship. Friendship presupposes that the individuals concerned know something about each other. The doctor is likely to know more about the patient than vice versa, so that the relationship may be unequal, but few GPs are so remote that patients do not know something about them—perhaps more than is realized!

It would sometimes feel easier if we could 'put on different hats' when fulfilling different functions. To a certain extent we do this, and it is necessary, but perhaps enough has been said about fragmentation and dissociation in this book to show that this option is unsatisfactory. We have to offer help to many patients whose lives we share, and yet live our own lives.

Balint has drawn attention to the importance of clarifying our own feelings when interacting with patients, and using our own human qualities and experience in assessing what is happening to them. Allowing our patients to see us as real people helps in therapy, but also puts burdens on us, making it difficult to remain remote, mysterious, or magical.

How these conflicting factors are reconciled is something that everyone has to work out for themselves. Decisions have to be made about the allocation of time and energy. Home life has to be protected, outside interests pursued. But for most GPs contact with patients will remain at the centre of their professional lives and will take up a large part of their time. Building up relationships with patients, based on honesty and openness, are helped by non-authoritarian, patient-centred consulting styles, and by shared decision-making. This leads to the establishment of trust—both ways. When this is coupled with the patient's acceptance of the doctor as a human being, progress can be made in offering help on a realistic basis, in whatever area the problem lies. The doctor is likely to find work more rewarding, and the patient to show genuine regard for the doctor, rather than awe born of the fear of an ill-understood technician. This, in our opinion, is a goal worth striving towards and one which we have tried to share with our readers while writing this book.

Appendix I

THE MENTAL HEALTH ACT (1983)

This act applies only to England and Wales. Those practising elsewhere will have to consult locally.

Over 95 per cent of people receiving treatment in mental hospitals or psychiatric units are there on an informal basis. The Mental Health Act of 1983 regulates the care of those who need compulsory detention. It is a large and complex act, which covers both civil and criminal admissions. Most GPs will make every effort to avoid a 'section', as even a brief deprivation of liberty carries stigma and may make the patient resentful on discharge. On the other hand, failure to arrange compulsory treatment, when it is needed, may result in allegations of negligence.

The sections likely to involve GPs are few and come under two main headings:

(1) emergency and short-term orders for assessment for up to 28 days (Sections 2 and 4);

(2) longer-term orders for treatment (Sections 3 and 7).

Short-term orders apply to *any* mental disorder, which does not need to be specified, while long-term ones cover four types of mental disorder:

- mental illness—not defined, but the Act states that a person should not be 'treated as suffering from mental disorder by reason only of promiscuity, or other immoral conduct, sexual deviancy or dependence on alcohol or drugs';

- severe mental impairment, associated with abnormally aggressive or seriously irresponsible conduct;

- mental impairment—similar to above but of lesser degree;

- psychopathic disorder with associated aggressive conduct.

The Act specifies the involvement of a number of people or agencies:

1. 'Nearest relative' is the nearest adult relative (in order: spouse, son, daughter, father, mother, sibling, grandparent, uncle or aunt, nephew or niece) with preference being given to a relative who cares for the patient. Cohabitees (of either sex) come last.

2. 'Approved social worker' (ASW), is one approved by the local authority as having special experience of mental illness.

3. 'Approved doctor', is one who has been approved under Section 12 of the Act as having special experience of mental disorder. This will usually be a psychiatrist.

Section 4   Admission for assessment in
cases of emergency

Duration of detention   Maximum 72 hours.

Application for admission   By ASW or nearest relative, either of whom must have seen the patient in the last 24 hours.

Procedure   Any one doctor (preferably one who is acquainted with the patient) must confirm that:

(1)   it is of urgent necessity for the patient to be admitted; and

(2)   waiting for a second doctor would cause undesirable delay.

The patient must be admitted within 24 hours of application or examination, whichever is earlier, or the application is null and void.

Section 4 expires 72 hours after hospital admission and cannot be renewed. If the patient needs continued admission and is unwilling to stay as an informal patient, detention may be necessary under Section 2.

Section 2   Admission for assessment

Duration of detention   Maximum 28 days.

Application for admission   by ASW or nearest relative who must have seen the patient within the last 14 days.

Procedure   Two doctors, one of whom one must be an approved doctor, and the other preferably a doctor who already knows the patient (e.g. a GP) must confirm that:

(1)   the patient is suffering from a mental disorder which warrants detention in hospital; and

(2)   the patient ought to be detained in the interests of their own health and safety, or with a view to the protection of others.

Section 2 expires after 28 days and cannot be renewed. If the patient requires further detention this has to be done under Section 3. Detailed reasons why informal admission is not appropriate must be given in writing for the benefit of the Review Tribunal to whom the patient can appeal.

Section 3   Admission for treatment

Duration of detention   Six months, renewable for a further six months and then for one year at a time.

Application for admission   By nearest relative, or by ASW when nearest relative consents or is displaced by a Court, or when it is not reasonably practical to consult the nearest relative.

Procedure   Two doctors (as for Section 2) must confirm that:

(1)   the patient is suffering from one of the four categories of mental disorder specified above, of a nature or degree which makes it appropriate for him or her to receive medical treatment in hospital; and that

(2) in the case of a psychopath, such treatment is likely to 'alleviate or prevent a deterioration' of his or her condition; and that

(3) it is necessary for the patient's safety or the protection of other persons that he or she should receive such treatment and that it cannot be provided unless he or she is detained under this section.

Guardianship

Sections 7 and 8 make it possible for patients to be given care, support and treatment in the community without the need for hospital admission.

The reasons for reception are:

(1) that the person is suffering from one of the four categories of mental disorder specified above; and

(2) that it is necessary in the interests of the person's welfare or for the protection of others that he or she be received into guardianship.

Application   is made on a form which has to be signed by an approved social worker or the patient's nearest relative.

Medical recommendation   needs to be made by two doctors, one of whom must be 'approved', and one who should, if possible, already know the patient (e.g. a GP).

Other sections, including those involving the police and criminal cases, rely on an 'approved' doctor for the medical recommendation, usually a psychiatrist and very rarely, therefore, a GP.

For further information on this act, the reader is referred to the Appendix of the *Oxford textbook of psychiatry* 2nd edn (Gelder, Gath, and Mayou, 1989) or to the four excellent leaflets prepared by MIND (for address see Appendix II), which also contain helpful information on patient's rights.

Appendix II

There follows a list of organizations that offer our patients additional advice and information, and which we hope our readers may find useful.

ACCEPT National Services
Addiction Community Centres for Education Prevention, Treatment, and Research Accept Clinic
200 Seagrave Road,
London SW6 1RQ.
Tel: 01 381 3155/2112

An independent national charity providing multidisciplinary team community services and treatment centres for problem drinkers, tranquillizer misusers, and their families.

ACCEPT also publishes a wide selection of literature on alcohol and tranquillizer problems, families, and so on. Price list available upon request.

Action on Smoking and Health (ASH)
5–11 Mortimer Street,
London W1N 7RH.
Tel: 01 637 9843

A registered charity set up by the Royal College of Physicians.

Age Concern
Age Concern England,
60 Pitcairn Road,
Mitcham,
Surrey CR4 3LL.
Tel: 01 640 5431

Age Concern Scotland,
33 Castle Street,
Edinburgh EH2 3DN.
Tel: 031 225 5000

Age Concern Wales,
1 Park Grove,
Cardiff CF1 3BJ.
Tel: 0222 371821

Age Concern Northern Ireland,
128 Great Victoria Street,
Belfast BT2 7BG.
Tel: 0232 245729

A network of 1400 independent local groups throughout the UK providing services for elderly people, e.g. visiting day care, clubs and a wide range of innovative projects.

AIMS

Action for Research into Multiple Sclerosis,
71 Grays Inn Road,
London WC1X 8TR.
Tel: 01 568 2255

This provides a telephone service by volunteers, themselves with MS, all of whom have had relevant professional training including case work/counselling.

Al-Anon Family Groups

61 Great Dover Street,
London SE1 4YF.
Tel: 01 403 0888 (24-hour service covering UK and Eire)

A self-supporting recovery programme for relatives and friends of problem drinkers whether or not the alcoholic seeks help.

Alateen (a part of Al-Anon) helps teenagers, aged 12–20, who have an alcoholic parent, brother, or sister.

Albany Trust

24 Chester House,
London SW1W 9HS.
Tel: 01 730 5871

A counselling service for people with sexual and relationship problems.

Alcohol Concern

305 Gray's Inn Road,
London WC1X 8QF.
Tel: 01 833 3471

A national agency dealing with problems related to alcohol abuse.

Alcoholics Anonymous

PO Box 1, Stonebow House,
Stonebow,
York YO1 2NJ.
Tel: 0904 644026; 01 352 3001

To contact AA look for Alcoholics Anonymous in the telephone directory, or phone the general service office for the UK at the address above.

Alzheimer's Disease Society

Bank Buildings
Fulham Broadway,
London SL6 1EP.
Tel: 01 381 3177

The Society aims to give support and advice to families of dementia sufferers by linking them through membership. It provides information about the disease and about services and aids which are of use to both the sufferer and carer.

Anorexic Aid
The Priory Centre,
11 Priory Road,
High Wycombe,
Bucks HP13 6SL.
Tel: 0494 21431

Anorexic Aid aims to support and advise sufferers (of anorexia nervosa, bulimia nervosa, and allied eating disorders) and their family and friends, and to offer friendship to dispel these people's feelings of isolation.

Association for Postnatal Depression
7 Gowan Avenue,
Fulham,
London SW6 6HR.

The association has four areas of activity: education, information, support, and research.

Beaumont Trust
BM Charity,
London WC1N 3XX.
Tel: 01 730 7453 (7–11 p.m.) (Trustline); 061 256 2521 (7–10 p.m.) (wives and partners)

Offers guidance and support to transvestites and transsexuals.

Body Positive
BM Aids,
London WC1N 3XX.
c/o Terrence Higgins Trust.
Tel: 01 833 2971

Support and advice for people who are HIV-antibody positive; with a telephone counselling service run by Ab+ volunteers, and individual and group counselling.

British Pregnancy Advisory Service
Ansty Manor,
Wootton Wawen,
Sullihull,
West Midlands B95 6BX.
Tel: Henley in Arden 3225

This organization offers information, counselling, and practical help to anyone with problems connected with pregnancy, contraception, sexuality, fertility, or sterilization. This is provided by paid professionals and trained counsellors. The information services are free, but fees are payable for other services.

Brook Advisory Centres
153A East Street,
London SE17 2SD.
Tel: 01 708 1234/1390

An advisory service for young people, mainly under 25, who require advice, treatment, and supplies for contraception, pregnancy diagnosis, pregnancy counselling, and counselling on emotional and sexual problems. Service is provided by doctors, nurses, and social workers with relevant professional training.

Catholic Marriage Advisory Council
15 Lansdowne Road,
Holland Park,
London W11 3AJ.
Tel: 01 727 0141

The council provides a remedial marital counselling service; an education service for those preparing for marriage; for parents and others involved in sex education; for married people to enrich their relationships; and a medical advisory service of instruction and support in the use of natural methods of family planning.

The Compassionate Friends
5 Lower Clifton Hill,
Clifton,
Bristol BS8 1BT.
Tel: 0272 292778

Offering mutual support by and for bereaved parents.

Cruse, the national organization for the widowed and their children
Cruse House,
126 Sheen Road,
Richmond,
Surrey TW9 1UR.
Tel: 01 940 4818/9047

Cruse is a registered charity with over 125 branches in Britain. Through national and branch membership it offers help through counselling for the individual and in groups, and provides advice and information on practical problems and opportunities for social contact.

Epilepsy Association (British)
Anstey House,
40 Hanover Square,
Leeds LS3 1BE.
Tel: 0532 439393

Established in 1950, the British Epilepsy Association is a registered charity. It specializes in social work and family services, epilepsy research, health education, and community activities.

Epilepsy Association of Scotland
48 Govan Road,
Glasgow G51 1JL.
Tel: 041 427 4911

Lothian Region Branch,
13 Guthrie Street,
Edinburgh EH1 1JG.
Tel: 031 226 5458

The association offers information and advice to men, women, and children with epilepsy, their families and friends, and all who come across epilepsy in the course of their work—doctors, nurses, social workers, teachers, health visitors, careers officers,community workers, employers, and so on.

Families Anonymous
88 Caledonian Road,
London N1 9DN.
Tel: 01 278 8805

A self-help support group for the families and friends of drug abusers.

Family Planning Association
Margaret Pike House,
27–35 Mortimer Street,
London W1N 7RJ.
Tel: 01 636 7866

Operates the family planning information service to inform people of free NHS family planning facilities. Runs a resource centre and personal information service for public and professionals, and a book centre. Also courses on sex education and personal relationships for professional groups.

Family Service Units
207 Old Marylebone Road,
London NW1 5QP.
Tel: 01 402 5175/6

Through its various family service units in different parts of the country it provides social work with families, including family case work, therapy, contractual work, family group work, playgroups, etc.

Fellowship of Depressives Anonymous
36 Chestnut Avenue,
Beverley,
N. Humberside HU17 9QU.

A national self/mutual help organization for all past and present sufferers.

Foundation for the Study of Infant Deaths (cot death research and support)
18 Belgrave Square,
London SW1X 8PS.
Tel: 01 235 1721; 01 235 0965

The foundation gives personal support to bereaved families and acts as a centre of information about cot death for parents and professionals.

Gamblers Anonymous
17/23 Blantyre Street,
Cheyne Walk,
London SW10.
Tel: 01 353 3060

The Gam-Anon meetings are designed to teach the family of the compulsive gambler to understand him and to live with, or without, him.

Help the Aged

St. James Walk,
London EC1R 0BE.
Tel: 01 253 0253

Help the Aged is a national charity dedicated to improving the quality of life of elderly people in need of help in the UK and overseas.

Huntington's Chorea

Association to Combat Huntington's Chorea,
c/o Mrs E. Reynolds,
108 Battersea High Street,
London SW11.
Tel: 01 223 7000

London Rape Crisis Centre

PO Box 69, London WC1X 9NJ.
Tel: 01 837 1600 (24 hours); 01 278 3956 (office hours)

A 24-hour telephone service for women and girls who have been raped or sexually assaulted.

The Medical Council on Alcoholism

1 St Andrew's Place,
London NW1 4LB.
Tel: 01 487 4445

A registered charity that acts as a consultative body on the medical problems of alcoholism.

MENCAP, The Royal Society for Mentally Handicapped Children and Adults

123 Golden Lane,
London EC1Y 0RT.
Tel: 01 253 9433

Among numerous services for mentally handicapped people and their families the society provides a counselling service for families with a mentally handicapped member.

Mental Health Foundation

8 Hallam Street,
London W1N 6HD.
Tel: 01 580 0145

The objectives are to promote, encourage, and finance research into mental disorders of every kind, and to promote the welfare, treatment, and the care of persons suffering as a result of mental disorder and handicap.

Metabolic Diseases in Children Research Trust

9 Arnold Street,
Nantwich,
Cheshire CW5 5QB.
Tel: 0270 629782

Supports research and prenatal diagnosis. Offers grants for treatment and care plus information for parents.

MIND (National Association for Mental Health)
22 Harley Street,
London W1N 2ED.
Tel: 01 637 0741

Miscarriage Association
18 Stoneybrook Close,
West Bretton,
Wakefield,
W. Yorks WF4 4TP.
Tel: 092 485515

Offers support and information to women and their families, and assists in setting up self-help groups.

Narcotics Anonymous
PO Box 246,
London SW10 0DP.
Tel: 01 351 6794/6066/6067

A fellowship of men and women, for whom drugs have become a major problem, who meet regularly to help each other to stay clear of mood-altering chemicals.

National Association for the Childless
Birmingham Settlement,
318 Summer Lane,
Birmingham B19 3RL.
Tel: 021 359 4887

A self-help support group offering advice and information to people experiencing infertility problems.

National Association for Citizens' Advice Bureaux
110 Drury Lane,
London WC2B 5SW.
Tel: 01 836 9231

Through over 900 local branches, the Citizens' Advice Bureau provides a free, independent, impartial, and confidential service on advice, help, and information to anyone on any subject.

National Association of Victims' Support Schemes
17a Electric Lane,
Brixton,
London SW9 8LA.
Tel: 01 737 2010; 01 326 1084

There are over 300 groups whose addresses are available from local police or citizens' advice bureaux.

National Autistic Society

276 Willesden Lane,
London NW2 5RB.
Tel: 01 451 3844

The aims of the society are to provide and promote day and residential centres for the care, education, and training of autistic children and adults.

National Council for Carers and their Elderly Dependants

Jill Pitkeathley,
29 Chilworth Mews,
London W2 3RG.
Tel: 01 724 7776

The council is a registered charity which helps and advises carers of the elderly and infirm at home.

National Federation of Gateway Clubs

MENCAP Centre,
117–119 Golden Lane,
London EC1Y 0RT.
Tel: 01 253 9433

A national voluntary youth and community organization providing for the leisure-time needs of 38 000 mentally handicapped children and adults, in 650 clubs throughout England, Wales, and Northern Ireland, through the involvement of some 20 000 volunteers.

The National Marriage Guidance Council
(recently re-named **'Relate'**

Herbert Gray College,
Little Church Street,
Rugby CV21 3AP
Tel: 0788 73241

National Schizophrenia Fellowship

78/79 Victoria Road,
Surbiton,
Surrey KT6 4NS.
Tel: 01 390 3651 (3 lines)

Its purpose is to act as a national organization for all matters concerning the relief of sufferers from schizophrenia and of their families and dependants.

National Society for the Prevention of Cruelty to Children

67 Saffron Hill,
London EC1N 8RS.
Tel: 01 242 1626

The National Society for the Prevention of Cruelty to Children is a national charity which aims to prevent child abuse in all its forms.

Phobic Action
Greater London House,
547/551 High Road,
Leytonstone,
London E11 4PR.
Tel: 01 588 6012

Support and advice for acute anxiety sufferers through local self-help groups.

Phobics Society
4 Cheltenham Road,
Chorlton-cum-Hardy,
Manchester M21 1QN.
Tel: 061 881 1937

The society is a national charity with the prime aim of promoting the relief and rehabilitation of sufferers from agoraphobia and other phobic illnesses.

Psychiatric Rehabilitation Association
The Groupwork Centre,
21a Kingsland High Street,
Dalston,
London E8.
Tel: 01 254 9753

The basic aim is to stimulate the patients to a greater initiative and awareness of their environment and society. By education it prepares and encourages them to return and re-adapt to the society they were once a part of.

Relate (see National Marriage Guidance Council)

RELEASE
1 Elgin Avenue,
London W9 3PR.
Tel: 01 289 1123

Provides advice for people in trouble or difficulty, particularly in the area of drugs, criminal law (including those arrested), and abortion. The service is provided by paid, full-time workers (including a pregnancy counsellor), and by volunteer doctors and lawyers.

The Richmond Fellowship for Community Mental Health
8 Addison Road,
Kensington,
London W14 8DL.
Tel: 01 603 6373/4/5

Operates a national network of therapeutic communities offering a supportive environment and expert help for those recovering from mental illness and emotional problems, including drug- and alcohol-related problems. Some houses offer long-term support, including places for retired people.

The Samaritans
17 Uxbridge Road,
Slough,
Bucks SL1 1SN.
Tel: 0753 32713

Schizophrenia Association of Great Britain
International Schizophrenia Centre,
Bryn Hyfred,
The Crescent,
Bangor,
Gwynedd LL57 2AG.
Tel: 0248 354048
A charity for the benefit of schizophrenics and their relatives.

Scottish Marriage Guidance Council
26 Frederick Street,
Edinburgh EH2 2JR.
Tel: 031 225 5006
This is a separate organization from the national council, although with similar aims.

Scottish Society for the Mentally Handicapped
13 Elmbank Street,
Glasgow G2 4QA.
Tel: 041 226 4541
The society was originally formed by parents of the mentally handicapped to help other parents in the same position. It now welcomes anyone who is concerned for the welfare of mentally handicapped people.

Self-Help Association For Transsexuals (SHAFT)
106, Barton Ave.,
Keyham,
Plymouth PL2 1NZ.
Tel: 0752 559939
The association endeavours to give support to established transsexuals.

Sigma
BM Sigma,
London WC1N 3XX.
Tel: 01 837 7324
Support for heterosexuals with homosexual or bisexual partners.

Spastics Society
12 Park Crescent,
London W1N 4EQ.
Tel: 01 636 5020
The society aims to provide care, treatment, education, and employment training for people with cerebral palsy. With its affiliated local groups, it has established more than 160 schools and centres throughout the country. A handbook of services is available along with other information pamphlets on cerebral palsy.

Spina Bifida And Hydrocephalus Association
22 Upper Woburn Place,
London WC1H 0EP.
Tel: 01 388 1382 (8 lines)

ASBAH, founded in 1966, has two main objectives: to provide individual support to children and young persons disabled in these ways, and to their families; and to promote research.

The Stillbirth and Neonatal Death Society
Argyle House,
29–31 Euston Road,
London NW1 2SD.
Tel: 01 833 2851

The society runs a network of support groups around the country for parents who have experienced stillbirths and neonatal deaths.

Stroke (Chest and Heart) Association
Tavistock House North,
Tavistock Square,
London WC1H 9JE.
Tel: 01 387 3012

65 North Castle Street,
Edinburgh EH2 3LT.
Tel: 031 225 6963

21 Dublin Road,
Belfast BT2 7FT.
Tel: 0232 220184

The CHSA works for the prevention of chest, heart, and stroke illnesses; and helps people who suffer from them. This is done through a continuing programme of health education, research, rehabilitation, counselling, and welfare services.

Terminal Cancer Care
The Hospice Advisory Service,
St Christopher's Hospice,
Lawrie Park Road,
London SE26 6DZ.
Tel: 01 778 9252

Terrence Higgins Trust
BM AIDS,
London WC1N 3XX.
Tel: 01 833 2971

Trained volunteers offer help and support to people who are HIV-antibody positive and those with AIDS, their friends and families.

Tranx
17 Peel Road,
Wealdstone,
Harrow.
Tel: 01 427 2065/2827

Self-help agency giving advice and support to people dependent on minor tranquillizers and sleeping pills.

Turning Point
4th Floor, CAP House,
9/12 Long Lane,
London EC1a 9HA.
Tel: 01 606 3947/9

Turning point is a registered charity offering rehabilitation and care to those experiencing a drug- or alcohol-related problem; and support to families and friends.

Index